Forensic Medicine
A Guide to Principles

Forensic Medicine
A GUIDE TO PRINCIPLES

I. Gordon MB ChB (Cape Town) FRSS Af Hon MD (Natal) Hon LLD (Unisa)
Hon F For. Path. (S.A.) MA (Natal)
Emeritus Professor of Forensic Medicine,
University of Natal,
Formerly Chief Government Pathologist, Durban, and
Dean, Faculty of Medicine,
University of Natal, 1955–1971

The Late **H. A. Shapiro** BA PhD MB ChB (Cape Town) FRSS Af
Hon LLD (Natal)
Professor of Forensic Medicine,
University of South Africa;
Visiting Professor of Forensic Medicine,
University of Natal;
Honorary Consulting Pathologist,
National Research Institute for Occupational Diseases, Johannesburg;
Former Government Pathologist, Cape Town;
Editor-in-Chief, *Forensic Science*;
Honorary Lecturer in Forensic Medicine, University of the Witwatersrand, Johannesburg

S. D. Berson MB BCh (Witwatersrand) DCP (London) DPath (RCP London,
RCS England) FF Path (S.A.) F For. Path. (S.A.) Hons BA (Unisa)
Forensic Pathologist to the Royal Swaziland Police, Swaziland;
Formerly Senior Lecturer in Forensic Medicine,
University of the Witwatersrand, Johannesburg, and
Senior State Pathologist, Johannesburg

THIRD EDITION

CHURCHILL LIVINGSTONE
EDINBURGH LONDON MELBOURNE AND NEW YORK 1988

CHURCHILL LIVINGSTONE
Medical Division of Longman Group UK Limited

Distributed in the United States of America by
Churchill Livingstone Inc., 1560 Broadway, New
York, N.Y. 10036, and by associated companies,
branches and representatives throughout the world.

First edition 1975
Second edition 1982
Third edition 1988

ISBN 0-443-03440-0

British Library Cataloguing in Publication Data
Gordon, I. (Isidor)
 Forensic medicine: a guide to principles.—3rd ed.
 1. Medical jurisprudence
 I. Title II. Shapiro, H. A. III. Berson, S. D.
 614'.1 RA1051

Library of Congress Cataloging in Publication Data
Gordon, I. (Isidor)
 Forensic medicine.
 Includes bibliographies and index.
 1. Medical jurisprudence. 2. Forensic pathology.
I. Shapiro, H. A. (Hillel Abbe) II. Berson, S. D.
III. Title. [DNLM: 1. Forensic Medicine. W 700 G662f]
RA1051.G66 1988 614'.1 87-23857

Printed at The Bath Press, Avon

Preface to the Third Edition

There was a favourable reception to the first and second editions of this work. However, valid criticisms of certain areas of the text led us to revise aspects of its former presentation. We have set as our objective the writing of a work on the principles of forensic medicine for use in English-speaking countries, and in non-English-speaking countries where English is used as the medium or the alternative medium of instruction in forensic medicine. The importance of English as the medium of communication in forensic medicine is shown in the success of its use at international congresses on forensic medicine and the forensic sciences. English is used in the major international journals in forensic medicine and forensic science. Many Scandinavian, Western European and South American journals, and journals of the Middle East, carry English summaries of their original and research articles on forensic medicine.

We have been encouraged by the use of the work for reference and research purposes at the international level. In order to fulfil the needs of the undergraduate medical student, graduate students, specialist pathologists and research workers in the field, we have sought to elaborate principles in forensic pathology in accordance with many significant advances which have occurred in recent years. The advances in medical research have become highly pertinent in present-day forensic pathology practice. Accordingly, we have deleted aspects of earlier presentations on different topics, where these have been overtaken by modern presentations. Apart from these specific aspects, which we will list here, the overall text has been brought up to date.

We have revised the section on the Clinical Aspects of Toxicology, for the purpose of providing practitioners with a guide to tangible access to sources of reference which can be applied in the preventive and the therapeutic management of cases of accidental poisoning. In particular, in the guide, we have drawn attention to active procedures which can be taken rapidly to save the lives of children and workers who accidentally ingest or inhale one of the daily-expanding variety of products used in the household, and in commercial, industrial and agricultural environments.

The important change effected in the chapter dealing with the phenomena that occur after death relates to rigor mortis. The physical and chemical changes involved in muscle contraction and rigor mortis have been extensively revised in the light of modern findings in analytical biochemistry and electron microscopy. Included in this presentation are three electron photomicrographs and three charts which depict the biochemical changes involved in different forms of muscle contraction. In the chapter dealing with deaths usually initiated by hypoxic hypoxia or anoxic anoxia, an entirely new section has been written on drowning. This section takes into account modern views at both the clinical and pathological levels. We have substituted new material in the section on exposure to high and low environmental temperatures.

We have made some minor changes in the section on acute neurogenic cardiovascular failure. We have added to this chapter the important entity of the adult respiratory distress syndrome (ARDS)—(the lung as target organ). An important addition to the chapter on the medical investigation of the causes of death is an elaboration of the causes of sudden death due to acute infections. In the past decade we have recognised the phenomenon of sudden deaths due to acute virus infections. Accordingly, as far as possible, we have indicated the criteria needed for laboratory confirmation. In addition, we have set out a new discussion of the possible causes and consequences of the sudden infant death syndrome (SIDS).

The chapter on deaths associated with anaesthetic procedures has been completely re-written and brought up to date in accordance with the sophisticated techniques which are applied in modern anaesthesia.

Apart from re-casting the chapter on poisoning, in the light of the importance of access to sources of information in the field of clinical toxicology, we have deleted many figures from this chapter as well as the detailed analyses of arsenical and barbiturate poisoning. In the chapter on regional injuries of medico-legal importance, we have re-written parts of the text on head injuries and have provided illustrations in order to stress the importance in diagnosis of CT scanning techniques. We have re-written the section on fat embolism. Its importance has been brought into focus by the significant contributions of recent investigations into the possible mechanisms of death due to fat embolism.

The chapter on firearm wounds has been completely re-written. This became necessary because there has been a change in the type of injuries with which surgeons and pathologists have to deal. Apart from the increasing use of high velocity hand firearms, reference is made to the explosive effects on tissues of various missiles.

Because of its increasing importance in the last decade, we have completely re-written the section on the battered child syndrome. In the chapter on the medico-legal aspects of acute alcoholic intoxication, we have deleted certain sections including detailed references to chemical analytical techniques.

Allied to forensic medicine are the legal aspects of medical practice. We have not referred to relevant aspects of specific legal systems in different countries, because of the variations which exist in these countries, and in different states, provinces, counties and cantons of particular countries. There is an increasing trend for lawyers to write books, treatises and monographs for the specific post-graduate requirements of medical practitioners working in the private and public sectors.

In our opinion, in the training of medical undergraduate students in forensic medicine, it is not desirable to provide them with relatively superficial analyses of legal medicine (or medical law); ethics, or subjects such as civics and preventive and community health. Medical practitioners find that, when faced with a legal problem, they have to consult members of the legal profession.

In sudden deaths caused by acute infectious diseases, medical practitioners must be guided by epidemiologists, hygienists and other public health workers.

We have recognised the need for the training of undergraduate medical students in the clinical examination of complainants and accused persons, but we have emphasised the importance of basic knowledge of traumatic pathology in forensic medicine.

Durban and Mbabane 1988   I. G.
                                                                     S. D. B.

Acknowledgements

We acknowledge our thanks to publishers, editors of medical journals and other publications, authors, research workers, our pathologist colleagues, technologists, ballistic experts and the Heads of University and State medico-legal laboratories for their assistance, and for their permission to reproduce the following illustrations, tables, graphs and diagrams:
Interscience Publishers, London and New York: Figs 1.1A–C from F. Schleyer, *Determination of the time of death in the early post-mortem Interval* in *Methods of Forensic Science*, vol. 2, 1963, pp. 257, 259 and 263.

The British Medical Journal: Figs 1.2A–B from Haider et al, 1968, 2, 314.

The Editor of the Star, Johannesburg: Fig. 1.3 from the publication on 22 January 1976, p. 23.

Veb Verlag, Volk and Gesundheit, Berlin: 0, Prokop, 1966 *Forensische Medizin*, 2nd ed., p. 43.

The Lancet: Fig. 1.5 from Mullan et al, March 1965 i, 705.

The Journal of Forensic Medicine: Figs 1.6 and 1.7 from H. A. Shapiro, 1953–4, 1, 144–169.

Dr H. Isaacs, Neuromuscular Research Unit, Department of Physiology, University of the Witwatersrand: Figs 1.8–1.13, and for assistance in the preparation of the section on rigor mortis.

Forensic Science: Table 1.1 from C. M. Tidy, reproduced from *Legal Medicine*, Part 1, London, Smith Elder: 1882, pp. 58–74, 1973, 2, 123.

Professor L. S. Smith, Emeritus Professor of Forensic Medicine and Toxicology, University of Cape Town: Figs 1.14, 6.1, 12.19 and 12.39. Successive Heads of the University of Cape Town and State Medico-legal laboratories: for the use of Figs 1.15, 4.1A–C, 4.2A–B, 4.5, 12.10, 12.22, 12.25 and 14.8.

The South African Medical Journal: Figs 2.1A–C and Figs 4.3, 4.4 from I. Prinsloo and I. Gordon, 25, 1951, 358–361.

Forensic Science: Fig. 2.1D from I. Gordon et al. 7, 1976, 161–170.

Lea and Febiger, Philadelphia: Fig. 3.1 from V. H. Moon, *Shock:its Dynamics Occurrence and Management*, 1942, p. 208.

Journal of Forensic Medicine: Figs 3.2–3.5, from I. Gordon et al, 2, 1955, 31–50.

Dr Frank E. Berkowitz of the Department of Paediatrics, Baragwanath Hospital, Johannesburg, and Dr Keith Klugman of the Department of Microbiology, School of Pathology, South African Institute for Medical Research, Johannesburg: Fig. 8.1, and for their assistance in the section of this work on acute infections in obscure causes of death from natural causes.

Journal of Forensic Medicine: Table 11.2 from I. Robertson and P. R. Hodge, 4, 1957, 2–10.

Journal of Forensic Medicine: Table 11.3 from H. A. Shapiro and I. Robertson, 9, 1962, 5–9.

Churchill Livingstone, Edinburgh: Figs 12.1, 12.2,, 12.4, 12.5, 12.7, 12.8, 12.11, 12.12, 12.20 and 12.24 from G. F. Rowbotham *Acute Injuries of the Head*, 4th ed., 1964.

Lea and Febiger, Philadelphia: Fig. 12.3 from A. R. Moritz, *The Pathology of Trauma*, 1942, p. 327.

The Journal of Neurosurgery, The American Journal of Surgery, Radiology and Churchill Livingstone, Edinburgh: Tables 12.1 and 12.2 and Figs 12.6A–G. from E. S. Gurdjian et al, as set out on p. 337.

Ms Margaret Nicholas, Johannesburg: Figs 12.9 and 12.23.

Dr V. D. Kemp, Head of the University of the Witwatersrand and State Medico-legal laboratories, Johannesburg for the use of Figs 12.13–18, 12.21, 13.1–6, 13.9–14.

Edward Arnold (Publishers) Ltd, London: Figs 13.7 and 13.8 from M. S. Owen-Smith, *High Velocity Missile Wounds*, 1981, p. 23.

Figure 13.8 is Crown Copyright and is reproduced with the permission of The Controller of Her Majesty's Stationery Office.

The British Medical Bulletin: Fig. 14.1 from H. S. Baar, *The post-mortem examination of the newborn infant*, 1946, 178–188.

Clinical Proceedings, Journal of Forensic Medicine and Legal Medicine Annual 1976: Figs 14.2–7, from H. A. Shapiro, as set out on p. 394.

American J Roentgenol. Rad. Therapy: Fig. 14.9 from J. Caffey 56, 1946, 163–173.

Chapter 15, 'Medico-legal aspects of acute alcoholic intoxication', is based largely on the original contribution by the Late Professor H. A. Shapiro to *South African Motor Law* by W. E. Cooper and B. R. Bamford published by Juta & Co. Ltd Cape Town and Johannesburg, 1965.

We appreciate the assistance which we received from members of staff of the University of the Witwatersrand Medical School/Johannesburg General Hospitals Complex as follows:
On rigor mortis: Dr H. Isaacs and Professor M. James. *On deaths from exposure to low and high environmental temperatures*: Dr Ralph Bernstein. *On*

deaths from acute neurogenic cardiovascular failure: Dr Colin Clinton. *On deaths associated with anaesthetic procedures*: Professor M. James. *On head injuries*: Mr R. Plotkin. *On injuries to the chest, abdomen, urogenital tract and limbs*: Mr H. Green and Mr K. Boffard. *On firearm wounds*: Professor Lewis Levien, Mr K. Boffard, Mr C. Macfarlane and Mr W. Ritchie. *On the sudden infant death syndrome*: Professor S. Levine and Professor J. K. Mason (of the United Kingdom).

We thank the photographic units of the University of the Witwatersrand and the National Research Institute for Occupational Diseases for their assistance. We are grateful to Successive Heads and members of staff of the Department of Medical Illustration of the University of Natal; we appreciate the assistance received from members of staff of the photographic units of the Johannesburg and Diepkloof Mortuaries.

We thank Claire Maguire, Senior Librarian in charge of the Medical Library of the University of Natal for her considerable assistance. For their secretarial and administrative assistance we are most grateful to Norma J. Beare (who also helped in the compilation of the index), Val A. Cohen, Colleen M. Emmerich, Marlene V. French, Hilary J. Ralph and T. Maureen Stroud (former Executive Assistant to the Late Professor H. A. Shapiro).

We are especially indebted to Mrs Elif Fincanci-Smith, the Editor at Churchill Livingstone, London, for her assistance and advice.

Soothsayer. In nature's infinite book of secrecy
           A little I can read.

      Antony and Cleopatra, Act I, Scene ii.

Contents

1

The diagnosis and the early signs of death: the phenomena that occur after death

THE SO-CALLED MOMENT OF DEATH

Death is an abstract noun which may be meaningful to laymen, lawyers, philosophers and priests but which is very inadequate as a biological description. It is, however, a useful and convenient shorthand term to denote a disintegrating biological process in which we may recognize a beginning and an end, with striking changes in between.

There is really no moment in time at which it occurs. The moment of death is a legal fiction and the biological truth is quite different. Biologically, we die in bits and pieces, so the moment of death can only have any scientific meaning if we use this phrase to describe the time when we can state, with reasonable certainty, that an irreversible disintegrating process has begun. Prediction is implicit in this diagnosis.

The need to define this so-called moment as soon and as precisely as possible, assumed a new importance on 3 December 1967, when Professor Chris N. Barnard carried out the first human-to-human heart transplant at Groote Schuur Hospital in Cape Town.

Although corneal and kidney transplants had been carried out, with organs removed from dead bodies, well before that date, the need for the shortest possible post-mortem interval (to ensure optimal survival and function of the donor graft) became very urgent once heart transplants were technically feasible.

But such therapeutic needs are not an adequate reason to abandon the criteria on which we have relied for centuries to determine the fact of death. Newer and better criteria may, of course, be developed; but their worth will be tested for their ability to describe or predict the onset of a disintegrating biological process, irrespective of whether the new criteria facilitate the availability of organs and tissues for therapeutic needs.

Most civilized countries, for a compelling variety of religious and moral reasons, would find it repugnant and unacceptable if any stratagems were adopted with the object of circumventing the established criteria for establishing the fact of death, merely to be able to snatch vital parts from a living body for a therapeutic purpose, however laudable that purpose may be.

1

We are concerned, then, with the biological properties of living matter. In this context death can best be defined as the irreversible loss of the properties of living matter. This may involve the organism as a whole or its component parts.

The irreversible loss of the integrating and co-ordinating functions of the organism as a whole is sometimes referred to as somatic death (soma = the body). This is the stage of biological disintegration in which the law is interested. Its recognition entitles a medical practitioner to certify that death has occurred.

The conventional criteria relied on to establish this condition are the evidence of permanent cessation of spontaneous respiration and of the circulation of the blood. These are the so-called principal signs of death, which are established by means of inspection, palpation, auscultation and the electrocardiogram. We know that when these two functions of the body have been in abeyance for some 4 or 5 minutes, irreparable damage has also occurred in those parts of the brain which maintain the respiration, the heart beat and the blood pressure.

Fatteh, in a paper presented at the Sixth International Meeting of Forensic Sciences in Edinburgh in September 1972, reported on a malpractice suit arising out of the first heart transplant carried out on 25 May 1968 at the Medical College of Virginia in Richmond, Virginia, USA. The condition of the prospective heart donor was maintained by artificial respiration; 5 minutes after the respirator was switched off the prospective donor was pronounced dead.

Dr Edward Stinson, formerly of Stanford University Medical Centre and who had carried out 22 heart transplants at the time of this law suit, said: 'After the heart stops the brain can be alive from 3 to 5 minutes.' Thus after an interval of the order of 4 to 5 minutes, no evidence of any function can be elicited in the central nervous system. This is seen clinically as a total areflexia. This cessation of function of the central nervous system is referred to as brain death, but it is clearly secondary to the permanent arrest of the respiration and the circulation. The areflexic condition of the body provides the concomitant signs of death and confirms the diagnosis made on the basis of respiratory and circulatory arrest.

Diagnostic programmes which require the absence of the signs of life for periods of 2 hours or longer, before death is certified, are of no practical value. They do not establish that death has occurred; they establish that the deceased has been dead for 2 hours or longer. Such diagnostic criteria are neither realistic nor helpful in the context of organ transplantation.

Resuscitation versus resurrection

The use of resuscitation machines has introduced a complex variable into the equation linking life and death and the state of suspended animation in between these two extreme limits. The criteria for abandoning the use of resuscitation machines are determined solely by the clinical assessment of the patient's condition. Apparently cerebral (brain) death, as evidenced by an electroencephalographic (EEG) record indicating electrical silence of the brain (i.e. a completely flat or isoelectric tracing) has been suggested as a sufficient basis for removing the beating heart from an unconscious potential donor still independently capable of maintaining his breathing and his heart beat. This assigns to brain death a primary role in certifying somatic death. It is, however, well known that an electrically silent brain may recover and be completely normal (see p. 7); so any attempt to make brain death a primary reason for certifying somatic death is unwarranted in view of the absolute certainty required in making the diagnosis that death has occurred. The most reliable criteria for the diagnosis of permanent electrical silence of the brain remain those which rely on the permanent arrest of the respiration and the circulation.

When the integrated, co-ordinated functioning of the organism as a whole has been lost irreversibly, the biological properties of the component parts may still be demonstrable. In the early hours after death, striated (skeletal or so-called voluntary) muscle can be made to contract in response to mechanical or electrical stimuli (Figs 1.1A and B). The sweat glands and the pupil can still respond to appropriate pharmacological stimuli (Fig. 1.1C). Every second-year medical student knows that rhythmic contraction is an inherent property of cardiac muscle and he has himself kept a frog's heart beating for hours after its removal from its body. He can make it beat faster or slower or stop it or start it, at will. But the time for which these properties persist soon runs out. There is a biological law of diminishing returns. Indeed, it is this very persistence of the biological properties of living matter in the component parts of an organism that makes organ transplantation possible. The donor organ can thus be resurrected to function in the body of the recipient.

The donor organ bank

When the patient's heart and breathing have stopped and he can no longer maintain these functions spontaneously and independently, somatic death can be certified if, after the lapse of 4 to 5 minutes, these facts are confirmed. However, if the heart is then restarted and respiration is maintained artificially, the result is a very elegant heart-lung preparation whereby the heart is really being maintained under optimal conditions of viability in an organ bank. In such circumstances there can be no objection to the removal of a beating heart from a donor previously certified to be dead according to the conventional criteria of permanent arrest of the respiration and the circulation.

Conclusions

The irreversible loss of the properties of living matter constitutes its death.

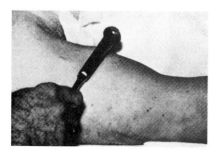
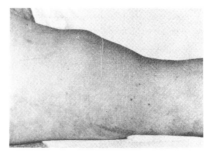

Fig. 1.1A Persistence of the muscular contraction after a mechanical stimulation applied 45 minutes after death.

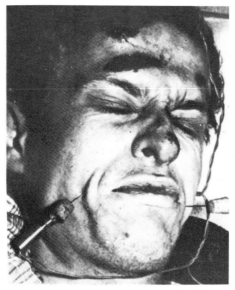

Fig. 1.1B Contraction of the muscles around the mouth after the application of a weak electric stimulus 45 minutes after death. Note the spreading of the reaction to involve the muscles around the eyes.

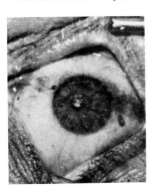
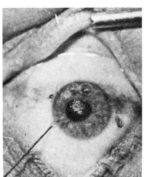
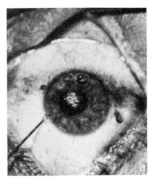

Fig. 1.1C Mydriasis on intraocular stimulation by homatropine 4 hours *post mortem*. (Same case as in Fig. 1.1A.)

Figs. 1.1A–C With acknowledgements to F. Schleyer's *Determination of the time of death in the early post-mortem interval*, in *Methods of Forensic Science*, Vol. 2, 1963, pp 257, 259, 263. London and New York: Interscience Publishers.

This may involve the integrated organism as a whole (the irreversible loss of its co-ordinated activities—so-called somatic death) or its component parts (organs, tissues, cells—so-called cellular death).

The legal certification of death depends on the diagnosis of somatic death. Organ transplantation depends on the persistence of the properties of living matter in the component parts of the organism even after somatic death.

The distinction between somatic and cellular death has become important because the removal of essential organs, e.g. heart, liver and kidneys, for transplantation is usually only permitted after somatic death has been established. Because of the relatively short time for which the biological properties of living matter persist in the component parts of the organism after its somatic death, the needs of organ transplantation have led to attempts to define more precisely the criteria for the diagnosis of somatic death at the earliest possible moment.

Somatic death occurs with the permanent cessation of the functions of the vital nerve centres of the brain-stem, after complete and permanent cessation of spontaneous breathing and the circulation of the blood. With somatic death there is complete generalized anoxia of the tissues and, as a consequence, there is ultimately a cessation of the metabolic processes carried out by the tissue cells, i.e. processes whereby substances are handled by organs and tissues after absorption from the gut or after injection into the body. There is a variation in the sensitivity of the different types of cells to a lack of oxygen. The most sensitive cells appear to be the ganglionic cells of the central nervous system which die from anoxia within a few minutes while the least sensitive cells, such as those of the connective tissues, may survive for some hours. The persistence of biological properties in the component parts for a few hours after somatic death is shown by the temporary persistence of such phenomena as muscular irritability, ciliary movements (of the pupil of the eye) and independent and spontaneous contractions of the excised heart.

After a varying period, however, all the cells undergo irreversible changes and total cellular death occurs. Anaerobic chemical processes carried out by tissue cells, i.e. processes carried out in the absence of oxygen, may continue for some hours after somatic death, e.g. the liver cells may break down alcohol to acetic acid and complex chemical changes may occur in the muscles. With the fall in body temperature and the accumulation of waste products, there is ultimately a cessation of these anaerobic processes.

THE DIAGNOSIS OF DEATH

Medical practitioners are often required to certify that death has occurred. In order to do this they rely upon certain so-called signs of death. The principal signs of somatic death are the cessation of the circulation and the cessation of the respiration. If the heart sounds and respiration are absent over a continuous period of several minutes, death may be certified.

Cessation of the circulation

Cessation of the circulation may be determined by palpation of the pulse, but this sign is not a reliable indication of death because the heart may continue to contract feebly without producing any palpable pulsation in the peripheral arteries. Auscultation is a more reliable method for detecting the absence of heart action, but the auscultation must be performed carefully over the whole precordial area (chest area overlying the heart), before it is decided that such cardiac action is absent. The heart sounds may be so feeble or—because of a thick chest wall—so distant, that they cannot readily be heard. Apart from auscultation, the absence of circulation may be demonstrated by other methods, such as the application of a ligature round a finger of the patient. If circulation is present, a pale zone will develop at the site of the ligature while the part of the finger beyond it will become congested (distended with blood which cannot pass beyond the obstruction created by the ligature). This test is known as the Magnus test. In cases of doubt, an incision may be made and an artery opened. A pulsating flow, not an even continuous escape of blood, will indicate cardiac action.

Electrocardiography, if available, will settle the issue.

Cessation of the respiration

Cessation of spontaneous breathing may be detected by a careful inspection of the chest and abdomen. Particular attention should be given to the inspection of the upper anterior abdominal wall for evidence of slight respiratory movements. The absence of air entry may be demonstrated by auscultation, and this examination should always include the placing of the stethoscope bell over the region of the larynx. Additional simple methods for detecting the cessation of breathing, such as the 'mirror test',* may be employed. It is advisable, however, to rely mainly upon auscultation for establishing the cessation of breathing.

Brain death

So-called brain death is a vague term. It does not, e.g. include death of cortical areas of the brain. It refers, in this context, to the death of those parts of the brain-stem concerned with the maintenance of breathing, the blood pressure and the circulation of the blood. These parts of the brain-stem are generally known as the vital centres. Brain death is secondary to the irreversible cessation of the function of the vital centres and cannot, therefore, be relied upon (e.g. electroencephalographically, i.e. by a record of the electrical activity of the brain) to establish somatic death, if the

---

* In the 'mirror test' a clean mirror is placed before the nostrils and mouth and if respiration is present the surface of the mirror becomes clouded over with moisture.

breathing, the circulation of the blood and the blood pressure are still being maintained spontaneously.

If, after somatic death, the beating of the heart is restored and maintained by artificial means, the heart may be regarded as part of a rather elegant heart-lung preparation which is being stored in an organ bank. It is in such circumstances that a beating heart may be removed for organ transplantation.

Haider and his co-workers[1] recorded complete electrical silence of the brain in five patients in drug-induced coma, unresponsive to any stimuli. This absence of any evidence of electrical activity of the brain (i.e. so-called brain death) lasted for up to 11 hours. One patient died and the remainder made a complete clinical recovery.

They cite the following illustrative case:

As an example, one 63-year-old female who had taken a large dose of sodium barbitone was admitted deeply unconscious and unresponsive to all stimuli. Her EEG showed complete electrical silence. Eight hours after her admission her EEG for the first time showed slight activity but continued flat (Fig. 1.2A). There was still no clinical response to stimuli. The EEG activity gradually increased to generalized slow waves, as shown in Fig. 1.2B. The EEG one month later was within normal limits.

They comment:

It is important to bear in mind that flat EEG records are not uncommon in patients who have ingested large quantities of drugs which depress the central nervous system, and that complete recovery can occur. It is also worthy of note that patients who at first have complete electrical silence may not show any clinical response to stimuli for as long as 15 hours, yet the

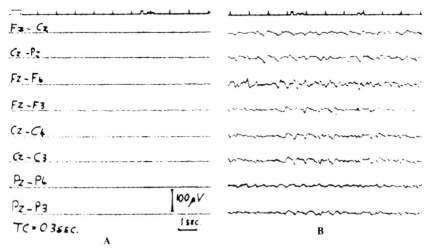

Fig. 1.2A Eight hours after admission the EEG continues almost flat.
Fig. 1.2B Twenty-six hours after admission the EEG shows generalized slow activity.
From Haider *et al*, Br. Med. J., 3 August 1968, p. 314.

EEG may show progressive increase in electrical activity. Such a record can be of predictive value.

Sament et al[2] review and report on the persistence of electroretinal potentials in isoelectric EEG records in patients on a respirator, showing no reflexes or spontaneous breathing and no response to noise or pinch, clinically or in the EEG.

These observations emphasize that the failure to demonstrate electrical activity in the brain does not prove that the properties of living matter have disappeared from tissues very intimately related, in this case, to the brain itself.

Juul-Jensen,[3] in an assessment of 76 patients to determine criteria of brain death for the selection of donors for organ transplantation, recorded the case of a 32-year-old woman (his Case 5) who, despite an isoelectric EEG (recorded after an anoxic episode and an intravenous Nembutal injection), recovered and survived.

Levin and Kinell[4] (and others) have also reported cases of complete recovery in spite of prolonged periods of isoelectric EEG tracings during anaesthesia.

Concomitant signs of death

Other signs of death include the loss of all reflexes (automatic reponses of the body to appropriate stimuli), the development of muscular flaccidity, changes in the eyes and the loss of skin translucency and elasticity.

The muscular limpness which develops at the time of somatic death is known as primary muscular flaccidity to distinguish it from the secondary muscular flaccidity which follows rigor mortis.

Figure 1.3 illustrates an interesting problem. The facts were reported in The Star, Johannesburg, on 22 January 1976 on page 23. The deceased was observed sitting on a bench in a public park in Johannesburg at about 7.00 a.m. on 21 January 1976, apparently asleep. At about 2.30 p.m. (i.e. some $7\frac{1}{2}$ hours later), as he was still 'asleep' in the same position, the manager of a nearby parking garage, who had observed him apparently asleep in the same position all day, approached him and, on shaking his shoulder, realized that he was dead. He was then stiff and cold. According to the attendant, the deceased was admitted to the mortuary 'stiff, in a sitting position'. It seems remarkable that the deceased did not collapse at the moment of death, when primary muscular flaccidity occurs. It is certainly inconceivable that a fully anaesthetized patient, for example, could be placed in this sitting position and maintain that posture unsupported.

In this case it is not known when the deceased died and how, despite a presumed primary muscular flaccidity at the time of death, the deceased maintained a sitting position; or whether, for reasons that are not clear, the whole body was involved in instantaneous cadaveric rigidity at the moment of death.

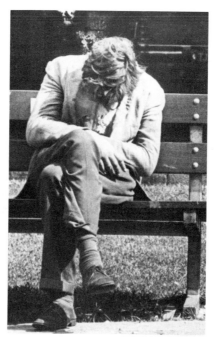

Fig. 1.3 *The Star*, Johannesburg, 22 January 1976, p. 23.

The maintenance of the posture in which the body was found is remarkable on either hypothesis.

Death was apparently due to natural causes (a cardiomyopathy).

In *Forensische Medizin*, Prokop describes and illustrates a similar case (Fig. 1.4).

In the eye, the corneal reflex is lost, the eyeball becomes flaccid and clouding of the cornea follows. As the pupils usually dilate at the time of death, and later become constricted through the development of rigor mortis, their state after death is no indication of their ante-mortem appearance. Sims and Bickford[5] have pointed out that bilateral dilation of the pupils is not characteristic of brain death. They presented photographic evidence that average-sized pupillary diameters (neither constricted nor dilated) can occur in human brain death.

Thus, in this respect, the post-mortem interval may also be very important as the size of the pupil may be influenced by the changes in the body occurring after somatic death.

The loss of skin transparency, which is indicative of the absence of circulation, may be demonstrated by inspecting the webs of the fingers in transmitted light.

All these concomitant signs of death may precede somatic death and do not, in themselves, establish that death has occurred. Final certification of

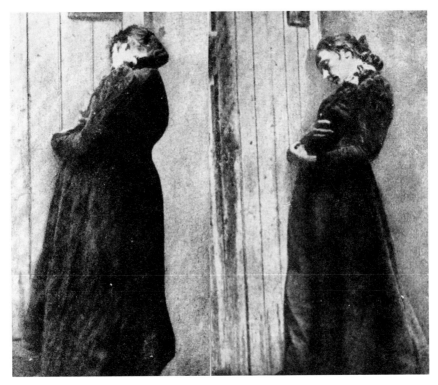

Fig. 1.4 (Prokop's Fig. 26): The famous Wahncau case. The corpse of a 45-year-old woman was found standing upright in a corner of an empty timber yard. There was a lump of faeces on the ground under her dress; the arms were folded. Death ostensibly occurred in uraemic coma. In this case it is difficult not to believe in cataleptic rigor mortis.
Comment: Prokop does not give the evidence for the diagnosis of uraemic coma and apparently refers to the condition known as flexibilitas cerea.
(Reproduced with acknowledgements to the author and the publishers, VEB Verlag Volk and Gesundheid, Berlin: O. Prokop 1966 *Forensische Medizin*, 2nd edn, p. 43.)

death should always depend upon the demonstration of a cessation of the circulation and of spontaneous, indepedent breathing.

Errors in the diagnosis of death

As a general rule there is no difficulty in the diagnosis of somatic death. In certain cases, however, the heart-sound intensity or the breathing movements may be greatly diminished. Errors of certification may arise in these circumstances if the examinations are undertaken hurriedly and superficially. Errors of this nature may occur in dying patients, e.g. in patients dying from kidney failure with associated Cheyne-Stokes respiration. Even though relatives and nurses may expect such patients to die, a premature diagnosis of death may prove most distressing. Errors in the diagnosis of death are more serious, however, when apparently healthy persons who have collapsed suddenly are wrongly diagnosed as having died of acute heart failure. Such errors are likely to occur in cases of apparent drowning, in electrical injuries, in hypoxic or anoxic newly born infants, and in certain types of collapse under anaesthesia. Particular care should be exercised in all these instances before it is decided that death has occurred. In all cases of doubt it is advisable to apply appropriate methods of revival. Such revival must be applied promptly in order to prevent, in the event of recovery, residual paralyses or other effects from hypoxia or anoxia of the central nervous system. In cases of acute breathing failure, e.g. after electrical injuries, it is important to persist with artificial respiration for a prolonged period. Such measures should only be abandoned when unmistakable signs of death are apparent.

Despite all care, erroneous death certification seems to occur all over the world, e.g. Stockholm,[6] Denver,[7] Bombay[8] and Rome,[9] to illustrate only a few examples reported in the lay press from time to time.

Mullan and his co-workers[10] described two cases of severe barbiturate poisoning in patients who had been certified dead by a medical practitioner, but who were subsequently found to be alive.

Their case 1 is very instructive:

A woman, aged 40, had taken an unknown quantity of Carbrital (pentobarbitone sodium and carbromal). On admission, she was deeply comatose and a mechanical respirator had to be used. Twelve hours later she became pulseless with an unrecordable blood pressure, inaudible heart sounds, and fixed dilated pupils. Her temperature was below 35 °C. She was therefore certified dead by a doctor.

Half an hour later, while she was being 'laid out' by the nursing staff, she made a shallow respiratory grunt. Although she appeared dead at the time, an electrocardiogram showed remarkably good complexes (Fig. 1.5). She was therefore put back on the mechanical respirator.

Nineteen hours after admission we were asked to see the patient and decided to haemodialyse her immediately. During the dialysis the systolic blood pressure rose to 80 mmHg, the pulse rate was 100 per minute, and the pupils began to react to light. Spontaneous respiration did not return, however, and she died.

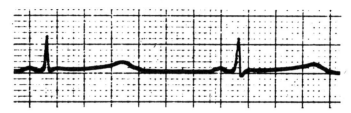

Fig. 1.5 Electrocardiogram. Lead II, normal standardization. Mullan *et al*, *Lancet*, 27 March 1965, *i*, 705.

Under normal conditions there is usually a relatively long delay between the diagnosis of death and the final disposal of the body. During this interval unmistakable signs of death, such as rigor mortis, usually appear. Although errors may arise in the diagnosis of death, there would appear to be little danger of premature burial under normal conditions. Under abnormal conditions, e.g. during war or during major epidemics, bodies may be buried soon after apparent death, and premature burials may take place. Such premature burials, however, are unlikely to occur even under abnormal conditions, when medical services are available. Smith[11] states that no instance of premature burial has been substantiated on investigation by competent authorities in cases where the body was examined by a medical practitioner before burial.

COOLING OF THE DEAD BODY

The normal oral temperature fluctuates between 35.9 °C (96.7 °F) and 37.2 °C (99 °F). The rectal temperature is from 0.3–0.4 °C (0.5° to 0.75 °F) higher (Wright).[12] This temperature range is maintained in health as there is normally a balance between the amount of heat produced in the body and the amount of heat lost to the environment. According to Sheard[13] there are three main ways by which the human body loses heat, namely, by radiation, convection and vaporization. Heat loss by conduction is not an important factor during life.

Heat production ceases soon after death, but the loss of heat continues. As a result, the body cools until the temperature of the body and that of the environment are the same. This fall in temperature mainly depends upon a loss of heat through radiation and convection, but a body lying on the cold ground might lose a considerable amount of heat by conduction. The surface cools more rapidly than the interior of the body, and within a few hours after death the body may feel cold to the touch. An estimation of the body temperature based upon such an examination, however, is completely unreliable. It is possible to register the skin temperature by special methods, but this is seldom done in practice. The most reliable method of determining the body temperature after death is to record the visceral temperature.★

In calculating the fall of temperature after death it is usually assumed that the body temperature was normal at the time of death. It is probable that there is no appreciable rise or fall in temperature in sudden deaths from natural causes and in rapid violent deaths. In certain cases the temperature may be subnormal or markedly raised at the time of death. The temperature

---

★ The visceral temperature is registered by making a small midline incision into the peritoneal cavity and placing the bulb of the thermometer in contact with the inferior surface of the liver. The thermometer should be graduated in degrees Fahrenheit from about 50° to 100° (or in corresponding centigrade degrees). The reading must be taken *in situ*. Rectal temperatures have also been used.[14]

may be subnormal in deaths from congestive cardiac failure, massive haemorrhage and secondary shock. The temperature may be raised at the time of death (even to levels as high as 43.3 °C (110 °F)) in deaths from certain infections, pontine haemorrhage and heat stroke. In deaths from fulminating infections, e.g. septicaemia, the body temperature may continue to rise for several hours after death.

When estimating the post-mortem interval from the rate of cooling of the body, all these possibilities must be considered.

THE RATE OF COOLING OF A DEAD BODY

As the body is not a mass of uniform composition but consists of a number of different tissues, each possessing different physical properties, the cooling of the body after death is a complex process which does not occur evenly throughout the body. As the body cools most rapidly on the surface and more slowly in the interior, the internal body temperature should be taken for the purpose of estimating the post-mortem interval (p. 12).

The post-mortem temperature plateau

The temperature of the body in the early post-mortem interval is generally regarded as providing one of the most reliable ways of estimating the time of death. Simpson[15] states: 'This is the only real guide to the lapse of time during the first eighteen hours after death, and its *early* measurement is often vital to the establishment of an approximate time of death.'

Various popular rules of thumb have been formulated for calculating the post-mortem interval. Simpson[16] gives the following formula:

Under average conditions the clothed body will cool in air at the rate of about $2\frac{1}{2}$ degrees an hour for the first six hours and average a loss of $1\frac{1}{2}$ to 2 degrees for the first twelve.

Taylor[17] states that soon after death the temperature may fall at the rate of 2.2–2.8 °C (4–5 °F) per hour. The rate of fall becomes progressively less, and after 20 hours less than 1 °F of temperature may be lost per hour. In a medium air temperature, 10–15 °C (50–60 °F), the clothed adult body takes about 24 to 30 hours to cool to the temperature of the environment.

Smith[18] whilst recognizing that the time for complete cooling is extremely variable, nevertheless claims that 'the rate of cooling may be slow for the first hour or two, but in general the temperature falls fairly rapidly for a few hours thereafter, then gradually becomes slower as the temperature of the air is approached'.

Glaister[19] also asserts that during a few hours following death 'the temperature falls comparatively quickly . . .'

These views about the cooling of a dead body appear to depend on Newton's law of cooling, according to which the rate of cooling is deter-

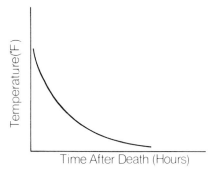

Fig. 1.6 Graph showing fall in temperature when a small inorganic body cools from a temperature of 98.4 °F to atmospheric temperature (see text).

mined by the difference between the temperature of the cooling body and that of its environment. Cooling would therefore be most rapid initially (when this temperature difference is greatest) and slow down progressively as the temperature of the cooling body approaches that of its environment. This relationship can be depicted graphically by a curve resembling a hyperbola (Fig. 1.6).

In forensic practice the temperature is never recorded as that of the surface of the body. One acceptable technique is to take the subhepatic or intrahepatic[20] temperature; another is the rectal temperature.[21,22]

In 1953, Shapiro[23] reported that apparently healthy persons who had died at known times were found to have normal temperatures for at least 4 hours after death, by which time (according to various rules of thumb) the body temperature should have dropped by some 3.3–5.6 °C (6 to 10 °F). This empirical observation of an initial plateau brought into question the validity of these formulae, certainly in the first few hours after death, when the need to apply them might be crucial. Shapiro pointed out that while Fig. 1.6 is undoubtedly an accurate representation of what happens to the temperature of a small inorganic body when it cools, this Newtonian graph does not fit the curve of the rate of cooling of a human cadaver, which has considerable mass and a particular shape. If we leave out the influence of complex and variable external environmental factors[24] (e.g. clothing, wind movement, humidity, etc.), the problem may be simplified by considering what happens when a solid sphere of uniform temperature cools to the temperature of its environment. From the centre of the sphere heat is lost by conduction to the surface, from where further heat loss occurs to the atmosphere by radiation and convection.

The rate of cooling will depend, among other things, on the heat conductivity of the material. Elaborate mathematical calculations can be made for the rate of cooling at points along the radius of the sphere. The surface will, at the beginning, cool more rapidly than the centre of the sphere, because of the greater temperature difference. Moreover, because the dead human body is a poor conductor of heat, it is to be expected that a similar state of affairs will take place in the human cadaver in the early hours after death . . . As the rate of cooling of the interior of a solid body will depend on conduction, the amount of heat at the centre of a large sphere or ovoid cylinder (which the human frame virtually is) can be expected to remain unchanged for some time. We know from actual observation that this period may be at least 4 hours.

It is possibly considerably longer.[25]

Fiddes[26] has pointed out that metabolic processes do not necessarily cease at the moment of somatic death. In so far as they may continue for a short while after clinical death, they may produce heat and so constitute an additional factor contributing to the maintenance of the initial plateau. Fiddes[27] also states that:

> Shapiro has usefully drawn attention to the initial plateau of sustained temperature which characterizes the cooling curve as it applies to the centre of a body, and to the heat conductivity of the body as a factor affecting the rate of cooling. Cooling at the centre of a body is delayed until, by conduction, a temperature gradient is established from the centre to the periphery.

He has relied on this plateau phenomenon to explain the curve observed in the plotting of his own data.[28]

> When the percentage cooling rates are projected on logarithmic graph paper, the result is a line which is straight, except in the first or top part of its extent where a slight flattening no doubt reflects the initial plateau of sustained central temperature referred to by Shapiro.

Hence an accurate representation of the relationship between the postmortem interval and the temperature of a dead body must incorporate the initial plateau. To fit the observed facts we must therefore derive a sigmoid curve (Fig. 1.7). The validity of Newton's laws is not thereby challenged. Indeed, it may truly represent thermal relationships at or very near the skin surface and explains the gradient set up along the 'radius', so to speak, from the centre to the surface of the body. Appreciation of the sigmoid relation-

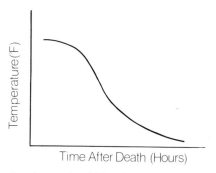

Fig. 1.7 Graph representing the way in which a dead body cools to atmospheric temperature. The graph incorporates the initial post-mortem temperature plateau (see text).

ship avoids the error of mistaking the Newtonian curve (which represents the *rate* of cooling) for the curve which represents the *resultant* of the many complex variable factors which influence the rate of cooling which still occurs according to Newton's law.

De Saram[29] and Fiddes[30] have devised formulae to express the rate of cooling mathematically. The use of these rules requires completely standardized conditions, and in such circumstances they can prove very useful indeed. Fiddes has calculated the limits of accuracy which can be expected and has also made the very important observation that many bodies may take 60 to 70 hours (or more) to reach the temperature of the environment.[31]

Marshall and Hoare[32] have confirmed the existence of the initial plateau described by Shapiro, stating that this plateau of slow cooling may last up to five hours. They also attribute to Rainy[33] and to Seydeler[34] the independent observation in 1869 of an initial lag in cooling. Schleyer[35] (in a critical review of the post-mortem temperature of the dead body as an index of the time of death) reproduces curves (based on rectal measurements) depicting the actual observations made by Schwarz and Heidenwolf[36] in 1953. These curves also demonstrate the presence of the initial plateau.

Schleyer concludes that there can be no reliable rule of thumb and that cooling rates per hour *post mortem* 'are useless and dangerous to rely upon (p. 266) . . . Errors of ± 2 hours are possible in spite of the mathematical analysis (advocated by Marshall (p. 269))'.

Marshall[37] himself states that despite a mathematical formula giving greater accuracy:

> Considerable errors . . . will still be introduced by changes in the environment during cooling, and the persistent limitation in the calculation of the time of death of all methods employing cooling is ignorance of the body temperature at death. This can vary considerably.
> It would seem that the timing of death by means of temperature can never be more than an approximation.

Despite the many sound objections to the use of the temperature of the cadaver in the early post-mortem interval for precisely estimating the time of death, it has nevertheless been the empirical experience of those who have relied on popular rules of thumb that they have occasionally been surprisingly correct, when the conclusion has been tested by other independent types of evidence. Why, then, does the rule of thumb sometimes work? It clearly cannot be accurate (even approximately) in the first 4–5 hours after death (especially on the basis of a single temperature reading), because of the initial post-mortem temperature plateau which imparts a sigmoid character to the curve of cooling. For the same reason it cannot be any useful guide when the cadaveric temperature approaches that of the environment. Fiddes[38] found that when the body temperature was within about 4 °C (7 °F) of the atmospheric temperature, '. . . the recording of that temperature could be of no value in assessing the time of death with any degree of accuracy'.

In the intervening period, however (as Fiddes[38] and Marshall and Hoare,[39] among others, have shown), the rate of loss of heat becomes more directly proportional to the excess temperature of the body over that of its environment 'and the rate of cooling per degree of temperature difference (the cooling factor) is then proportional to the ratio of the effective radiating surface of the corpse to its mass (the size factor)'.[39]

Therefore any formula which involves an *averaging* of the temperature decline per hour may well give a reasonably reliable approximation to the correct answer, if the estimate happens to be made in this intermediate zone. If a particular body takes 24 hours to cool to the temperature of its environment, a rule of thumb calculation (while hopelessly inaccurate at the beginning or the end of this period) may well be approximately correct around the mid-point (or half-cooling time), e.g. 12 hours *post mortem*. The difficulty in a particular case will be to know the region of the half-cooling time; but the calculation may have some merit, in these circumstances, in providing collateral support for an opinion on the time of death based on other evidence. It is in this limited way that the cadaveric temperature may assist in estimating the time of death in the early post-mortem interval, provided the sigmoid nature of the relationship between the temperature of the cooling body and that of its environment is kept in mind.

The rate of cooling of a body exposed to air after death

The main factors which influence the rate of cooling of a body which is exposed to air after death may be summarized as follows:

1. The mean atmospheric temperature during the period of cooling;
2. The presence or absence of clothing or other coverings on the body after death;
3. The movement and humidity of the atmospheric air; and
4. The state of nutrition and development of the body.

1. The atmospheric temperature during the period of cooling. The rate of cooling depends on the difference in the body and atmospheric temperatures. When the difference between these temperatures is relatively great, the rate of cooling is rapid. For this reason a body cools more rapidly on a cold day than on a hot day.

The rate of cooling is also influenced by the fact that the atmospheric temperature is not uniform during the period of cooling, e.g. the nocturnal atmospheric temperature may be considerably lower than the diurnal temperature.

As the body temperature falls, the rate of cooling becomes progressively slower as the temperature of the body approaches that of the environment. For this reason the temperature fall in all cases is at its greatest during the first few hours of cooling after the period of the initial post-mortem temperature plateau, and it is very slow in the later hours.

2. The presence or absence of clothing or other coverings on the body after death. The presence of clothing or some other covering, by insulating the body from the air, materially affects the flow of heat from a body. Cooling is therefore relatively slow in clothed or covered bodies.

3. The movement and humidity of the atmospheric air. Air movement accelerates cooling by promoting the convection of heat from the body. A body cools more rapidly in the open than in a small badly ventilated room. Moist air is a better conductor of heat than dry air, so that cooling is more rapid in a humid temperature than in a dry atmosphere.

4. The state of nutrition and development of the body. The cooling of a large body is relatively slower than the cooling of a small body. The rate of cooling of a large body as compared with a small body depends not only upon the absolute mass of the body but also upon the size of the surface area of the body relative to its mass. Bodies of infants cool much more rapidly than the bodies of adults, not only because they are smaller but because the surface area of the body of a child relative to its mass is proportionately larger than in the adult.

Fat is a poor conductor of heat and therefore the transfer of heat from the interior of the body to the surrounding atmosphere is greatly retarded in obese as compared with thin subjects.

The condition of muscular activity immediately before death and the manner of death are factors of minor importance in the cooling of the body. If the glycogen content of the muscles has been exhausted by muscular activity immediately before death, heat production by glycogenolysis during the stage of molecular death will be minimal. If death is caused by haemorrhage, the loss of blood will cause loss of body heat immediately prior to death.

It is often difficult to assess the influence of the various factors which affect the rate of cooling of the body. For this reason it is not possible to determine the post-mortem interval accurately from an estimation of the rate of cooling alone.

The rate of cooling of a body immersed in a fluid medium after death

Water is a far better conductor of heat than is air. The rate of cooling of a body immersed in water is therefore much more rapid than the rate of cooling in air. The main factors which influence the rate of cooling in water are:

1. The temperature of the water; bodies cool more rapidly if immersed in cold water than in warm water.

2. The nature of the fluid medium; bodies cool more slowly in water containing sewage effluent or other putrefying organic material than in fresh water or sea water.

3. The movement of the fluid; bodies cool more rapidly in running fluids than in stagnant fluids.

RIGOR MORTIS

Rigor mortis is a post-mortem stiffening of the voluntary and involuntary muscles of the body which develops at a variable period after death and succeeds the state of primary muscular flaccidity.

Its physical characteristics have been investigated experimentally by Forster,[40,41] who has demonstrated two properties (plasticity and elasticity) and evaluated quantitatively the deformation undergone by striped and cardiac muscle during the stiffening which occurs soon after death. No measurable shortening of muscle occurs during rigor mortis unless the muscles are subjected to tension. Muscle shortening in these circumstances only occurs when the muscle is, within certain limits, being stretched. In physiological terms, this means that rigor mortis may be equated with what is virtually the last stretch reflex of which the recently dead muscles are capable. It represents the final biological response of striped muscle. In the case of the heart, it represents the last systole.

When rigor mortis is fully developed the joints of the body become fixed, and the state of flexion or extension of these joints depends upon the position of the trunk and limbs at the time of death. If rigor mortis develops when the body is in the supine position, the large joints of the limbs become slightly flexed. The joints of the fingers and toes are often markedly flexed. This is due to the shortening of the muscles of the forearms and legs.

The position of the joints can be altered if the rigidity of their related muscles is overcome by force. When rigor mortis is 'broken down' in this manner, the rigidity does not recur. If the rigidity is not overcome by force, rigor mortis passes off spontaneously. This occurs after a variable period of time and is followed by secondary muscular flaccidity.

Rigor mortis causes contraction of the heart muscle, and this should not be mistaken for myocardial hypertrophy. Secondary muscular flaccidity may result in distension of the atria or ventricles and this should not be mistaken for ante-mortem dilatation of the chambers or myocardial 'degeneration'.

In view of these post-mortem changes it is not possible to determine at autopsy whether a heart has stopped in systole or diastole.

During rigor mortis the arrectores pilorum muscles contract and this contraction may result in a condition of puckering of the skin known as 'cutis anserina' or 'goose skin'. This condition is also seen in cases of drowning, and it is believed that in such cases the phenomenon is caused by an agonal contraction of the arrectores pilorum muscles. There is no means of distinguishing between these two forms of 'cutis anserina' (p. 117). Rigor mortis affects the iris muscles, and the degree of the change may vary in each eye, giving rise to irregularity and inequality of the pupils. For this reason, the state of the pupils after death is no indication of their ante-mortem appearance (p. 9).

The physiology of muscle contraction and rigor mortis

Figure 1.8 is a diagrammatic representation of the physical and chemical changes which occur in muscle contraction.

To appreciate the changes that occur prior to and during the onset of rigor mortis, a working knowledge of the functioning of skeletal muscle and its structure is necessary.

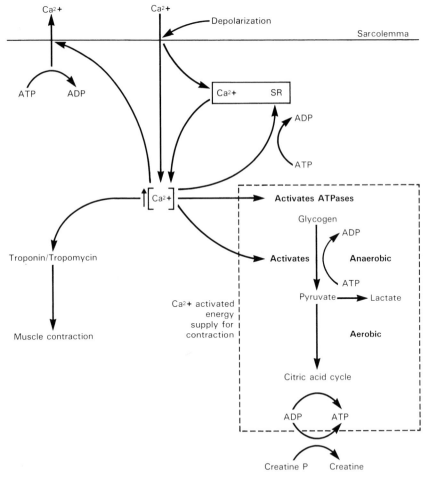

Fig. 1.8 Physicochemical changes in normal muscle contraction.
Ca^{2+} = Concentration of free cytosolic ionized calcium.
SR   = Sarcoplasmic reticulum.

The basic functioning unit in muscle is the sarcomere and this is seen to be the area between two Z-lines. The Z-lines are the densest of the striations and serve as a plate to which the actin filaments attach. Actin filaments are arranged in a hexagonal fashion around each myosin molecule. The overlap between these filaments gives rise to the dark and light zones which contribute to the striated appearance of muscle. Each fibre is a multinucleated cell which may vary in cross-section from 10 to 100 μm, largely dependent upon the site of the muscle, the longitudinal measurements may vary from millimetres to several centimetres and possess a Golgi apparatus. Non-contractile functioning units which are found throughout the sarcomere are the intermyofibrillar and subsarcolemmal mitochondria, the sarcoplasmic reticulum (SR) and the T tubule which is in continuity with the cell membrane or sarcolemma. The sarcoplasm also contains glycogen granules, lipofuscin and lipid droplets. Recent histochemical studies have revealed that the muscle fibres are functionally varied and have been classified by Dubowitz[42] as Type 1 and Type 2. The Type 1 fibres which have a fundamentally oxidative function and represent the bulk of the fibres commonly found in muscles maintaining posture, are capable of long sustained activity, are relatively slow contracting fibres and depend largely on fat as fuel. The Type 2 fibres are the faster contracting fibres which mainly utilize glycogen as fuel.

Proteins constitute 75–80% of dry muscle weight and consist of one or combinations of polypeptide chains. Polypeptides are made up of amino acids which are linked together by peptide bonds. There are also linkages between the polypeptides which involve disulphide cross bridges. Some proteins consist of more than one polypeptide chain which may have been synthesized as separate units while others form multiple units by means of proteolytic splitting of the original single chain. The sequences of the various amino acids which form the basis of the primary structure have been determined for most of the known proteins. Proteins can be divided into two groups, namely the globular and the fibrous. Those of globular configuration have shapes close to being spherical whereas the fibrous have a much longer length to width ratio. The three-dimensional structure of proteins is determined fundamentally by the way the polypeptide chains are folded and this folding is referred to as the secondary structure. The secondary structure is dependent on the regulation and relationship with neighbouring amino acid residues and the overall shape of the chain including the bends and turns, accounts for the tertiary structure. Where proteins consist of more than one chain, interactions between the subunits determine the quaternary structure of the protein. The secondary structures are divided into two forms. One of the most significant is the α helix[43] and the polypeptide presents as a long coil. When polypeptides form B structures or chains, they may bond with adjacent B structures running either in parallel or in the opposite direction resulting in pleated B sheets. These structural elements pack together by interaction of the side chains on both α and β forms to produce a final structure possessing a great deal of flexibility which is particularly important in the myosin and actin interaction as the myofibrils consist entirely of proteins.

The contractile proteins make up 60% of the muscle protein and of these the main proteins myosin and actin account for 60 and 20% respectively. Other proteins present are tropomyosin, troponin, α-actinin as well as proteins of ill-defined function known as C protein, M protein, desmin and connectin which together acccount for 11.5%. Myosin forms the thick filament in the myofibril, actin the thin filaments and tropomyosin and troponin are found on the thin filaments and exert a regulatory capacity. Tropomyosin is situated as two long strands in the groove of the double helix of F-actin[44] and the troponin is attached to the tropomyosin strains with a periodicity of 40 nm.[45]

Myosin is divided into light and heavy meromyosin,[46] the light meromyosin having an α helix configuration. The heavy meromyosin has an α helical fragment and this head region of the molecule containing polypeptide chains[47] is the enzymatically active part of the molecule. Myosin ATPase situated at this site is capable of hydrolysing the terminal phosphate of ATP producing ADP and inorganic phosphate; this reaction is stimulated by Ca^{2+} and inhibited by Mg^{2+}.[48] A myosin filament represents a bundle of many myosin molecules. The rod-like, light meromyosin portions make up the body of these filaments and the enzymatically active heavy meromyosin heads correspond to the bridged portion seen on electron micrographs between the myosin and actin filaments.[49]

Actin consists of a double helix of globular actin units.[50] The combination of actin and myosin forms actomyosin and Ca^{2+} plays an active role in maintaining the association of these two proteins.[51]

Tropomyosin, first shown to be present in muscle[52] has a high α helical content and acts as a regulatory protein. Troponin, a second regulatory protein,[53] has three components whose activity confers Ca^{2+} sensitivity to actomyosin in the presence of tropomyosin. The separate components have the ability to combine with tropomyosin, to inhibit actomyosin ATPase activity and to bind Ca^{2+} respectively. Three troponin subunits form a troponin complex and there is a troponin complex for each tropomyosin molecule. Ca^{2+} activates the actin–myosin interaction by combining with the specific troponin subunit. The subunit for binding calcium is referred to as the TnC subunit and possesses four Ca^{2+} binding sites, each site with a differing degree of affinity. The high affinity sites competitively combine Mg^{2+} while those with low affinity are specific for Ca^{2+}.

Proteins may also act as enzymes so that they are capable of regulating the rate at which metabolic processes take place. These proteins possess an active site which has a definite relationship to the compounds whose reaction it regulates. The enzymatic activity of proteins is frequently linked to the presence of smaller molecules or to coenzymes which are generally derivatives of the vitamins. Metal ions also play an important part in many enzymatic reactions. Enzyme activity may be regulated by the substrate concentration or by combination with 'effectors' which are generally of small molecular size. These moderate with the enzyme and change its activity towards the substrate. Regulation may also be biosynthetic in which the products of a reaction influence the biosynthesis of the enzyme which is catalysing a particular reaction, an important example of this type of control is seen in the phosphorylation of enzymes by protein kinases.

Early attempts to understand the control of muscle contraction and relaxation began with the postulation of a relaxing factor by Marsh in 1951.[54] This factor inhibited the ATPase of the myofibrils and was thought to be present in granules in the sarcoplasm. It is now accepted that these granules were fragments of sarcoplasmic reticulum. The sarcoplasmic reticulum commences in a triad-like structure when viewed electron microscopically.[55] The central or lacunar component of the triad is in contact with the transverse tubule (T tubule) and extends laterally into longitudinally running sacs. The triad is the site of initiation of the excitation process within the fibre and relates to the point of contact between the T tubule and the SR. The sarcoplasmic reticulum stores Ca^{2+} in the presence of ATP. The splitting of ATP is the energy source of all active transport of Ca^{2+} into the inside of the sarcoplasmic reticulum and into the sarcoplasm through the sarcolemma. This calcium pumping action may also be seen to reverse when ATP is synthesized on efflux of Ca^{2+} from the Ca^{2+}-loaded vesicle.[56] The sarcoplasmic reticulum has several protein components. One of these is an ATPase which contains three calcium-combining sites. Calciquestrin, a second protein, is also capable of binding Ca^{2+} [57] and there are also proteins whose functional capacity is not clearly understood though capable of calcium binding.[58] With depolarization of the sarcoplasmic membrane and consequently the T tubules, Ca^{2+} is released into the sarcoplasm from the SR which reaches the actin–myosin overlap zone where its attachment to troponin initiates the contraction process. The actin filaments slide over the myosin and thus reduce the sarcomere length. This Ca^{2+} activation occurs by removal of the inhibitory effect of the tropomyosin–troponin system and once removed, cross bridge formation between actin and myosin is activated while the muscle shortens by progressive attachment. At the same time Ca^{2+} activates the phosphorylase system[59] and in this way begins to mobilize energy from glycogen.

Energy kinetics

The main sources of fuel in muscle are glycogen and fat.

The glycogen is broken down during muscle work and this may occur either anaerobically, where the degradation proceeds as far as lactic acid, or in the presence of oxygen where breakdown will be complete and the end result will be carbon dioxide and water. When great demands on energy supply occur the breakdown is largely anaerobic and the lactic acid is then partially oxidized in the liver and partly resynthesized to glycogen. The breakdown of glycogen is initiated by the enzyme phosphorylase. The phosphorylase is present at rest in an inactive form referred to as phosphorylase b. This is transformed into the active phosphorylase a by ATP phosphorylation catalysed by the enzyme phosphorylase kinase. Phosphorylase kinase has four sub-units one of which identified by Cohen et al[60] has the Ca^{2+} binding protein calmodulin, this subunit is the binding site for the activating Ca^{2+}. Many of the enzymes (e.g. phosphorylase kinase) exist in both an active and an inactive form, inactivation being brought about by phosphorylation which is catalysed by a cyclic-AMP-dependent protein kinase. The production of AMP from ATP is catalysed by the enzyme adenylcyclase which is influenced by hormones such as glucagon and neurally produced agents such as epinephrine.

ATP synthesis in the anaerobic glycolytic process depends upon the reaction between glyceraldehyde-3-phosphate and the coenzyme nicotinamide adenine dinucleotide (NAD), a reaction which leads to the esterification of the phosphate residue which is eventually transferred to ADP to form ATP. Synthesis of ATP also occurs utilizing the phosphate residue that originated in the phosphorolytic breakdown of glycogen by the activity of phospho-enylpyruvate-ADP. With these reactions, the anaerobic breakdown of one glucose component of glycogen produces the formation of three molecules of ATP.

In the presence of oxygen (aerobic metabolism), breakdown of glycogen proceeds beyond the point of pyruvic and lactic acid formation, e.g. with the oxidative breakdown of pyruvate the NADH formed in the reduction of glyceraldehyde phosphate is unable to react with the pyruvate and is itself oxidized. The metabolism of pyruvate and the oxidation of NADH are effected by the enzyme complexes in the various compartments of the mitochondria. The mitochondria, more numerous in the slow-acting fibres, possess an outer membrane separated by a gap from the inner membrane and have a large number of protrusions from the inner membrane into the interior of the mitochondria. These are the so-called cristae. Most of the mitochondrial enzymes are located within this inner membrane and in the cristae and effect the electron transfer for oxygen and control the kinetics for the phosphorylation of ADP to ATP. The pathway controlling the breakdown of pyruvic acid is known as the Krebs cycle, the citric acid cycle or the tricarboxycyclic acid cycle. Pyruvate is oxidized to acetate and coenzyme A. The acetyl residue is then linked with an SH group and the acetyl-CoA interacts with oxaloacetic acid to form citric acid. In the course of these reactions both NAD and NADP are reduced and the removal of two molecules of carbon dioxide and water results in the complete breakdown of the acetate residue. In the citric acid cycle, the NADH and other coenzymes which have been reduced in this reaction are reoxidized by enzymes whose active groups are mainly flavines and iron-containing compounds known as cytochromes. In the mitochondria the participation of a coenzyme Q, copper and non-haem iron form what is commonly known as the respiratory chain. These undergo cyclic reduction and reoxidation with the formation of three ATP molecules for each pair of electrons. This electron flow effects the combination of inorganic phosphate with various acceptors and finally the rephosphorylation of ADP to ATP and in the normal process of oxidative phosphorylation three phosphate moieties are transformed into ATP for each oxygen atom used. The ADP produced by muscle contraction acts as a receptor for rephosphorylation and thus serves as a regulating link between energy conservation and the energy-producing process.[61]

Fat is the other main source of fuel for muscle and fatty acid oxidation performs a vital function. Fatty acids are broken down by the repeated pair-wise removal of carbon residues starting at the carboxyl end of the molecule leading to the formation of an acetate residue in the even-numbered fatty acids and propionic acid in the odd-numbered fatty acids. Both of these substances are linked to coenzyme A and acetyl-CoA enters the citric acid cycle, propionyl-CoA is converted into succinate which is another intermediate in the tricarboxylic acid cycle and water and CO_2 are liberated as discussed in the metabolism of carbohydrates.

High energy compounds

There are number of substances present in muscle which fall into this category and they include ATP, phosphenolpyruvate, creatine phosphate, 1-phosphoglycerol-3-phosphate, acetyl phosphate and acetyl-CoA. There are also low energy compounds such as glycero-1-phosphate, glucose-6-phosphate, fructose-6-phosphate and glucose-1-phosphate. These substances are largely divided into high and low depending upon the amount of energy that becomes available for work by cleaving of the phosphate bond[62] or as in the case of acetyl-CoA where hydrolysis liberates the same free energy as do the high energy phosphates.

In ATP the bond between the terminal and the middle phosphate and between the middle phosphate and the bond nearest the ribose ring are high energy. There are several enzyme systems capable of transferring phosphate from one compound to another such as creatine kinase[63] which catalyses the reaction.

$$CrP + ADP \rightleftharpoons Cr + ATP$$

Myokinase catalyses, as already stated, the transfer of phosphate from ATP to AMP resulting in the formation of two molecules of ADP which in the reverse action supplies further energy. ATP has a purine ring which when reduced to ADP or AMP may be deaminated releasing the NH_2 group. The energy for muscle contraction can be accounted for by the breakdown of ATP and creatine phosphate.[64] These chemical changes require the presence of Ca^{2+}. The concentration of calcium in the sarcoplasmic reticulum as previously discussed involves an active pumping process, i.e. an active transporting process where ions are transported against the gradient of the membrane's electrochemical potential. In muscle the excitability of the membrane depends upon such gradients and there is a potential difference of approximately -90 mV between the internal and external environment of the muscle fibre. The negativity of the inner aspect of the sarcolemma is maintained by the constant pumping out of Na^+ while the high inside K^+ and low Cl^- establish the resting membrane potential.[65] When this membrane is depolarized by the action of acetylcholine which allows Na^+ intrusion, a change in Na^+, K^+ and Cl^- gradients occurs, Ca^{2+} is released into the sarcoplasm and thus the process of excitation contraction coupling begins.

Muscle and death

Figure 1.9 is a diagrammatic representation of the physiochemical changes which occur in rigor mortis.

With cessation of myocardial and respiratory function, the muscle tissue becomes anoxic and all oxygen-dependent processes cease to function. Within a certain period after death, the muscle fibres contract and retain this shortened state for a variable period of time before passively relaxing. This state of muscle contracture depending entirely on physicochemical changes and devoid of electrical excitation is known as rigor mortis. The persistence of this rigid inextensible state depends upon both external and internal factors. The external factors are those such as environmental heat or strenuous physical exertion before death which will hasten the depletion of ATP and glycogen producing early onset of the rigor state. The absence of exertion before death and the cooling of the body after death delay the onset and prolong the period of rigor. The internal changes responsible for the development of rigor relate to the muscles' ability to maintain an adequate level of ATP as ATP inhibits the activation of the linkages between actin and myosin. The major areas for resynthesis of ATP depend on the supply of phosphocreatine in the muscle and also on anaerobic glycolysis. Anaerobic glycolysis continues until most of the glycogen is depleted and results in increasing levels of pyruvic and lactic acid. Production of lactic acid and breakdown of glycogen remains linear until the pH reaches 5.8 after which the process of glycolysis slows down at which time very little glycogen remains. As the level of ATP decreases beyond a critical level the process of rigor proceeds rapidly. Rigor under these circumstances, associated with a low pH, is known as acid rigor. On the other hand where the individual was exhausted or starved before death, the glycogen stores are minimal and rapid or precipitated rigor may occur. Pyruvic and lactic acid are not formed and the muscle remains alkaline and is commonly known as the 'alkaline rigor' of Bernard.[66] The processes of ATP reconstitution and of ATPase activity have been referred to in earlier paragraphs. Mitochondrial activity ceases abruptly at death while myofibrillar ATPase activity is active at normal pH and becomes very active at high pH levels. With a fall in pH the sarcoplasmic ATPases become hyperactive and ultimately ATP is degraded. At this time nucleotide changes occur and the

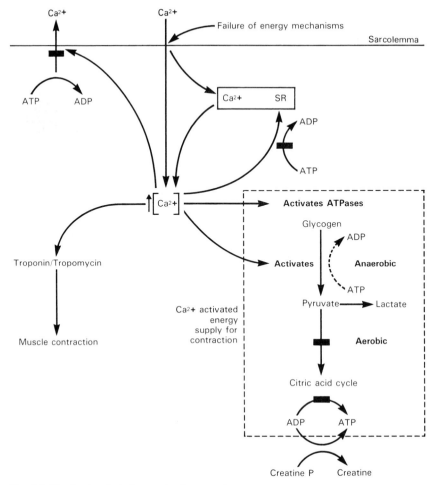

Fig. 1.9 Physicochemical changes in rigor mortis.

formation of inosine monophosphate can be demonstrated chromatographically. Other changes that occur largely as a result of the phosphorylation and deamination are increasing levels of inosine and hypoxanthine and accumulation of phosphate of non-nucleotide origin. At this stage bonding between actin and myosin can no longer be maintained as all energy supplies are exhausted and the muscle passively relaxes. Of the ultrastructural changes that take place during rigor mortis, the early loss of mitochondrial cristae has been noted.[67] This was seen to occur before any observable change in the myofibrillar protein. Other observable changes are the disappearance of matrix and with this the gradual disappearance of glycogen granules. After several days the presence of intramitochondrial inclusions can be seen and it is likely that these are derived from the original cristae and take on the form of rod-like structures, curved structures and concentric spiral bodies.[68] Small dense inclusions appear in the sarcoplasmic space which have the appearance of clumped glycogen granules and occasionally may be seen as glycogenosomes

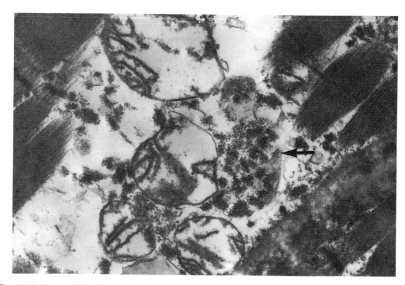

Fig. 1.10 Dense inclusions in sarcoplasmic space ($\times$ 14 600)

(Fig. 1.10). The myofibrils show little alteration when maintained at 4 °C and even after 72 hours show no significant change in some regions while in other sections there is widening and rupture of the I-bands indicating that the actin filaments are the first of the myofibrillar proteins to rupture (Fig. 1.11).[68] The mitochondrial inclusions mentioned are identical to many of the inclusions seen in live muscle (Fig. 1.12).[68]

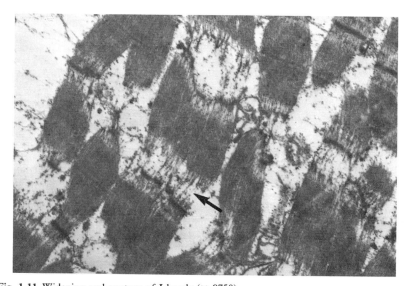

Fig. 1.11 Widening and rupture of I-bands ($\times$ 9750)

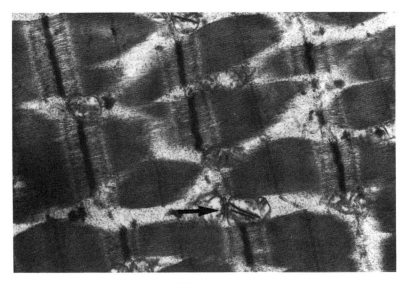

Fig. 1.12 Mitochondrial inclusions ($\times$ 9750)

Though early disruption of mitochondria is noted, mitochondria extracted at 12 hours have been found to be still capable of oxidative phosphorylation *in vitro*.[69]

Rigor associated with malignant hyperthermia

Though many cases of hyperthermia occuring during anaesthesia date back to 1922 or earlier the major publication leading to the recognition of hyperthermia was that of Denborough and Lovell.[70] Ten deaths occurred in a family, accelerated metabolism occurred during anaesthesia resulting in muscle rigor and death in approximately 70% of those afflicted. Britt, Locher and Kalow[71] subsequently described this condition as an autosomal dominantly inherited trait. Isaacs and Barlow[72] identified the problem as being primarily muscular and demonstrated that the creatine kinase level in carriers was elevated in approximately 70%. The clinical events leading up to rigor in susceptible patients are tachycardia, tachypnoea, pyrexia, acidosis and because of muscle breakdown, a large quantity of potassium, creatine kinase, ionized calcium and myoglobin is released into the circulation. These changes are the result of an uncontrolled marked increase in muscle metabolism. The fundamental cause of malignant hyperthermia is still not clear but the most likely hypothesis is that various anaesthetic agents alter the control of intracellular Ca^{2+} by the sarcoplasmic reticulum (SR). The SR fails adequately to reaccumulate Ca^{2+} (Fig. 1.13) and this results in an abrupt rise in the intracellular concentration which triggers the process of aerobic and anaerobic metabolism in a runaway fashion. Malignant hyperthermia may not express itself fully when the patient is challenged by anaesthesia but all rises in temperature of unexplained aetiology following on anaesthesia must be investigated to eliminate the possibility of malignant hyperthermia.

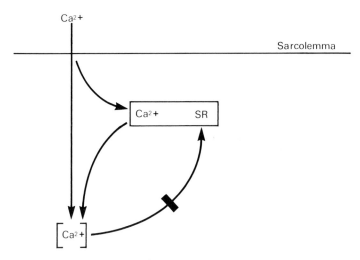

Fig. 1.13 Malignant hyperthermia. Ca^{2+} uptake defect.

An antidote to the heat reaction in malignant hyperthermia has been produced by way of a substance known as sodium dantrolene. This chemical which is close in structure to sodium hydantoinate antagonizes further Ca^{2+} release within the muscle. It is obviously essential that every operating theatre has Dantrium available. A less satisfactory therapeutic measure is IV procainamide or procaine. The intravenous requirements consist mainly of sodium bicarbonate to counteract the lactic acidosis and restore the circulating blood volume. Cooling procedures are carried out and the potassium level may require the use of ion-exchange resins.

Once a malignant hyperthermia patient is identified, the members of the family must be investigated and the carrier status established. This diagnosis is confirmed by muscle biopsy whereby strips of muscle are attached to a specially constructed tension-measuring apparatus in which the muscle is exposed to varying concentrations of halothane and caffeine.

The neuroleptic malignant syndrome

This syndrome (NMS) has some features in common with malignant hyperthermia. NMS is characterized by a pyrexia that may be fatal in susceptible individuals who are treated with various antipsychotic agents and major tranquillizers. NMS differs from malignant hyperthermia as the cause of the rapid rise in fever is mediated via the central nervous system. The most important drug interactions occur with drugs possessing antidopaminergic potency. Sudden withdrawal of anti-Parkinson agents or the use of dopamine-depleting agents such as reserpine may also cause the NMS. Though centrally mediated, the skeletal muscular stimulus to thermogenesis ultimately gives rise to tonic contraction of the skeletal muscles. NMS has responded to treatment with dantrolene and dopamine agonists such as bromocryptine mesalate and amantadine hydrochloride.

Order of appearance of rigor mortis in striated (voluntary) muscles

Rigor mortis is commonly described as commencing in the muscles of the neck and lower jaw and then spreading throughout the muscles of the body.

It is generally accepted that rigor mortis passes off in the same order in which it develops.

Shapiro[73] states that rigor mortis does not follow the anatomical sequence usually described. He has often observed 'in bodies which have not been disturbed and in which rigor mortis has developed to a sufficient degree to involve the wrists and ankles, that, although there may be no more than about 5 to 10 degrees of movement at the elbow or the knee, there is a much greater degree of movement in flexion or extension at the shoulder or the hip.' He suggests that as rigor mortis is a physicochemical process, it is mostly likely to develop simultaneously in all the muscles and to involve completely small masses of the muscles much more rapidly than large masses. Therefore, 'variations in the sizes of different joints, and in the muscles which control them, determine the development of fixation and produce on superficial study an apparent proximo-distal progression of the rigor.' This hypothesis would explain why a relatively small joint (e.g. the elbow joint) surrounded by a moderate amount of muscle becomes immobilized sooner than a large joint (e.g. the shoulder joint) surrounded by a relatively greater mass of muscle. It also explains why rigor mortis appears to affect the relatively small temporo-mandibular joint at an early stage. This hypothesis is important as it emphasizes the difficulty of estimating the post-mortem interval from the distribution of rigor mortis.

The rate of onset and the duration of rigor mortis

There is great variation in the rate of onset and the duration of rigor mortis. As a general rule when the onset of rigor mortis is rapid the duration is relatively short.

The two main factors which influence the onset and duration of rigor mortis are: (1) the environmental temperature; and (2) the degree of muscular activity before death.

1. *The environmental temperature.* When the environmental temperature is high, the onset of rigor mortis is accelerated and the duration is shortened. A low environmental temperature retards the onset and prolongs the duration of rigor mortis. As long as bodies are exposed to environmental temperatures below 10 °C, it is exceptional for rigor mortis to develop, but when the environmental temperature is raised rigor mortis sets in in the normal manner.

Factors such as the movement of the atmospheric air and the presence or absence of clothing or coverings on the body probably influence the development of rigor mortis indirectly by their effects on body temperature (p. 18).

2. *The degree of muscular activity before death.* The degree of muscular activity before death is an important factor in determining the rate of onset of rigor mortis. It has been observed that rigor mortis is rapid in onset and of short duration after prolonged muscular activity, e.g. in deaths after exhaustion in battle and in deaths following convulsions. A relative absence of muscular activity before death might account for the delay in the onset of rigor mortis in many sudden deaths.

Apart from the environmental temperature and muscular activity, the onset and duration of rigor mortis are apparently influenced by several factors such as age and muscular development and nutrition. Rigor mortis is relatively rapid in onset and of short duration in the fetus and stillborn babies. In infants and children and in aged persons, the onset is relatively more rapid than in adults. *It is not possible to deduce any general rule for the rate of onset, duration and disappearance of rigor mortis because of the number and variability of the factors which influence its development.*

Tidy[74] quotes the observations of Niderkorn, 'whose observations on rigor mortis appear to have been made with scrupulous exactness', as shown in Table 1.1.

Table 1.1 Time required for completion of rigor mortis

Number of cases	Hours post-mortem at which rigor was complete	
2	2	
14	3	
31	4	In 79 of 113 cases post-mortem rigidity was
14	5	complete between the third and the sixth hour
20	6	
11	7	
7	8	
4	9	
7	10	
1	11	
2	13	
Total: 113		

Glaister,[75] however, states that in the adult, under average conditions rigor mortis commences within three to four hours after death, spreads throughout the skeletal muscles in 10–12 hours and disappears about 36 hours after death.

Movement of a body before the onset of rigor mortis

When a body is moved before the onset of rigor mortis, the joints become fixed in the new position in which the body is placed. For this reason, when a body is found in a certain position with rigor mortis fully developed, it cannot be assumed that the deceased necessarily died in that position. On the other hand if a body is found in a certain posture with the joints fixed in positions which they do not normally assume in that posture, it can be presumed that the body or portions of the body were moved after death.

The same presumption may be raised if it can be shown that the rigidity in certain groups of muscles has been mechanically 'broken down'.

CADAVERIC SPASM OR INSTANTANEOUS CADAVERIC RIGIDITY

Cadaveric spasm (described by many early writers, e.g. Tidy[74]) is a condition in which those muscles which are in a state of normal contraction at the actual moment of somatic death persist in this state throughout the period of molecular death when the other muscles are in the state of primary flaccidity. Cadaveric spasm continues until rigor mortis is developed in the other muscles and only passes off in the stage of secondary flaccidity.

Cadaveric spasm is said to develop in cases in which somatic death occurs with extreme rapidity. Such cases are usually also associated with great emotional tension at the time of death. The spasm is primarily a vital phenomenon in that it is originated by normal nervous stimulation of the muscles. It would appear that the persistence of the contraction after death is due to the failure (for some obscure reason) of the chemical processes required for active muscular relaxation to occur during molecular death (but see p. 8–10).

Cadaveric spasm may affect all the muscles of the body but it most commonly involves groups of muscles only, such as the muscles of the forearms and hands. When some object is held in the hand of a person at the time of death, the development of cadaveric spasm may result in this object remaining firmly grasped after death. An object cannot be grasped in this manner during the ordinary development of rigor mortis. Cadaveric spasm of this nature can be stimulated if an object is placed in the hand of the deceased during the stage of primary muscular flaccidity, and if the fingers are then tied into position around the object until rigor mortis is fully developed. For practical purposes, however, if an object is firmly grasped in the hand of a deceased it is strong presumptive evidence that the object was in his hand at the time of death.

Cadaveric spasm is seen:

1. In a small proportion of suicidal deaths from firearm and cut-throat wounds when the revolver, pistol or knife is firmly grasped at the moment of death;

2. In certain cases of drowning when grass or weeds or other objects in the fluid medium are clutched by the deceased (Fig. 1.14);

3. In certain mountain fatalities when branches of shrubs or trees are seized by the deceased; and

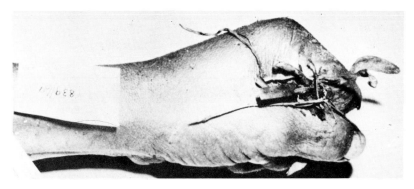

Fig. 1.14 Instantaneous cadaveric rigidity involving the hand in a case of drowning. Note the prominence of the volar tendons. All the other limbs were flaccid. (Prof. L. S. Smith's case.)

4. In certain cases of homicide when some portion of clothing or hair belonging to the assailant is found in the deceased hands.

HEAT RIGOR OR HEAT STIFFENING

Heat rigor is a condition of post-mortem stiffening or rigidity of the muscles. It is caused by a coagulation of the muscle proteins when the body is exposed to a very high temperature. Heat rigor is often seen in bodies removed from burned-out buildings, motor cars or aircraft, and in these cases the stiffening usually develops immediately after death. This rigor may develop, however, at some period after death in those cases where bodies are deliberately burned after death in order to conceal the cause of death or the identity of the deceased.

Rigor mortis does not develop in muscles that have undergone heat stiffening, but this stiffening can occur after the development of rigor mortis. Heat rigor persists until the muscles undergo softening during the process of putrefaction.

There is a marked degree of shortening of the muscle fibres in heat rigor and this shortening results in flexion of the joints of the upper and lower limbs.

The contraction of muscles by heat stiffening may be sufficiently forceful to cause tearing of the affected tissues. Such post-mortem lacerations must be distinguished from ante-mortem wounds (p. 242). When the whole body is burned, the flexion of the joints gives rise to the so-called pugilistic attitude in which such bodies are often found (Fig. 1.15). The flexion of the limbs occurs after death. In certain cases the position of the body or an obstruction may prevent the flexion of limbs. The medico-legal significance of this fact was illustrated in the case of Rex v. Rouse (Northampton Winter Assizes, 31st January, 1931):[76]

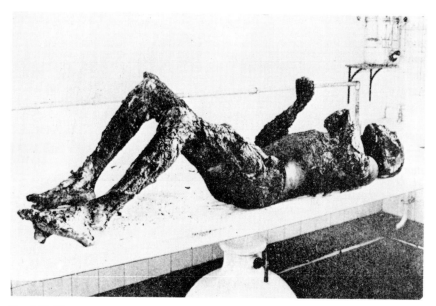

Fig. 1.15 The pugilistic attitude in heat rigor.

The Crown alleged that on the night of 5th November, 1930 (Guy Fawkes night), the accused met a man (whose identity was never established), gave him a lift in his motor car, and stopped in a small country lane near Northampton. It was alleged that he then struck his passenger on the head with a mallet and rendered him unconscious, placed him on the front seat of the car in a prone position and then poured petrol over him and set the car alight. At the time of the murder Rouse was in difficulties, and it was believed that he intended that the burned body should be mistaken for his own. The defence contended that the fire had arisen accidentally. The accused stated that he stopped the car on the roadside, and, as he noticed that his petrol was running low, he asked his passenger to fill the tank from a spare petrol can which he opened himself and placed on the driver's seat. He then walked down the road for a short distance, and when he turned round he saw that the car was in flames.

The bodywork of the car was completely burned out and only the chassis remained. The charred body of the deceased was found across the front seat of the car. The head was on the driver's seat, face downwards, and the body was on the passenger's seat. The left lower limb was bent up underneath the body with the leg flexed on the thigh and the thigh flexed on the abdomen. The right thigh was extended and the right leg was burned off below the knee. The defence maintained that this position of the body suggested that the deceased has been trapped in the blazing car and had made a violent attempt to get to the off-side door of the car. The medical witnesses called by the prosecution said that the position in which the body was found was consistent with the Crown's allegation. They explained that the muscles of the limbs had undergone heat rigor, and that although the left leg and thigh were free to bend as the limb projected beyond the edge of the seat, the right thigh could not become flexed because it was in contact with the seat. The accused was found guilty.

STIFFENING DUE TO FREEZING

Under very cold climatic conditions the tissues of a body are frozen after death. The muscles become rigid and hard and the condition simulates rigor mortis. The extreme coldness of the body, the marked rigidity and the crackling of ice in the synovial fluid when the joints are forcibly flexed distinguish this condition from rigor mortis. Freezing usually occurs before the onset of rigor mortis and, if thawing takes place, the initial rigidity passes off and rigor mortis develops in the usual manner.

POST-MORTEM HYPOSTASIS OR LIVIDITY

After death the blood, while it is still fluid, gravitates to the dependent portions of the body and the dependent capillaries and veins become distended. This capillovenous distension is known as post-mortem lividity or hypostasis.

Post-mortem lividity occurs in all the tissues and viscera. Areas of lividity are readily observed in the lightly pigmented skin and appear as mottled patches which gradually extend and coalesce. In certain cases, isolated patches of lividity remain separate from the large areas of lividity and such patches can resemble bruises. The method of distinguishing between areas of lividity and bruises is dealt with at page 38. The colour of the areas of lividity in the skin is usually purplish-blue. The intensity of this colour depends upon the amount of reduced haemoglobin in the blood. When there has been a marked reduction of haemoglobin before death, the colour of the blood is a deep purplish-blue. In certain conditions the areas of lividity are pink, cherry-red or brown in colour. In acute cyanide poisoning the patches of lividity in the skin are at first a bright pink colour (p. 132). In acute carbon monoxide poisoning the areas of lividity have a characteristic cherry-red colour (p. 129). A chocolate-brown appearance is observed in cases where methaemoglobin is formed in the blood during life, e.g. in potassium chlorate poisoning. Areas of bright pink mottling of the skin are seen in deaths from exposure to cold (p. 144). This form of mottling is also seen in bodies placed in cold storage after death. Franchini[77] has observed that patches of lividity change from a purplish-blue to a bright pink colour at an early stage during refrigeration after death. The reason for this change at low temperatures is not known.

The distribution of post-mortem lividity

External appearances

The distribution of lividity depends upon the position of the body after death. Most persons die in the supine position and are left in this position after death. In these cases the lividity is distributed externally over the dorsal aspect of the trunk, the posterior aspects of the head and neck, the extensor surfaces of the upper limbs and the flexor surfaces of the lower limbs. In the supine position lividity is not observed over the back of the crown of the head, the backs of the shoulders, the buttocks and the backs of the heels as pressure prevents the filling of the veins and capillaries of the skin in these areas. Pressure on the skin capillaries may also prevent the appearance of lividity under tight portions of clothing.

Lividity is usually well marked in the lobes of the ears and in the tissues under the nails of the fingers. In the supine position isolated areas of lividity may be observed over the front and sides of the neck. These areas result from an incomplete emptying of tributaries of the superficial veins of the neck, e.g. the external jugular and common facial veins. The internal jugular veins are usually found to be markedly engorged at autopsy with blood which has drained from the head. The heart prevents this blood draining away below, and the valves in the subclavian veins prevent the drainage of blood into the upper limbs. As a result of this engorgement of the internal jugular veins, the blood cannot be effectively drained from the superficial veins, and there is a distension of the tributaries of the superficial veins in the skin. In this way isolated areas of lividity may develop on the front and sides of the neck and such patches should not be mistaken for bruises, particularly in putrefied bodies (p. 53).

A ventral distribution of lividity is seen externally when a body is left in a prone position after death.

The site of distribution of lividity often depends upon the posture that is assumed in certain forms of deaths. In deaths from hanging lividity is usually observed in the dependent lower limbs, the external genitalia, the lower parts of the forearms, and the hands (p. 111). In deaths from drowning, as the body usually floats face downwards, with the back of the chest at the highest level, lividity is most marked in the face, over the front of the trunk and in the limbs.

Internal appearances

The site of distribution of hypostasis in the viscera depends upon the position of the body. When a person is left in the supine position, hypostatic engorgement is seen in the posterior portions of the cerebrum and cerebellum, the dorsal portions of the lungs, the posterior wall of the stomach, the dorsal portions of the liver, the kidneys, and the lowermost coils of the intestine in the pelvic cavity. It is important to differentiate post-mortem hypostatic engorgement from congestive changes produced before death in certain pathological conditions, e.g. hypostatic engorgement of the dependent portions of the lungs must not be mistaken for the inflammatory congestion of pneumonia, and hypostatic engorgement of the mucous membrane of the stomach must not be regarded as evidence of irritant poisoning. It may be possible to differentiate a zone of inflammatory reaction in a viscus from an area of hypostatic engorgement by certain

naked-eye changes such as the presence of an exudate. In cases of difficulty, portions of the tissue should be examined histologically. Histological
examinations are also necessary in cases where pathological lesions in the
dependent portions of viscera are obscured by hypostatic engorgement.

Patterns of lividity

The pattern of lividity may be modified by local changes in the configuration of the body, e.g. if, for some hours after death, the head remains
turned to one side and slightly flexed on the neck, blood may gravitate into
a linear distribution determined by the folds formed in the skin and
subcutaneous tissues of the neck resulting from the posture of the deceased.
When the body is inspected subsequently after the neck has been straight-
ened, the linear discolorations due to post-mortem lividity may be confused
with the results of trauma applied to that part. Any doubt about the
interpretation of the observations can be resolved by a microscopic examination of the areas of linear discoloration. In certain areas of the body, for
reasons which are anatomically not clear, the distribution of lividity may
be patchy, e.g. on the sides of the neck, when the body is in the supine
position, irregular areas of lividity may be formed. These must be
distinguished from sites of trauma by the appropriate investigations, e.g.
inspection after section, microscopy, etc.

The extent and the time of appearance of post-mortem lividity in the skin

The extent and the time of appearance of lividity mainly depend upon (1)
the volume of blood in circulation at the time of death, and (2) the length
of time that the blood remains fluid after death.

1. When the total blood volume is decreased, e.g. in deaths from acute
massive haemorrhage, the lividity is usually limited in its extent. When the
total blood volume is increased, e.g. in congestive cardiac failure, the extent
of lividity is usually marked and the time of its appearance is accelerated.

2. The fluidity of the blood at autopsy depends upon the rate of intravascular coagulation after death and the concentration of fibrinolysin
(p. 89). When the fibrinolysin is active and the rate of coagulation is slow,
the blood remains fluid and gravitates relatively rapidly into the dependent
capillaries and veins over an extensive area. The blood remains fluid in
deaths from a wide variety of causes, and for this reason the rapid development of hypostasis over an extensive area of the body is not characteristic
of any special cause or mechanism of death (p. 90).

Patches of post-mortem lividity are observed in the skin at a variable
period after death. Taylor[78] states that lividity appears within a few hours
of death and usually reaches its maximum extent about twelve hours after
death.

Medico-legal significance of the distribution of post-mortem lividity

The blood usually remains fluid for a prolonged period after death, except for clots already formed. When the position of a body is changed before the pattern of lividity is established, fresh ares of lividity develop in the new dependent areas, but patches of lividity persist in the old site of distribution. When the position of a body is changed after the distribution pattern of the blood in the dependent vessels has been fixed, the pattern of lividity cannot be altered. Therefore, if a body is found in a certain posture with post-mortem lividity distributed over a region of the body which is not the most dependent part in that posture, careful consideration has to be given to the possibility of the body having been moved after death.

Method of distinguishing between areas of lividity and bruises

An area of lividity may be distinguished from a bruise if putrefactive changes have not developed in the tissues.

A bruise may be found in any region of the body while lividity occurs in the dependent parts but may be seen on the sides of the neck. Abrasions of the overlying skin and swelling of the tissues often accompany bruises. If an incision is made into the area of discoloration the blood is confined to the vessels in the case of lividity whereas it is extravasated into the tissues in the case of a bruise. This distinguishing feature may be demonstrated by a histological examination of the affected tissue. Bruises may occur in dependent parts of the body, and in these cases their presence should be confirmed by histological examination.

Areas of lividity undergo changes at a relatively early stage in the process of putrefaction. The red cells soon haemolyse and the escaped blood pigment diffuses out of the vessels into the surrounding tissues where it may undergo secondary changes, e.g. sulphaemoglobin formation. The capillary endothelium and the surrounding cells undergo lytic changes. On microscopic examination the cellular outlines are obscured and the capillaries are not identifiable. Similar putrefactive changes occur in bruised areas and it may be impossible to determine whether the pigment in a stained putrefied area originated from an intravascular or an extravascular localized collection of blood, i.e. from a patch of congestion or from a bruise.

Haemorrhage may occur from post-mortem wounds when a large vessel in a dependent portion of the body is injured. This possibility is considered at page 245.

The liquidity of the blood after death

Within a short period after death (30–60 minutes),[79,80] the blood in most bodies dead from natural or non-natural causes becomes permanently incoagulable. This is due to the release of fibrinolysins, especially from small-calibre vessels (e.g. capillaries) and serous surfaces (e.g. the pleura). Clots are formed when the mass of the clot is too large to be liquefied by the fibrinolysin available at the site of the clot formation; also in certain deaths associated with infection and cachexia, this fibrinolysin may fail to develop, thus explaining the presence of abundant clot in the heart as well as in the limb vessels in such cases.

Many reputable reference works on forensic pathology state that the blood remains liquid longer in asphyxial deaths and this is claimed to be a valuable autopsy sign confirming the view, in a particular case, that death was due to some mechanical interference with the ability of the tissues to use oxygen.

It is also generally claimed that this increased liquidity of the blood, due to a prolonged clotting time, results from the increased amount of carbon dioxide which accumulates in the circulation during asphyxia or, as it should more properly be called, hypoxic or anoxic anoxia.

In the past, eminent exponents in the forensic field held these views. In the trial of Dr Buck Ruxton for the murder of his wife and a servant, Professor John Glaister expressed the opinion that 'in asphyxial death there is an increased interval of time during which fluidity of blood may remain—up to 12 hours or thereabouts, but I would not be certain'.[81]

Taylor,[82] recognized in many countries as an authority in matters of medical jurisprudence, states (in connection with post-mortem appearances of simple asphyxia) that 'the blood is found fluid for an unusually long time after death; it coagulates very slowly, owing amongst other factors, to excess of carbonic acid (H_2CO_3) contained in it, and for the same reason is very dark in colour.'

That fluid blood has been observed *post mortem* in cases of asphyxial death will not be disputed, but there is every reason to doubt whether this fluid blood is a sign pathognomonic of asphyxia as the cause of death. But this same kind of liquid blood occurs in cases in which death was clearly not due to asphyxia. While the observation of fact is not doubted, the interpretation which has been placed upon it is certainly very suspect. No difference in clotting time is recognized between normal venous and arterial blood. This alone should give cause for caution. Moreover, the matter has been put to the test of experiment. Ponka and Lam,[83] who produced asphyxia in dogs under experimental conditions, concluded that severe asphyxia did not have any effect on the clotting properties of canine blood: 'There was certainly no tendency for the second specimen, obtained during asphyxia, to show a prolongation of clotting time which would have indicated a breakdown of the coagulation mechanism.'

A very adequate review of the whole problem has been published by Mole[79] who states: 'Emphasis on the fluidity of the blood as characteristic of any special cause or mechanism of death is probably misplaced . . .' These conclusions are in accord with the earlier observations reported by the Russian investigator Yudin[80] in his work on the use of cadaver blood for transfusion, and confirms what Hunter wrote as long ago as 1794: 'In many modes of destroying life the blood is deprived of its power of coagulation, as happens in sudden death produced by many kinds of fits, by anger, electricity or lightning; or by a blow on the stomach, etc. In these cases we find the blood, after death, not only in as fluid a state as in the living vessels, but it does not even coagulate when taken out of them'.[79]

Mole concluded that the liquidity of the blood was a feature of 'sudden' death associated with 'shock or collapse' during life. The mechanism appears to be the production of fibrinolysin (p. 90).

Mole also makes the important observation that 'fluid and coagulable blood was also found, whatever the cause of death, when the autopsy was carried out within an hour or so of death.' It is clear that in cases of 'sudden' death the blood remains spontaneously coagulable 'only during a brief period after death and then becomes completely free from fibrinogen';[79] hence it will never again clot, whether asphyxia has contributed to the fatal outcome or not. Indeed, this incoagulability of the blood is a commonplace at autopsy.

This approach to the problem of liquid post-mortem blood was appreciated in the case in which Donald Hume pleaded guilty to being an accessory after the fact in connection with the murder of Stanley Setty, whose torso was disposed of by being dropped into the sea from an aeroplane.

Camps, who gave evidence in that case, recognizing that the blood of the cadaver could remain permanently liquid, stated: 'This must modify previous teaching that clotting is complete after death in 12 hours'.[84]

It seems that many forensic pathologists have mistakenly come to regard the common occurrence of the liquid and incoagulable blood found at autopsy in a great variety of different kinds of death as a diagnostic sign of the anoxic type of death occurring in asphyxia. This completely disregards the properties of cadaver blood, which are in great measure determined by the post-mortem interval. This erroneous view is no longer tenable.

Misuse of the term 'cyanosis'

'Cyanosis' means a bluish colour of the skin, the mucous membranes or the internal organs. It is usually most easily seen in the lips, the tip of the nose, the ears, the cheek and the digital extremities. The word was coined to describe such an appearance in the living body due to certain changes in the oxygen-carrying capacity of the blood.

Oxygen is carried in the blood in a fairly loose combination with haemoglobin. When this compound gives up its oxygen to the body tissues it loses its bright red colour and becomes a purplish blue. When there is a sufficient amount of this deoxygenated blood in the arterial side of the circulation, the skin will take on this blue colour. Normally, the contribution which the blood makes to the colour of the skin is by virtue of the presence of oxygenated blood in the capillaries. Consequently, when this 'blue' blood circulates in the surface capillaries the patient's appearance also becomes bluish and can properly be described as cyanotic. The cyanotic colour of the blood will not usually be detected unless there is at least 5 g of reduced haemoglobin per cent in the capillary blood.

Anything, therefore, that interferes with the oxygenation of the blood (e.g. in the lungs) or that short-circuits blood from the venous to the arterial circulation will produce an appearance of cyanosis, particularly of the ears and the lips and the tips of the extremities, sites in which the cyanosis is usually detected very easily.

We need not consider the numerous causes of cyanosis, but the fundamental principle involved in its production should be understood clearly, because to diagnose cyanosis correctly is to appreciate certain important physiological possibilities underlying this appearance.

In the dead no dynamic chain of events such as has been described can take place. The arterial blood all over the body (including the capillaries) will begin to yield up the oxygen which has been loosely combined with the haemoglobin. But the whole animal body does not die at a particular moment in time. The precision of the moment of legal death is a fiction devised to satisfy statutory requirements. Biologically we die in bits and pieces, and tissue respiration continues for a short time after legal death can be certified. Oxygen dissociation, therefore, continues in the recently dead or dying tissues and this process will go on until equilibrium has been reached between the tension of the oxygen in the capillaries and that in the neighbouring tissues.

In addition, there may be reflux of venous or 'blue' blood from the venular end of the capillaries, thus adding to the blueness of the blood *post mortem*.

For these reasons the colour of the blood in the dead becomes purplish blue and not as a result of some interference with the physiological processes whereby oxygen is bound to the haemoglobin of the blood in the lungs, e.g. throttling, strangling, drowning, etc.

A second important point is that, as a result of the force of gravity, after death the liquid blood gravitates to the most dependent parts, a phenomenon known as the development of post-mortem lividity. (*The Concise Oxford Dictionary* defines 'lividity' as 'of bluish leaden colour'. This is a very accurate, non-committal and objective description of the appearance commonly seen in the recently dead.) Two factors are, therefore, important:

1. The post-mortem diffusion of oxygen gas until equilibrium has been reached with the neighbouring tissues (together with possible venular reflux) will produce a blood bluish in colour irrespective of the cause of death. (We except certain special instances such as carbon monoxide poisoning, cyanide poisoning, etc., which do not concern the point at issue.)

2. By the physical law of gravitation this bluish coloured blood will gravitate into the dependent parts of the body.

The supine position is the commonest in which dead bodies are found and the position of the hands is such that the finger tips are also usually in the dependent position. The head may or may not be turned to one side and the result established in the earlier hours after death is a distribution of bluish coloured blood into the very areas in which cyanosis is looked for in the living, namely, the face, the ears, the tips of the fingers.

The detection of bluish coloured blood in these situations is not, therefore, to be regarded as evidence of the manner in which the deceased person met his death. The pathologist is inspecting no more than the normal appearance of post-mortem lividity and he can easily be misled into making major assumptions about the cause of death if, without any justification, he infers that the bluish colour of post-mortem lividity has the same connotation as cyanosis produced during life. It is not uncommon to find in post-mortem reports a statement that there was cyanosis of the face and the finger nails, because of this confusion between cyanosis and lividity.

In a recent case of alleged asphyxial death (submersion and throttling) a medical practitioner described in his autopsy report that the face and the finger nails of the deceased were cyanosed (blue). At the preparatory examination he argued from this evidence that the word 'cyanosed' used in the post-mortem report indicated that the nails and the face were blue and that this in turn indicated asphyxia.

It is quite clear that evidence about cyanosis, if the word is used in its proper clinical sense, must come from other quarters (i.e. the practitioner who examined the patient when he was alive) and not from the pathologist performing an autopsy.

As it is not possible to distinguish the discoloration seen in dead bodies from that produced by a cyanotic process in the living, the use of cyanosis to describe appearances in the dead is strongly to be deprecated.

Taylor,[85] gives the following list of synonyms for post-mortem lividity: '*Post-mortem* hypostases, subcutaneous hypostases, cadaveric lividities, suggilations, vibices, *post-mortem* stains'.

It is noteworthy that 'cyanosis' is excluded and that it is not used either by Smith or by Glaister as an alternative to 'hypostasis' or 'lividity' in the chapters of their textbooks dealing with post-mortem lividity; and Polson, Brittain and Marshall[86] also avoid the use of the term 'cyanosis' when dealing with the post-mortem appearances of the dead.

As we know, the normal colour of areas of post-mortem lividity is a 'cyanotic' hue and this appearance will, therefore, be seen in areas such as the face, the ears and dependent extremities such as the finger tips and the heels. It is commonplace to see so-called cyanosis under the finger nails at autopsy even in cases of death not due to asphyxia resulting from obstruction of the airway. The use of the term 'cyanosis' in such circumstances reveals an entirely unwarranted presumption about the cause of death and a prejudice in favour of a diagnosis of asphyxia. It is unjustifiable to invest a non-committal, chromatic appearance with such a diagnostic significance which the observation must lack because of the non-specific way in which the bluish colour of the blood is brought about after death.

Evidence about cyanosis must be adduced from other sources than those of a post-mortem inspection several hours after death. Fallacious inferences may otherwise be drawn from what is a normal development of post-mortem lividity.

PUTREFACTION

The body ultimately undergoes a process of putrefaction which results in the gradual dissolution of the tissues into gases, liquids and salts. This transformation is caused mainly by proteolytic and other enzymes produced by bacteria.

Bacteria and putrefaction

A systematic study of the post-mortem bacteriology of human tissues has been undertaken by Burn.[87] Burn found that bacteria which can be isolated from organs and body fluids after death can be classified into two groups. The first group consists of organisms which are frequently found in the tissues at autopsy, and the second group consists of bacteria which are less frequently found. The first group includes anaerobic spore-bearing bacilli (e.g. *Clostridium welchii*), coliform organisms, micrococci, diphtheroids and proteus organisms. It is known that these organisms are normally present in the respiratory or intestinal tracts and it is probable that they penetrate the mucosae and rapidly invade the tissues shortly after death (Burn).[88] Frequently these organisms are widely disseminated in the tissues by a terminal bacteraemia which commonly occurs in protracted deaths.

The second group of bacteria includes a wide variety of pathogenic and non-pathogenic strains. When pathogenic bacteria of this group are found at autopsy they are usually present in association with some lesion or disease process caused by such bacteria. Burn suggests that the physicochemical changes which occur shortly after death during the process of autolysis determine the kind and the number of bacteria which grow in the tissues after death. The marked increase in hydrogen ion concentration and the rapid loss of oxygen in the tissues after death favour the growth of anaerobic organisms.

Tissue changes in putrefaction

Three main changes develop in tissues undergoing putrefaction. These are: (1) changes in the colour of the tissues; (2) the evolution of gases in the tissues; and (3) the liquefaction of the tissues.

1. *Changes in the colour of the tissues.* Haemolysis occurs within the vessels at an early stage of putrefaction. When the haemoglobin is released from the red cells it diffuses through the walls of the vessels and stains the surrounding tissues a red or reddish-brown colour. In the tissues the haemoglobin undergoes chemical changes and various derivatives of haemoglobin are formed. These derivatives include sulphur-containing compounds and the tissues gradually change to a greenish-yellow, greenish-blue or greenish-black colour.

The earliest external change is a greenish discoloration of the skin over the region of the right iliac fossa. This discoloration gradually extends over the whole of the anterior abdominal wall. At the same time prominent reddish-brown arborescent markings appear in the skin in various parts of the body. These markings are caused by the diffusion of haemoglobin into the tissues along the lines of the superficial veins.

The earliest internal change is a reddish-brown discoloration of the inner surfaces of the vessels, especially of the aorta. This change is followed by a progressive discoloration of the internal viscera. Bloodstained fluid is often extravasated into the body cavities.

2. *The evolution of gases in the tissues.* A number of gases are formed in the tissues during putrefaction. These gases include sulphuretted hydrogen, phosphoretted hydrogen, methane, carbon dioxide, ammonia and hydrogen. The offensive odour of putrefaction is caused by some of these gases and by small quantities of mercaptans.

Gases formed in the intestines cause early distension of the abdomen. As the pressure within the abdominal cavity rises, faeces may be forced out of the rectum and stomach contents may be forced through the mouth and nose. Smith[89] states that a fetus may be expelled from the uterus by the pressure of putrefactive gases. A case of this nature has been reported to one of us: A woman who died in childbirth before the delivery of the infant was exhumed some two weeks after burial. There was marked putrefaction present, and the fetus, still attached by the cord, was found between the thighs. The abdominal cavity ultimately bursts open.

Gases form in the subcutaneous tissues and the face and neck become bloated. The eyes are often proptosed and the tongue becomes swollen and protrudes beyond the line of the teeth. Bloodstained froth often appears at the mouth and nostrils. The external genitalia are often markedly distended. Bullae form in the dermis, and when they rupture, large portions of the epidermis become desquamated.

On internal examination, small bubbles of gas are often found in the solid viscera and give rise to the well-known 'foamy' appearance of such organs in putrefaction.

3. *The liquefaction of the tissues.* The tissues of the body gradually undergo a process of softening and liquefaction. The rate at which the

organs become liquefied varies. Glaister[90] states that the eyeballs liquefy at an early stage of putrefaction, and that the brain, the stomach, the intestines, the liver and the spleen putrefy more rapidly than the heart, the lungs, the kidneys, the bladder and the uterus. He believes that the rate of softening depends, to some extent, upon the amount of muscle and fibrous tissue in an organ.

The capsules of the liver, the spleen, and the kidneys resist putrefaction longer than the parenchymatous tissues and these organs are often converted into bag-like structures filled with thick turbid diffluent material. At a later stage in the process the capsules rupture, and it is impossible to recognize the individual viscera in the abdominal cavity.

Factors which influence the rate of putrefaction of a body exposed to the air after death

There is great variation in the time of onset and the rate of progress of putrefaction. As a general rule, when the onset of putrefaction is rapid the progress is accelerated.

The time of onset of putrefaction depends upon the following conditions:

1. *The atmospheric temperature.* This is an important factor. At very low atmospheric temperatures, i.e. at temperatures below 10 °C, bacterial growth is inhibited, and as long as bodies are exposed to such temperatures putrefaction will hardly occur. When the environmental temperature is raised putrefaction sets in in the normal manner.

The optimum temperature for the growth of many of the organisms which can be isolated from decomposing tissues is 37.5 °C (or 99.5 °F). The growth of these organisms is promoted and the rate of putrefaction is accelerated when the environmental temperature approximates this temperature. This fact probably accounts for the rapid development of putrefaction in the tropics during the summer months.

2. *The humidity of the atmosphere and the movement of air in the atmosphere.* Putrefaction is accelerated when there is free access of warm and humid air to a body after death. When there is little movement of the air and atmospheric conditions are warm and dry, the development of mummification is favoured (p. 54).

3. *The state of hydration on the tissues.* Moistures is essential for bacterial growth. Putrefaction is accelerated when the tissues are oedematous, e.g. in deaths from congestive cardiac failure. Putrefaction is delayed when the tissues are dehydrated, e.g. in deaths which are preceded by severe vomiting and diarrhoea. Dehydration is a possible factor in delaying the onset of putrefaction in acute arsenical poisoning and is dealt with at page 48.

4. *Age and nutrition.* The onset and progress of putrefaction are relatively slow in unfed newborn infants and in these cases putrefactive changes may be delayed for a week or longer. This fact must be borne in mind at the investigation of cases of alleged infanticide (p. 387).

Putrefaction tends to be more rapid in children than in adults, and proceeds more rapidly in obese subjects than in thin persons.

5. *Cause of death.* Putrefction is accelerated in deaths from acute infections, especially in deaths from septicaemia. In cases of dismemberment, the rate of putrefaction may vary in the different parts of the body, e.g., the process is usually more rapid in the trunk than in the isolated limbs. This probably depends upon an initial absence of organisms in the tissues of the limbs.

The average rate of putrefaction of a body exposed to the air after death

It is impossible to deduce any general rule for the rate of putrefaction of a body exposed to the air because of the number and variability of the factors which influence its development.

Under average conditions in temperate climates, i.e. with a mean atmospheric temperature between 15.5 °C (60 °F) and 21 °C (70 °F), early putrefactive changes may be seen within 36 to 48 hours after death. At the end of one week the evolution of gases in the tissues is usually well marked and it is often not possible to recognize the features of the deceased. The abdominal wall is discoloured and distended, arborescent markings have developed and bullae have formed in the dermis. The internal viscera are softened and discoloured and the solid organs may have a foamy appearance.

After a few weeks the abdominal cavity bursts open, individual organs are no longer recognizable, and the thoracic and abdominal contents are reduced to a mass of soft diffluent material. Within a few months most of the soft tissues have disappeared and only the skeleton remains. Small residual portions of blackened skin or putrefied tissues may be attached to some of the bones. The skeletal remains may take several years to disintegrate.

Putrefaction of a body immersed in a fluid medium after death

The putrefaction of a body immersed in a fluid medium is relatively slower than the decomposition of a body in air.

When a body is immersed in a fluid medium it often floats face downwards, and putrefactive changes first appear in the face and the front of the neck. The changes advance more rapidly in the face than in any other part of the body. For this reason, even though the rest of the body shows relatively little putrefactive change, it is often impossible to identity the features of bodies removed from fluid media.

Bodies which have been submerged in fluid media may float to the surface because of the evolution of gases in the tissues. This may occur even in cases where heavy weights have been attached to the body at the time of immersion.

The rate of putrefaction of a body immersed in a fluid medium depends upon the following conditions:

1. *The temperature of the medium.* Putrefaction is more rapid in a warm medium than in a cold medium.

2. *The nature of the medium.* Putrefaction is more rapid in a medium containing the products of decomposition of organic matter, e.g. sewage effluent, than in fresh water. On the other hand, putrefaction of a body is more rapid in fresh water than in salt water.

3. *The movement of the fluid.* Putrefaction proceeds more rapidly in stagnant water than in running water.

The rate of putrefaction is often accelerated after a body has been removed from a fluid medium.

Putrefaction after burial

There is considerable variation in the rate of putrefaction of bodies after burial.

It has been shown that the rate of putrefaction of a body buried directly in the soil is relatively slower than the rate of putrefaction in air or in a fluid medium.

If a body is buried in the soil within a short period of death and before changes of decomposition have developed, the rate of putrefaction may be considerably delayed. The rate of putrefaction is more rapid if changes of decomposition are already present at the time of burial. The rate of putrefaction in soil is also influenced by the nature of the soil and the depth of burial. Putrefaction is more rapid in moist soil than in dry soil and is more rapid in porous sandy soil than in soils with an excess of clay. Putrefaction is more rapid when bodies are buried in superficial layers of the soil than when they are buried several feet below the surface of the ground.

Bodies buried in coffins tend to putrefy more slowly than bodies which are buried directly in the soil. The nature of the soil and the depth of burial also influence the rate of putrefaction of bodies buried in coffins. Bodies that are buried soon after death in solid coffins in well-drained deep graves may remain sufficiently well preserved to permit of their identification for many months after burial.

After World War II, Mant carried out a large series of exhumations in

Europe. The bodies were exhumed after burial for periods varying from a few months to several years. The principal factors which influence the changes occurring after burial have been described by Mant.[91]

Putrefaction and arsenical poisoning

It has been stated that decomposition is retarded or prevented in deaths from arsenic and antimony poisoning. It is doubtful whether this is true. In dealing with this question, Copeman and Kamerman[92] state that it is difficult to see how amounts of arsenic, such as are usually found in the viscera in arsenical poisoning, can have any significant effect in preventing decomposition. Only three of the thirty-five cases investigated by them showed any state of preservation after burial. In one of these cases the evidence showed that before death the deceased vomited excessively. It was also known that the cemetery in which the deceased was buried was very well drained. Copeman and Kamerman emphasize that the cause of preservation may well be sought elsewhere than in the presence of arsenic in the body.

Special investigations in putrefied bodies

Bacteriological investigations

The overgrowth of pathogenic organisms by organisms associated with the processes of decomposition often vitiates bacteriological investigations in deaths caused by bacterial diseases. Such organisms may also interfere with biological tests for virus infections.

Biochemical investigations

After death, biochemical investigations may be carried out on blood, the vitreous, cerebrospinal fluid and urine. Because of the glycogenolysis and other chemical changes which may occur in the liver and muscles during the process of somatic death, and because of the redistribution of the electrolytes which occurs between the intracellular and extracellular fluids during the process of and after death, biochemical determinations on samples of post-mortem blood are of limited value and sometimes may give misleading results. If such samples are to be collected, e.g. for 'sugar determinations', they should be collected within a few hours of death, and they should be taken from the left ventricle of the heart so that they will not be influenced by post-mortem chemical changes which occur in the liver.

Plueckhan and Ballard[93] estimated the blood sugar concentration in post-mortem samples taken from non-diabetic persons. The blood sugar concentration was often markedly raised. Samples taken from the right chambers of the heart were most consistently elevated. Overall, the values ranged from 19 mg per 100 ml to 1050 mg per 100 ml.

Tonge and Wannan[94] have also reviewed the value, if any, that is to be attached to post-mortem blood sugar data.

Coe[95] has reviewed the value of biochemical analyses of human vitreous humour and the care required in the collection of specimens. His paper also surveys the significance of the biochemical results obtained from the post-mortem examination of the blood, the cerebrospinal fluid and the urine.

Naumann[96] has shown that post-mortem cerebrospinal fluid examinations are often of more value than blood examinations, but the period during which such examinations can be relied upon is limited. It is seldom practicable to undertake biochemical investigations at times later than 24 hours after death.

Histopathological examinations

Histopathological studies are extremely difficult when autolysis has occurred. Autolytic changes in the viscera affect the parenchymatous tissues and the tissues of the supporting stroma. The dissolution of parenchymatous cells is usually more rapid than the destruction of fibrous tissue, but after a period of 48–72 hours after death it may not be possible to recognize individual structures within an organ.

Toxicological examinations

Organic poisons are gradually destroyed in bodies undergoing putrefaction, but in the early stages of decomposition such poisons may be isolated, e.g. ethyl alcohol has been recovered (without any substantial reduction in its concentration) from peripheral blood 72 hours and longer after death.[97]

Inorganic metallic poisons cannot be destroyed by putrefaction, and poisons such as arsenic may be detected in residual portions of putrefied tissues or skeletal remains many years after burial.

In cases of suspected homicidal poisoning, toxicological examinations should always be carried out even when the tissues show advanced putrefactive changes.

Difficulties in the detection of lesions in putrefied bodies

A thorough examination of a body may reveal the presence of a gross traumatic or pathological lesion even when the body is in an advanced state of decomposition. In a putrefied body the skin is discoloured, but it may be sufficiently intact to show the presence of a gross external injury such as a bullet wound or a large incised wound. As bones are resistant to the processes of decomposition for a prolonged period after death, fractures may be readily detected in putrefied bodies.

It is often impossible to detect lesions in putrefied soft tissues, but gross pathological lesions may be found, particularly in viscera containing a large amount of muscle or fibrous tissue, e.g. valvular lesions may be found in the heart.

Discolorations produced by post-mortem changes may resemble decomposed bruises or decomposed areas of soft-tissue inflammation. In every case portions of the affected tissue must be examined histologically. The main value of such an examination, however, is that it often shows that an opinion cannot be given because of the advanced nature of the putrefactive change. The case of A. G. Carr *v* Rex (1949 (2) S.A.L.R., p. 693)[98] illustrates the difficulty in the diagnosis of bruises in putrefied bodies.

The body of a 2-year-old child was exhumed nine months after its burial.

The child died on 9th December, 1947. An autopsy was held by a medical practitioner on 10th December, 1947. The following changes were found:

1. There was a small bruise measuring 19 mm by 13 mm ($\frac{3}{4}$ in. by $\frac{1}{2}$ in.) on the left side of the neck about 13 mm below the lobe of the left ear.
2. There was a small bruise on the left cheek near the angle of the mandible. No bruise or any other lesion was observed on the right side of the neck.
3. There was a small abrasion in the middle of the upper lip and some minor recent abrasions below the left knee, on the outer surface of the right foot and on the left buttock.
4. An area of bruising was noted in the tissues of the scalp in the region of the vertex in front.
5. The brain and lungs were congested. Subpericardial petechial haemorrhages were seen over the anterior surface of the heart at the base and a limited number of subpleural petechial haemorrhages were noted over the lower lobes of the lungs.
6. The peritoneal cavity contained a quantity of blood which was not measured. At the trial the medical practioner estimated that the quantity amounted to half a pint of fluid blood.
7. A laceration measuring 25 by 6 mm (1 by $\frac{1}{4}$ in.) and from 3 to 6 mm ($\frac{1}{8}$ to $\frac{1}{4}$ in.) in depth was observed on the anterior surface of the liver between the right and left lobes, and a laceration similar in size was seen on the inferior surface of the right lobe.

On the basis of these findings the medical practitioner formed the opinion that the child's death was caused by shock and haemorrhage due to a lacerated liver.

A preparatory examination on an allegation of culpable homicide was opened against the father of the child. It was alleged that he had assaulted the child and that her death was due to laceration of the liver. On 21st September, 1948, during the preparatory examination, the body was exhumed and examined on behalf of the Crown by a senior medical practitioner.

The skin of the upper part of the body was described as being intact, green to greenish-black in colour, and 'dry mummified' in appearance. The tissues of the neck had not been dissected at the time of the autopsy and on reflection from a midline incision an isolated area of brown discoloration was found on the under surface of the skin on the right side. The discoloration was at the level of the upper part of the larynx below the lobe of the right ear. The deeper tissues of the neck showed advanced putrefactive changes and it was not possible to identify the muscles or the vessels of the neck, the thyroid gland or the structures of the larynx.

The senior medical practitioner stated that he considered that the discoloration was a bruise and that the child's death was caused by asphyxia through manual strangulation or throttling. As a result of these observations a charge of murder was substituted for the allegation of culpable homicide and the accused was commited for trial.

At the trial the main contentions for the Crown were contained in the evidence of the senior medical practitioner. He stated that he was convinced that the right-sided discoloration was a bruise. He considered that the bruise on the left side of the neck 'supported' the view that the death of the child was caused by asphyxia, but that the finding of the bruise on the right side of the neck 'confirmed' this view. He regarded the visceral congestion and petechial haemorrhages as pathognomonic signs of asphyxia. He said that the liver lacerations were caused shortly before or at the time of death. The main reason advanced for this contention was the fact that the medical practitioner who performed the autopsy did not record any naked-eye colour change of vital reactions at the margins of the liver lacerations.

The defence disputed the Crown's contentions and maintained that the child died of shock and haemorrhage due to a lacerated liver. On behalf of the defence, evidence was led to establish the fact that the child had fallen off a swing a few hours before her death. It was suggested that the abrasion of the upper lip, the bruising of the scalp and the abrasion of the left knee were the type of injuries which might be expected in a fall from a swing.

Two pathologists were called to give evidence on behalf of the defence. Their general contentions were that the right-sided discoloration was not proved to have been a bruise, that the age of the bruise on the left side of the neck had not been determined, and that even if the right-sided discoloration could be accepted as a bruise, there was no proof that both bruises were caused simultaneously; that the general pathological changes of traumatic shock may be indistinguishable from those of asphyxia; and that the intraperitoneal haemorrhage was caused by ante-mortem bleeding, and that this haemorrhage, combined with shock, afforded an adequate explanation for the death of the child.

In regard to the Crown's contention that the right-sided discoloration was a bruise, the defence medical witnesses maintained that this opinion should not have been given without microscopic confirmation. They stated that the discoloration was consistent with a bruise, but suggested that it was also consistent with a patch of localized decomposition or a decomposed subcutaneous capillary haemangioma or naevus. Authorities were quoted to show that capillary naevi are common and occur on the sides of the neck along the lines of the branchial clefts. It was pointed out that such naevi are not necessarily observed during life. As they consist of a mass of coiled capillaries, it was unlikely that blood would drain from these capillaries after death.

In his evidence the medical practitioner had stated that the external injuries which he had observed were of a minor nature and could have been sustained in the course of the child's ordinary activities. He had included the bruise on the left side of the neck in this observation, and had agreed that this bruise could have been caused several hours or longer before the death of the child. Accordingly it was not possible to prove that it was inflicted at the same time as the 'alleged' bruise on the right side. The defence medical witnesses maintained that in the absence of information about the condition of the deeper tissues of the neck and the larynx, such proof was essential before an inference of throttling could be drawn, particularly as there was evidence of a possible alternative cause of death.

The view that a colour change of vital reaction becomes visible at the margins of liver wounds within five minutes of their infliction was contested by the defence medical witnesses. They stated that vital reaction proceeds initially at a microscopic level and could not be recognized by the naked eye within such a short period of time.

The trial Court held that the discoloration on the right-hand side of the neck was a bruise and concluded that this bruise must have been made simultaneously with the bruise on the left-hand side of the neck. Accordingly, it was found that the child had been murdered by throttling. The accused was sentenced to death.

Leave to appeal to the Appellate Division of the Supreme Court was granted and on 31st March, 1949, the appeal was heard before three Appellate Court Judges. Because of the special circumstances connected with the appeal, the Court took the exceptional course of allowing the defence to lead new medical evidence on the question as to whether the patch of discoloration on the right side of the deceased's neck was an ante-mortem bruise.

The new medical evidence was given by a pathologist who had not given evidence at the trial. He stated that the stains on both sides of the neck were probably caused by degraded haemoglobin. He drew the inference that at some time shortly after death localized collections of blood had undergone decomposition in these sites. He stated that if the red cells had been outside the vessels at the time of death (as in a bruise) they would have rapidly undergone haemolysis and the tissues would have been stained with the freed haemoglobin pigment, which would gradually have undergone degradation changes. Autolysis of the capillary endothelium and other tissue cells would also have occurred and the microscopical architecture would have become completely obscured. The same putrefactive changes would have occurred if the red cells had been inside the vessels. The final appearances would have been the same and quite indistinguishable, whether the original localized collection of blood had been of intravascular or extravascular origin. He did not think that a microscopical examination of the putrefied stained skin would have been of any direct value, but it might have been of indirect value in demonstrating that a decision as to the origin of the stain could not have been given as all structural detail would have been destroyed by the putrefactive processes. Apart from the possibility of an ante-mortem bruise, the witness stated that there were four possible causes for intravascular engorgement at the site of the right-sided discoloration, namely, active hyperaemia, passive hyperaemia, fissural haemangioma, or a patch of post-mortem lividity. (The occurrence of areas of lividity on the sides of the neck is described at page 36.)

The Appellate Division of the Supreme Court found that it was impossible to exclude the reasonable possibility that the patch of discoloration on the right-hand side of the neck was not due to ante-mortem bruising. The Court therefore held that the Crown had failed to prove its contention that the child had been throttled. The appeal was allowed and the conviction and sentence were set aside.

SAPONIFICATION OR ADIPOCERE FORMATION

Saponification or adipocere formation is a modification of putrefaction which is characterized by the transformation of certain of the fatty tissues of the body into a substance known as adipocere. Adipocere is a yellowish-white, greasy, wax-like substance which has a rancid odour.

Adipocere is not common. It is seen occasionally in the tissues of bodies which have been buried in moist soil or have been immersed in fluid media. Adipocere develops in the subcutaneous tissues and is most commonly found in the fatty tissues of the cheeks, breasts and buttocks. On rare occasions, and particularly in infants, the process may involve all the subcutaneous tissues of the body. The process does not affect the viscera.

The time required for the formation of adipocere varies greatly. It usually develops over a period of many months. Under warm climatic conditions, e.g. in the tropics, the process may develop within a few weeks in bodies that are immersed in fluid media. Adipocere may persist for several years after its formation.

The importance of adipocere depends upon the fact that when the process involves the fatty tissues of the cheeks, the features of a deceased may remain identifiable many years after burial or immersion. Similarly, the anatomical form of wounds caused at the time of death may be recognizable many months or years after burial.

The origin of adipocere, the mechanism of adipocere formation and the external conditions necessary for adipocere formation have been described by Mant.[99,100]

MUMMIFICATION

Mummification is a modification of putrefaction which is characterized by the dehydration or desiccation of the tissues and viscera after death.

Mummification is not a common condition but is seen occasionally in bodies that have been buried in dry soil, e.g. in the desert sand. It is also occasionally seen in bodies that have been exposed to warm and dry atmospheric conditions shortly after death, e.g. it is seen in the bodies of newborn infants which have been concealed in boxes or trunks.

Marked dehydration before death favours the development of mummification. Mummified tissues are hard, dry and shrivelled and often black in colour. A striking feature of the process is the preservation of the anatomical features of the deceased.

The time required for the complete mummification of a body varies greatly from a period of several months to a year or longer. The condition may persist for many years once it has developed.

MACERATION

This is a form of decomposition which occurs when a fetus dies in utero and remains enclosed within the amniotic sac.

On external examination large moist bullae may be found in the skin. As these bullae often rupture, reddish-brown areas denuded of epithelium appear over the surface of the body. The internal viscera become soft, moist and discoloured. The process involves the soft tissues of the limbs, and gradually the bones are loosened from their muscular and tendinous attachments.

As the signs of maceration take time to develop, these changes are only seen when a fetus has been dead for several days before delivery.

POST-MORTEM WOUNDS PRODUCED BY ANIMALS, BIRDS AND FISHES

In urban areas, exposed bodies may be attacked by rats and dogs, while in rural areas bodies may be mutilated by hyenas and vultures. In the sea, crustaceans and fishes, including species of large fish such as barracuda and sharks, may ingest parts of bodies. Wounds produced in these ways may simulate ante-mortem injuries, or they may be superimposed upon ante-mortem injuries. In post-mortem mutilations, indentations resembling teeth marks are often found along the edges of the wounds. In a post-mortem rat bite, the teeth marks may be seen along the edges of the wound. In a shark bite, the indentations made by the rows of the shark's teeth may be seen along the edges of the wound. Vultures often wound the soft tissues of the face, and under these conditions personal identification may be difficult.

EROSIONS OF THE SKIN PRODUCED BY ANTS

Ants may be found on bodies after death. These insects produce characteristic brown linear erosions of the superficial layers of the skin. These erosions are most commonly found at muco-cutaneous junctions, about the eyelids, the nostrils, the mouth and the genitalia. They also occur in moist folds of the skin. Under certain conditions, ant erosions may be localized and may simulate ante-mortem abrasions. When ante-mortem abrasions are covered with coagulated serum or blood they may be distinguished from ant erosions. In cases of difficulty histological examination of the skin may show evidence of tissue reaction in an ante-mortem abrasion. Tissue reaction may be absent, however, if the death was too rapid for the development of such reaction.

DEVELOPMENT OF MAGGOTS IN TISSUES

Under favourable conditions certain species of flies may lay their eggs or deposit larvae on exposed bodies. Among the egg-laying species are houseflies (*Musca domestica*), greenbottles (*Lucilia cuprina*), bluebottles (*L. sericata, L. caesar*) and blowflies (*Chrysomyia albiceps* and *C. chloropyga*). Among the larviparous flies are several species of the carrion-fly (genus *Sarcophaga*).

In the case of the egg-laying species, after a variable period, depending mainly upon the atmospheric temperature, the eggs hatch and the larvae feed upon the tissues. In this manner a considerable amount of tissue may be lost after death.

As will be shown at pages 58–59 the identification of maggots may be of value in estimating the post-mortem interval. Accordingly, medical practitioners should be aware of the procedure which must be followed in submitting specimens of larvae and pupae for entomological examination. In order to ensure that the entomologist will be able to examine specimens representative of the different stages of development of the larvae and pupae, the medical practitioner should send several specimens of each kind of larva and pupa. It is also essential to send to the entomologist specimens of the soil around or beneath the body, as the soil may contain pupae. In all cases a description of the locality in which the body was found, together with any information about the temperature, shade and humidity which may be available, should be provided. Live specimens as well as specimens killed in 70% alcohol should be submitted for examination.

ESTIMATION OF THE POST-MORTEM INTERVAL

The period that elapses between death and the time of examination of a body is referred to as the post-mortem interval. It is often of medico-legal importance to estimate this interval, especially in cases of suspected homicide.

Estimations of the post-mortem interval within 36 to 48 hours after death are mainly based on the rate of cooling of the body, the rate of onset and disappearance of rigor mortis, and the time of appearance of post-mortem lividity. The factors which influence these conditions have been dealt with in detail in this chapter (pp 17, 30, 37).

Another factor which has been considered to be of value in estimating the post-mortem interval is the emptying time of the stomach.

Emptying time of the stomach

After an ordinary mixed meal the normal adult stomach empties in 3–4 hours. Accordingly, if undigested food is found in the stomach at a post-mortem examination it is often claimed that the deceased must have died within 3 to 4 hours of his last meal. This claim is of limited value as there are great individual variations in the emptying time of the stomach. Best and Taylor[101] state that the main factors which influence the emptying time of the stomach are: (a) the motility of the stomach; (b) the consistency of the gastric contents; (c) the osmotic pressure of the gastric contents; and (d) the quantity of material in the duodenum. A meal consisting mainly of carbohydrate leaves the stomach more rapidly than one containing protein, while a meal containing protein leaves the stomach more rapidly than one containing fat. Fluids and semi-fluids leave the stomach almost immediately after being swallowed. Best and Taylor consider that the shorter emptying time of carbohydrate food as compared with protein is due to the rapidity with which carbohydrate food is reduced to a semi-fluid state. Fat inhibits gastric motility and this accounts for the delayed emptying time after the ingestion of fatty foods. Emotion, e.g. fear, is also an important factor in prolonging the emptying time of the stomach.

State of digestion of food in the stomach

As the rate of digestion is variable and as it is not possible to determine the degree of digestion of various foods from a naked-eye examination of the stomach contents, little reliance can be placed upon estimates of the post-mortem interval which are based on the apparent state of digestion of the gastric contents. Gastric digestion may continue *post mortem*. This may create further difficulties.

Ilustrative cases

The determination of the exact time of death may become of major importance in the course of a criminal trial. The medical witness should clearly explain to the Court that any estimate of a post-mortem interval can only be an opinion based upon probabilities and must therefore be subject to limitations. The medical witness should not create the impression that determinations of the post-mortem interval can be made with scientific accuracy. In many cases, however, if the factors that influence the various post-mortem phenomena are analysed in relation to the known circumstances of death, an approximate estimate of the post-mortem interval can be given.

The type of analysis which can be undertaken may be illustrated by our findings in the cases of Rex *v.* Godwin Goodman and Rex *v.* Lineveldt.

Rex v. Godwin Goodman. At approximately 7 a.m. in the morning the accused reported the death of his wife to his employer. He said that his wife was perfectly well when she went to bed on the previous evening, and had died suddenly shortly before dawn (at about 6 a.m.). He suggested to his employer that she might have died from the 'fumes' of a coal brazier which he had taken into their room for warmth during the night. (At that time the public had been warned through the press of the danger of sleeping in rooms with coal braziers.) At the initial examination at 9 a.m. it was observed that the body was 'cold' and that rigor mortis was fully developed. At autopsy undigested food was found in the stomach. (It was known that at about 7 p.m. on the previous day the deceased had taken a meal containing food similar to that found in the stomach.) These observations strongly suggested that the accused's statement that the deceased had died at about 6 a.m. was untrue. The fact that the accused had suggested that his wife might have died of carbon monoxide poisoning was viewed with suspicion. Although the accused said that he had spent the night with his wife in the room, he apparently had not been affected by the 'fumes'.

At the post-mortem examination carboxyhaemoglobin was not found in the blood. There was no external evidence of injury on the neck, but dissection showed fairly extensive bruising of the connective and muscular tissues over the lower part of the neck. The hyoid bone and the laryngeal cartilages were not fractured. No other lesions were found. On the basis of these observations it was suggested that the deceased had probably died before midnight of the previous evening, and a post-mortem report was issued stating that the findings were consistent with throttling. After he was found guilty and sentenced to death, the accused confessed that shortly after his wife had fallen asleep in the evening he had placed a thick towel over her neck and had throttled her through the towel.

Rex v. Lineveldt. During a period of seven weeks from the 3rd October to the 25th November, 1940, four women were murdered by a young man.

The fourth victim in this series of murders was found dead at 7 p.m. on the 25th November, 1940. The 25th November was a fairly warm day with a maximum temperature of approximately 33 °C (91 °F). The deceased was found in a small, fairly well-ventilated room. She was clothed in a thin dress and was found lying exposed across a bed which was covered with a soft mattress, sheets and blankets. Her skull was fractured and she had several deep incised wounds on the neck. These injuries and the other findings at the scene of the crime suggested that there had been no opportunity for struggling.

A post-mortem examination was held at 10.30 p.m. and the temperature of the body as registered under the liver was found to be 31.7 °C (89 °F). On the assumption that the body temperature was normal at the time of the death, there had been a fall of body temperature of about 5 °C (10 °F). Rigor mortis was fully developed and areas of post-mortem lividity were found over the dorsal aspect of the body. No fluid or solid material was found in the stomach of the deceased.

At the trial the Crown advanced the theory that the deceased had been killed before midday on the 25th November. The last time that she was seen alive was at approximately 11 a.m. on that day, and there were signs in the kitchen that she had commenced the preparation of her midday meal.

On the basis of the body temperature fall of 5 °C (10 °F) and the full development of rigor mortis, it was suggested that the woman had died at least six to eight hours prior to the post-mortem examination at 10.30 p.m. This estimate of the post-mortem interval and the absence of food in the stomach were compatible with the theory of the Crown as to the time of death.

ESTIMATION OF THE POST-MORTEM INTERVAL IN DECOMPOSED BODIES

The estimation of the post-mortem interval becomes increasingly difficult with the onset and development of putrefaction. An approximate estimate of the interval may be made in cases of early putrefaction after all the factors influencing its rate of development have been analysed (p. 45). It is usually impossible, however, to estimate the interval in cases of advanced putrefaction. In recent years attention has been drawn to the value of maggot identification in the estimate of the post-mortem interval in certain of these cases.

In the British case of Rex v. Ruxton (Manchester Assizes, 13th March, 1936)[102] this method of investigation was followed. The salient factors relating to the post-mortem interval were as follows.

Mrs Ruxton and her nurse disappeared from their home between the 14th and 15th September, 1935. On the 29th September, 1935, the dismembered remains of two human bodies were found in a ravine 100 miles from the home of Dr Ruxton. The remains were in a state of advanced putrefaction and the larvae found on the tissues were submitted to an entomologist who was able to show that they belonged to a species of the common bluebottle fly. He was also able to show that the state of development of the larvae was compatible with the tissues having been placed in the ravine twelve to fourteen days prior to their discovery.

It was contended by the prosecution that Dr Ruxton had murdered his wife and nurse during the night of the 14th to 15th September, and had deposited their dismembered bodies in the ravine during the night of the 15th to 16th September. The entomologist's findings supported this theory and also corroborated the opinion as to the length of the post-mortem interval which was deduced from other grounds.

EXHUMATIONS AND THE POST-MORTEM INTERVAL

In most cases where exhumations are necessary for medico-legal purposes the time of death and the date of burial are known. Under certain conditions, however, these facts are not obtainable, e.g. in cases where bodies or skeletons have been discovered lying buried in the soil. In these cases factors such as the nature of the soil and the depth of the burial below the ground have to be considered in estimating the post-mortem interval (p. 54). In practice, however, it is usually impossible to estimate the interval from the autopsy findings in these cases with any degree of accuracy.

REFERENCES

1 Haider I, Oswald I, Matthew H. EEG signs of death. B Med J 1968; 2:314.
2 Sament S, Alderete G F, Schwab R S. The persistence of the electroretinogram in patients with flat isoelectric EEGs. Electroenceph Clin Neurophysiol 1969; 26: 117–121.
3 Juul-Jensen P. Criteria of brain death: Selection of donors for transplantation. Copenhagen: Munksgaard. 1970.
4 Levin P, Kinell J. Successful cardiac resuscitation despite prolonged silence of EEG. Arch Intern Med 1966; 117: 557–560.
5 Sims J K, Bickford R G. Non-mydriatic pupils occurring in human brain death. Bull Los Angeles Neurol Soc 1973; 38: 24–32. Abstracted in Excerpta Medica, Section 5, General Pathology 1973; 28:611.
6 Rand Daily Mail. Johannesburg, 14 August 1969: 'Dead' Woman is much better.
7 Sunday Express, Johannesburg, 15 December 1968: 'Dead' woman comes back to life.
8 The Star, Johannesburg, 19 November 1968: Boy left for dead is alive.
9 The Star, Johannesburg, 20 February 1969: Let me out of here, yelled the 'corpse'.
10 Mullan D, Platts M, Ridgeway B. Barbiturate Intoxication. Lancet 1965; 1:705.
11 Smith S. Forensic Medicine 9th ed. London: Churchill. 1949: p 19.
12 Wright S. Applied Physiology. 7th ed. Oxford University Press. 1945: p 592.
13 Sheard C. Temperature of skin and thermal regulation of the body. In: Glasser O. ed. Medical Physics. Chicago: Year Book Publishers. 1944: p 1523.
14 de Saram G S W. Estimation of the time of death by medical criteria. J Forens Med 1957; 4: 47–57.
15 Simpson K. Forensic Medicine. 5th ed. London: Arnold. 1964: p 7.
16 Simpson K. op. cit. p 7.
17 Taylor A S. Principles and practice of medical jurisprudence. 10th ed. Vol. 1. London: Churchill. 1948: p 177.
18 Smith S. Forensic medicine. 10th ed. London: Churchill. 1955: p 19.
19 Glaister J. Medical jurisprudence and toxicology. 11th ed. Edinburgh: Livingstone. 1962: p 110.
20 de Saram G S W. Estimation of the time of death by medical criteria. J Forens Med 1957; 4: 47–57.
21 de Saram G S W. op. cit 47–57.

22 Fiddes F S. A percentage method for representing the fall in body temperature after death; its use in estimating the time of death with a statement of the theoretical basis of the percentage method by T. D. Patten. J Forens Med 1958; 5: 2–15.

23 Shapiro H A. Medico-legal mythology—some popular forensic fallacies. J Forens Med 1953–4; 1: 144–169.

24 Shapiro H A. op. cit. 144–169.

25 Shapiro H A. op. cit. 144–169.

26 Fiddes F S. op. cit. 2–15.

27 Fiddes F S. op. cit. 2–15.

28 Fiddes F S. op. cit. 2–15.

29 de Saram G S W. op. cit. 47–57.

30 Fiddes F S. op. cit. 2–15.

31 Fiddes F S. op. cit. 2–15.

32 Marshall T K, Hoare F E. Estimating the time of death; the rectal cooling after death and its mathematical expression. Forens Sci 1962; 7: 56–81.

33 Rainy H. On the cooling of dead bodies as indicating the length of time that has elapsed since death. Glas Med J (New Series) 1868–69; 1:323. (Cited by Marshall and Hoare.[32])

34 Seydeler R. Nekrothermometrie. Vjschr prakt Heilk Prague 1869; 104:137. (Cited by Marshall and Hoare.[32])

35 Schleyer F. In Lundquist F. ed. Methods of forensic science, Vol. 2, London: Interscience. 1963: p 268.

36 Schwarz F, Heidenwolf F. Postmortem cooling and its relation to the time of death. Int Crim Pol Rev 1953; 31:256. (Cited by Schleyer.[35])

37 Marshall T K. Estimating the time of death; the use of body temperature in estimating the time of death. J Forens Sci 1962; 7: 211–221.

38 Fiddes F S. op. cit. 2–15.

39 Marshall T K, Hoare F E. op. cit. 56–81.

40 Forster B. The plastic and elastic deformation of skeletal muscle in rigor mortis. J Forens Med 1963; 10: 91–110.

41 Forster B. The contractile deformation of skeletal muscle in rigor mortis. J Forens Med 1963; 10: 133–147.

42 Dubowitz V. Enzyme histochemistry of skeletal muscle II. Developing human muscle. J Neurol Neurosurg Psychiat 1965; 28:519.

43 Pauling L, Corey R B, Bronson H R. The structure of proteins: Two hydrogen bonded helical centrifugations of the polypeptide chain. Proc Nat Acad Sci USA 1951; 37:205.

44 Hanson J, Lowy J. The structure of F actin and of elements isolated from muscle. J Mol Bio 1963; 6:46.

45 Ebashi S, Endo M, Ohtsuki I. Control of muscle contraction. Quart Rev Biophys 1969; 2:351.

46 Szent-Gyorgyi A. Meromyosins, the sub-units of myosin. Arch Biochem 1953; 42:305.

47 Lowey S, Slayter H S, Weeds A G, Baker H. Substructure of the myosin molecule I. Subfragments of myosin by enzymatic degradation. J Mol Biol 1969; 42:1.

48 Szent-Gyorgyi A. Studies on muscle. Acta Physiol Scand 1945: Suppl XXV.

49 Huxley H E. Muscle cells. In: Brachet J, Mirsky A E. eds. The cell, Vol. IV. New York: Academic Press. 1960: p 36.

50 Rice R V, Brady A C, Depue R H, Kelley R E. Morphology of individual macromolecules and their ordered aggregates by electron microscopy. Biochem Z 1966; 345:370.

51 Ebashi S. Calcium binding activity of vesicular relaxing factor. J Biochem 1961; 50:236.

52 Bailey K. Tropomyosin: A new asymmetric protein component of the muscle fibril. Biochem J 1948; 43:271.

53 Greaser M, Gergely J. Reconstitution of troponin activity from three protein components. J Biol Chem 1971; 246:4226.

54 Marsh B B. A factor modifying muscle syneresis. Nature 1951; 167:1065.

55 Porter K R, Palade G E. Studies on the endoplasmic reticulum III. Its form and distribution in striated muscle cells. J Biophys Biochem Cytol 1957; 3:269.

56 Makinose M. Calcium efflux-dependent formation of ATP from ADP and orthophosphate by the membranes of the sarcoplasmic reticulum vesicles. Fed Eur Biochem Soc Lett 1971; 12:269.

57 MacLennan D H, Wong P T S. Isolation of a calcium-sequestering protein from sarcoplasmic reticulum. Proc Nat Acad Sci USA 1971; 68:1231.

58 Ostwald T J, MacLennan D H. Isolation of a high affinity calcium-binding protein from sarcoplasmic reticulum. J Biol Chem 1974; 249:974.

59 Krebs E G, Beavo J A. Phosphorylation–dephosphoryĺation of enzymes. Ann Rev Biochem 1979; 48:923.

60 Cohen P, Burchell A, Foulkes G, Cohen P T W, Vanaman T D, Nairn A C. Identification of the Ca^{++}-dependent modulator protein of the fourth sub-unit of rabbit skeletal phosphorylase kinase. Fed Eur Biochem Soc Lett 1978; 92:287.

61 Chance B, Mauriello G, Aubert X M. ADP arrival in muscle mitochondria following a twitch. In: Rodahl K, Horvath S M. eds. Muscle as a tissue. New York: McGraw Hill. 1960: p 128.

62 Burton K. In: Krebs H A, Kornberg H L. eds. Energy transformation in living matter. Berlin: Springer. 1957.

63 Lohman K. Uber die enzymatische aufspaltung der kreatin-phosphorsaure: zugleich ein beitrag zum chemiismus der muskelkontraktion. Biochem Z 1934; 271:264.

64 Rall J, Homsher E, Mommaerts W F H M. Heat production and phosphocreatine hydrolysis with unloaded shortening in rana pipiens semi-tendinosus muscles. Fed Proc Fed Am Soc Exp Biol 1973; 32:730.

65 Horowicz P. Influence of ions on the membrane potential of muscle fibres. In: Shanes A M. ed. Biophysics of physiological and pharmacological actions. Washington: American Association for the Advancement of Science. 1961: p 217.

66 Bernard C. Lecons sur la diabete et la glycogenese animale. Paris: Bailliere. 1877: p 429.

67 Hegarty P V J, Dahlin K J, Benson E S. Ultrastructural differences in mitochondria of skeletal muscle in the pre-rigor and rigor states. Specialia In Experientia 1977; 34/8: 1070–1071.

68 Isaacs H, Badenhorst M. Personal communication: 1986.

69 Isaacs H, Whistler T. Personal communication: 1986.

70 Denborough M A, Lovell R R H. Anaesthetic deaths in a family. Lancet 1960; 2:45.

71 Britt B A, Locher W G, Kalow W. Hereditary aspects of malignant hyperthermia. Can Anaesth Soc J 1969; 16: 89–98.

72 Isaacs H, Barlow M B. Malignant hyperpyrexia during anaesthesia: possible association with subclinical myopathy. Br Med J 1970; 1:275.

73 Shapiro H A. Rigor mortis. Br Med J 1950; 2:304.

74 Tidy C M. Legal medicine, Part I. London: Smith, Elder. 1882: pp 58–74. Reprinted in Forens Sci 1973; 2: 113–123.

75 Glaister J. Medical jurisprudence and toxicology, 9th ed. Edinburgh: Livingstone. 1950: p 132.

76 Normanton H. Trial of Alfred Arthur Rouse. Edinburgh: Hodge. 1931: pp·49 and 95.

77 Franchini A. Anatomo-histological changes in the cadaver kept in the refrigerator. Boll Soc Ital Biol Sper 1946; 22: 149–150.

78 Taylor A S. op. cit. p 181.

79 Mole R H. Fibrinolysin and the fluidity of the blood post mortem. J Pathol Bact 1948; 60: 413–427.

80 Yudin S S. Transfusion of stored cadaver blood; practical considerations: first one thousand cases. Lancet 1937; 2: 361–366.

81 Blundell R H, Wilson G H. Trial of Buck Ruxton. 2nd ed. London; Hodge. 1950: p 157.

82 Taylor A S. op. cit. p 520.

83 Ponka J L, Lam C R. Effect of asphyxia on blood coagulation in dogs. Proc Soc Exp Biol Med NY 1948; 68: 334–336.

84 Camps F E. The case of Stanley Setty. Med-Leg J 1951; 19: 2–15.

85 Taylor A S. op. cit. p 181.

86 Polson C J, Brittain R P, Marshall T K. The disposal of the dead. London: English Universities Press. 1953: pp 222 and 257.

87 Burn C G. Post-mortem bacteriology. J Infect Dis 1934; 54: 395–403.
88 Burn C G. Experimental studies of post-mortem bacterial invasion in animals. J Infect Dis 1934; 54: 388–394.
89 Smith S. op. cit. p 29.
90 Glaister J. Medical jurisprudence and toxicology. 9th ed. Edinburgh: Livingstone. 1950: pp 135–136.
91 Mant A K. Factors influencing the changes occurring after burial. In: Simpson K J ed. Modern trends in forensic medicine. London: Butterworth. 1953: pp 84–91.
92 Copeman P R v d R, Kamerman P A E. Poisoning by arsenic in South Africa. S Afr Med J 1940; 14: 379–384.
93 Plueckhan V D, Ballard B. Factors influencing the significance of alcohol concentrations in autopsy blood samples. Med J Austral 1 June 1968: p 939.
94 Tonge J I, Wannan J S. The post-mortem blood sugar. Med J Austral 1949; 1: 439–447.
95 Coe J I. Postmortem chemistry of blood, cerebrospinal fluid and vitreous humour. In: Wecht C H. ed. Legal medicine annual 1976 . New York: Appleton-Century-Crofts. 1977: pp 55–92.
96 Naumann H N. Studies on post-mortem chemistry. Am J Clin Path 1950; 20: 314–324.
97 Bowden K M, McCallum N E W. Blood alcohol content: some aspects of its post-mortem uses. Med J Aus 1949; 2: 76–81.
98 Carr A G v Rex., Medico-legal aspects of the trial and the appeal. S Afr Med J 1949; 23: 647–651.
99 Mant A K. Adipocere—a review. J Forens Med 1957; 4: 18–35.
100 Mant A K. Adipocere. In: Simpson K ed. Modern trends in forensic medicine, 2. London: Butterworth. 1967: pp 152–158.
101 Best C H, Taylor N B. The physiological basis of medical practice. 4th ed. Baltimore: Williams & Wilkins. 1945: p 487.
102 Glaister J, Brash J C. Medico-legal aspects of the Ruxton case. Edinburgh: Livingstone. 1937: pp 261 and 263.

2

Autopsy technique*

The technique is described for a right-handed dissector who commences his dissection standing on the right-hand side of the body.

GENERAL INSPECTION

After the relevant history of the case has been obtained, the body is weighed, measured and identified. (The identity of the body is usually established by relatives or close friends.) In the case of unidentified bodies, it may be necessary to make anatomical (i.e. physical anthropological), radiological and dental observations to establish the sex, age, stature and personal identity of the deceased. It is preferable that such observations should be confirmed by experts in these various fields and that the observations should be interpreted by them. Details of the techniques and procedures which can be followed in the identification of bodies have been provided by Krogman[1]. The development and nutrition of the body are noted, and a careful general inspection of the external surface of the body, its orifices, and the mucous membranes, is made. The exact position of scars, tattoo marks, abrasions, bruises and other wounds must be noted. Wounds must be examined in a good light with a hand-lens if necessary, to determine whether they are incised or lacerated. Their exact dimensions should be measured with a ruler. The extent of rigor mortis, the distribution of post-mortem lividity and the degree of putrefaction, if any, must be recorded.

THE HEAD

It is an advantage to open the skull first because observations which depend on the sense of smell will be interfered with to a lesser extent by competing odours from the body cavities, their organs and their contents.

* This chapter describes the technique to be adopted at an ordinary adult autopsy and at exhumations (p. 78). For the post-mortem examination of infants, see p. 376. For the post-mortem procedure in the detection of poisons and the submission of specimens for toxicological analysis see pages 197 and 214.

The scalp is divided down to the bone across the vertex from ear to ear at a level just behind the ears. With the aid of a retractor the anterior half of the scalp is pulled forwards and dissected free from the skull, attention being paid to any haemorrhages in the scalp tissues and their size and position noted. The scalp is separated well forward down to the eyebrow ridges. The posterior half is next dissected free well down to below the occipital protuberance. The skull holder is now applied over the parietal eminences.

The skull is opened with a saw, beginning with a horizontal division an inch or so above the eyebrow ridges. It can be felt when the inner table of the bone is reached. The temporal muscles are divided down to the bone, and the division of the frontotemporal region of the skull bone is carried out in a line above the ears to meet the first line of division in the frontal region. Care must be taken to saw through the inner table, but to avoid dividing the dura mater. After the temporal divisions have been completed the saw line is carried obliquely downwards and backwards to the lambdoid suture.

It is convenient to make sure that the bone has been divided completely by applying a chisel along the line of sawing. With the aid of an elevator inserted into the frontal saw line, the cap of the skull is raised, and with the hands the whole skull cap is pulled backwards and removed. The external surface of the dura is now inspected.

The superior sagittal sinus is opened along its length with a sharp scalpel and carefully examined for signs of an ante-mortem thrombus. This is of medico-legal importance, as ante-mortem thrombosis in this situation can lead to back pressure in the bridging veins crossing the subdural space, and so to subdural haemorrhage. The dura mater is grasped anteriorly with a forceps, and with scissors or scalpel the dura mater is divided from before backwards at the level of the skull division. This is done on both sides. The scalpel is now passed vertically downwards alongside the falx cerebri at its anterior extremity, and the knife turned medially to divide the falx. With the aid of forceps the dura and the falx are pulled backwards. The exposed surface is now inspected. It is also advisable to smell the brain at this stage.

The anterior poles of both frontal lobes are mobilized with the left hand, and the optic nerves brought into view and divided. The exposed cranial nerves and the pituitary stalk are divided, and the knife is carried along the superior petrous temporal border through the attachment of the tentorium cerebelli. The remaining cranial nerves are divided, and the whole brain is pulled back and the medulla oblongata exposed and divided. The brain is freed and removed from the cranial cavity.

With a pair of lion forceps the dura mater is detached from the base and the sides of the skull, which can then be examined for signs of fracture. Fractures are best seen after the dura has been stripped, and the bones of the skull must also be tested for any signs of abnormal mobility.

OPENING THE CHEST AND THE ABDOMEN

The line of the primary incision is marked out with a cartilage knife. It extends from the level of the thyroid cartilage down the midline to the pubis. It is customary to avoid the umbilicus. The incision is deepened halfway between the xiphoid and the umbilicus, all the tissues, including the peritoneum, being divided. The middle and the forefinger of the left hand are inserted through the wound into the peritoneal cavity and spread out on either side of the incision and used as a guide to complete the division of the abdominal muscles along the line of the primary incision down to the pubis. The incision is also carried upwards to the xiphoid process.

The next stage is to remove the coverings of the chest wall. With the aid of a retractor in the line of the primary incision, the skin and muscles are retracted firmly laterally. While this is being done long incisions are made with the dissecting knife at right angles to the ribs. If oblique incisions are made on to the ribs, the chest muscles will not be removed cleanly, and a clear view of the ribs will not be obtained. The position of the retractor is altered from time to time, as the tissues are cleaned well up to the clavicle and well down to the lower rib cartilages.

The abdominal muscles can be divided on their inner aspect along the lower rib cartilages by turning the muscles back over the this border. If the dissection is carried well laterally, a clear exposure of the front and side of the chest is obtained. It is useful to turn the lower abdominal muscles outwards and to make two or three incisions transversely through the muscles on their inner aspect, taking care not to divide the skin. This procedure acts as a retractor by keeping the abdominal flaps open. When one side of the chest dissection has been completed, the dissector should cross to the opposite side of the body and repeat the dissection on the opposite side of the chest.

The abdominal contents should be inspected, including the mesentery and the mesenteric glands. A finger must be passed through the foramen of Winslow into the lesser sac and the common bile duct and its related structures palpated.

The dissector should now proceed to open the chest cavity. The rib cartilages may be divided with a cartilage knife. In older bodies where the rib cartilages have become calcified, it may be necessary to use a pair of rib shears.

The rib cartilages are divided in a slanting direction towards the dissector on the right side and away from him on the left side, beginning at the second rib cartilage and working downwards, carrying the knife from one cartilage to the next below it. By opening the chest through the rib carti-lages, dangerous spicules of bone are avoided, but the division must be carried out near the costal ends of the cartilages so as to make as big an opening in the chest as possible. The diaphragm is divided at its attachment to the lower ribs and sternum. The knife is carried up close to the under surface of the sternum and through the divided rib cartilages to the level of the first rib.

The dissector passes to the head of the body and divides the right first rib cartilage posterolaterally. He lifts up the sternum by its lower end and manipulates it so as to see the sternoclavicular joint. He carries the knife through the divided first rib cartilage into the joint. This procedure is repeated on the opposite side. The sternum is detached by dividing the remaining tissues attached to it. This technique ensures that no vessels of any size are divided and that no bleeding occurs into the pleural cavities as a result of the dissection.

The chest contents are now inspected and examined, the condition of the lungs being noted. The pericardial sac is opened with scissors and forceps and its contents inspected.

Where a pulmonary embolus is suspected, the right ventricle and the pulmonary artery should be opened in situ.

The lungs are now mobilized. With both hands the lateral, posterior and inferior surfaces of the lungs are palpated, pleural adhesions being broken down and the lung brought out of its bed so that it is demonstrated to be free. The pleural cavity and the region of the posterior mediastinum are inspected.

THE NECK

The dissection of the neck can now be undertaken. The back of the neck should be supported on a rest. This produces extension of the neck and facilitates the subsequent dissection. The dissection should be immediately deep to the skin, through the platysma, the skin being held with a toothed forceps and the dissection carried out with a sharp, long-handled scalpel.

If the skin is flayed from the body in this way and care is taken not to divide any of the great veins in the neck, a clear exposure of the subcutaneous tissues and the ventral surfaces of the anterior muscles of the neck is obtained. The subcutaneous dissection should be carried up to the lower border of the lower jaw, well laterally on the side of the neck and downward to meet the reflection of the tissues at the base of the neck and the clavicle. The general appearance of the dissection at this stage is shown in Fig. 2.1A.[2]

After inspection, the investing layer of deep cervical fascia is incised and reflected from the ventral surfaces of the anterior cervical muscles and the submandibular gland (Fig. 2.1B). The right sternomastoid muscle is inspected, freed from its clavicular and sternal attachments, separated from its underlying fascia and reflected. The same procedure is adopted on the left side followed in sequence by the exposure, inspection and reflection of the omohyoid, sternohyoid, sternothyroid and thyrohyoid muscles on each side. These reflections expose the lateral lobes of the thyroid gland and the

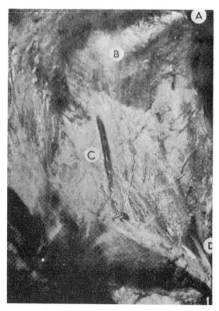

Fig. 2.1A Dissection of neck (right side). A, Point of chin; B, Angle of the lower jaw; C, External jugular vein; D, Sternal head of sternomastoid muscle. **Figs. 2.1A, B, C** from Prinsloo and Gordon (1951).[2]

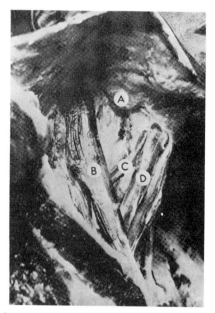

Fig. 2.1B Dissection of neck (right side). A, Submandibular gland; B, Sternomastoid muscle; C, Omohyoid muscle; D, Sternohyoid muscle.

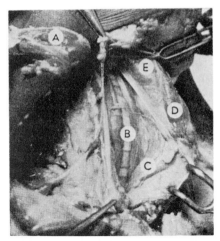

Fig. 2.1C Dissection of neck (right side). A, Reflected sternomastoid muscle; B, Anterior surfaces of bodies of cervical vertebrae; C, Oesophagus; D, Lateral lobe of the thyroid gland; E, Lateral wall of the pharynx.

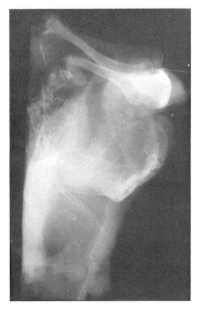

Fig. 2.1D Radiological appearance of a geniculate fracture of the hyoid bone in a case of suicidal hanging. The fracture is on the side opposite to the ligature knot.

carotid sheaths. These structures are then freed by blunt dissection from their investing connective tissues. By blunt dissection, the larynx and trachea and the pharynx and oesophagus are mobilized, raised and retracted from the prevertebral tissues (Fig. 2.1C). This technique of dissection of the neck muscles permits inspection of these medico-legally important areas before the position can be confused by bruises resulting from dissection artefacts.

Gordon *et al*[3] stressed the value of radiological studies of the excised hyoid-larynx complex. They have also described a geniculate fracture of the greater cornu of the hyoid bone in cases of suicidal hanging, blunt trauma to the neck and as a post-mortem artefact (Fig. 2.1D).

After all the cervical tissues have been examined *in situ* in this manner, the mouth is opened and the tip of the tongue pushed upwards and backwards with a forceps. The long-handled scalpel is passed horizontally in the midline deep to the symphysis menti. The palm of the free hand is placed on the outside of the lower jaw to steady it while the knife is carried along the inner border of the mandible in the direction of the ear, dividing the neck muscles attached to the lower jaw.

When both sides of the neck have been dealt with in this way, the fingers should be passed into the mouth from below and the tongue brought down into the upper part of the front of the neck through the floor of the mouth. The long-handled scalpel is passed horizontally through the floor of the mouth, and the junction of the hard and the soft palate divided. The knife is carried backwards and laterally on both sides of the midline to divide the posterior pharyngeal wall. The dissection should be carried well laterally in the direction of the ear.

The middle finger of the left hand is passed over the back of the tongue into the larynx, and with the scalpel in the right hand the pharyngeal tissues are dissected from behind forwards and laterally so that the pharynx is brought down to the upper part of the neck. The dissection is then carried distally, downward traction being exerted on the upper part of the neck tissues. The dissection is made right down through the prevertebral muscles on to the anterior surfaces of the cervical vertebrae. It is important to divide the tissues of the neck well outwards, taking care to cut through the carotid vessels. In this way the pharynx, larynx, oesophagus and the surrounding tissues are brought down to the level of the clavicles. The knife is passed under the ribs with its blunt edge uppermost over the apex of the lung to the under surface of the medial end of the clavicle. When this position is reached the knife is turned with its cutting edge uppermost and the stump of the neck tissues is divided. This manoeuvre is repeated on the opposite side.

The neck structures are now grasped *en masse*, and by strong downward traction the chest contents are pulled down to the level of the diaphragm. Unless the pleural adhesions have previously been freed, this will not be possible. The oesophagus is defined. It is the most left structure passing through the diaphragm, and a ligature should be tied around it as low down as is conveniently possible. The neck tissues and the chest contents are now thrown over to the right, and the pedicle formed by the dissection is divided above the oesophageal ligature.

After the neck structures have been removed, the anterior surfaces of the cervical vertebrae may be examined. The location of fractured ribs can then easily be determined by incisions dividing the intercostal muscles from before backwards.

THE ABDOMEN

The abdominal contents are dealt with next. The greater omentum with the transverse colon is thrown upwards, and the duodeno-jejunal flexure is defined. The assistant holds up a loop of the upper jejunum, and the dissector divides the mesentery of this loop horizontally close to the mesenteric border of the intestine. This portion of the gut is ligatured as high up as possible with two ligatures about an inch apart. The dissector holds the root of the mesentery in his left hand, and as the assistant pulls the coils of the intestines towards himself the mesentery is divided close to the mesenteric border of the gut. The assistant must inspect and palpate the intestines as he handles them. In this way gut is separated until the terminal ileum is reached, when the appendix is inspected.

The assistant grasps the caecum and the ascending colon and pulls them towards himself. The dissector frees the peritoneal reflections binding down the colon up to the hepatic flexure. The next step is to grasp the stomach with the left hand while the assistant holds the transverse colon. The dissector divides the transverse mesocolon and the greater omentum, thus exposing the cavity of the lesser sac, until the splenic flexure is reached. At this stage the gut can be divided between the two ligatures already tied. The descending colon is freed by dividing its attachment from above downwards, and the large bowel is mobilized in this way down to the pelvis. The contents of the rectum are massaged into an upper portion of the bowel and a ligature tied round the lower portion of the rectum, which is divided below the ligature. The whole of the small and the large bowel is now freed and is removed from the abdominal cavity.

The dissector takes the spleen and the tail of the pancreas in his left hand and mobilizes these organs by dissecting behind them to the midline. This procedure exposes the left suprarenal gland, which it is convenient to divide and inspect at this stage. The assistant pulls laterally on the ribs of the left side, while the dissector puts the left dome of the diaphragm on the stretch. The diaphgram is divided up to the midline in a slanting direction to the same point to which the spleen and the pancreas were mobilized. The assistant holds the liver, and the dissector pulls on the ribs on the right side to tense the diaphragm, which is divided to the same point in the midline as before. This manoeuvre is aided considerably if the assistant rotates the liver upwards so as to bring its posterior border next to the dissecting knife. The right suprarenal gland is brought into view, inspected, divided *in situ*, and examined.

The stump of the root of the mesentery is held in the left hand, and it is dissected free from below upwards in front of the great vessels until the superior mesenteric and the coeliac arteries have been divided. All the lines of dissection have converged to the same point in the midline, and so a pedicle has been produced. The abdominal contents are pulled to one side to expose the pedicle, which is divided, and the organs are removed from the abdominal cavity.

The genito-urinary organs remain to be removed. The cave of Retzius is defined, and the anterior surface of the bladder is freed with the fingers from the pubic bone. If the bladder is full its contents should be expressed. In the male the prostate is palpated. The urethra is divided distal to the prostate. The incision is carried through the rectum and into the ischiorectal fossae.

The procedure is the same in the female except that when the cave of Retzius has been exposed and the urethra cut, the vagina is divided. The sexual organs are also inspected *in situ*.

The left kidney is grasped in the left hand and mobilized towards the midline by dissection behind it to the midline, freeing it from the anterior surface of the iliopsoas muscle. The right kidney is freed in the same way. Both kidneys are then taken in the left hand, and the knife is carried down the midline behind the aorta to the pelvis. The pelvic contents have been freed above and below. The knife is carried around the side wall of the pelvis, dividing the lateral attachments of the bladder, each half of the pelvis being dissected downwards to the midline. In this way the pelvic contents are freed completely and removed.

The exposed vertebral column is inspected and palpated.

EXAMINATION OF THE ORGANS REMOVED AT AUTOPSY

The brain

The outer surfaces and the superficial vessels are first carefully inspected in a good light. The brain is placed in its normal anatomical position, with the orbital surfaces of the frontal lobes, the inferior surfaces of the temporal lobes, and the anterior surfaces of the midbrain, pons and medulla resting on a flat wooden board. With a long knife the two halves of the brain are separated by a single incision which passes through the corpus callosum, and through the midline of the midbrain, pons and medulla. If the incision is carried out in the median plane it should pass through the cavity of the septum lucidum and expose the internal surfaces of its two laminae which form part of the medial walls of the lateral ventricles on each side. The incision passes through the third ventricle, the aqueduct of Sylvius, and the fourth ventricle. The lateral ventricles are opened by dissection of the anterior, posterior and inferior horns, and the ependymal lining examined in a good light. The aqueduct of Sylvius and the fourth ventricle are inspected.

The half of the cerebellum with the attached brain stem is separated from the rest of the brain substance and held with the cut surface in contact with the palm. The cerebellum is halved with a single incision of the long knife carried down towards the palm. A good view is thus obtained of the cut surface and of the dentate nucleus. The cerebrum is placed on its lateral surface and long incisions are made antero-posteriorly, about a quarter of an inch apart, but not dividing the brain substance completely. This makes it easier to reconstitute the layers of the brain tissue in order to localize accurately the position of any lesion that may be found. This method of section exposes the grey matter in the base of the cerebral hemispheres.

Neck and chest contents

The tissues of the neck and the contents of the chest have been removed *en masse*. The neck tissues should be held in the hand, and with the long knife the lateral lobe of the thyroid gland is divided longitudinally and the cut surface inspected. Where fractures of the hyoid bone and thyroid or cricoid cartilages are suspected, it is not enough to palpate for the fracture. These structures should be exposed by dissection and the fracture seen. Where the facilities are available radiological records are advisable before the dissection of this region is begun.

The chest contents are placed upon their ventral aspect so that the oesophagus lies uppermost with its upper end nearest the dissector. After the tongue and the surrounding parts have been inspected, a blunt-pointed scissors is introduced into the upper end of the oesophagus, which is then opened along its whole length. Its inner surface is examined. The mass of chest contents is now turned round so that the oesophagus can be freed by dissection from below upwards, thus exposing very clearly the tracheal bifurcation and the lymph glands in this region. These glands are divided and inspected.

The respiratory tract

A pair of scissors is introduced into the upper end of the respiratory tract and the division is carried down the larynx and trachea into each main bronchus. Where a foreign body impaction is suspected, the division of the bronchi must be carried carefully down the branches of the bronchi. Specimens of mucus taken from the respiratory passages may be examined microscopically for carbon particles in appropriate cases. After the lungs have been washed, their outer surfaces are inspected. The long knife is passed with its blunt edge uppermost along the medial border of the lung at the hilum. The knife is then turned so that the cutting edge is uppermost and the lung is separated. The other lung is removed in the same way. Each lung is placed upon the dissecting table with the cut surface undermost. The long knife is placed on the convex surface of the lung in a line from apex to base. The free hand is placed in the form of an arch over the blunt edge of the knife to steady the lung tissue, which is divided with a single sweep of the knife so as to produce an even cut surface, which is inspected. The lung tissue is then grasped and squeezed firmly for signs of oedema.

The heart

The trachea and the bronchi are separated from the heart, the examination of which is now proceeded with. After inspection of its outer surfaces, the heart is placed on its ventral aspect with the atria towards the dissector. The openings of the great veins draining into the right atrium are defined, and with scissors and forceps an incision is made connecting both openings. Another incision is made horizontally through the posterior atrial wall into the atrial appendix. The tricuspid valve is inspected from above. The heart is now placed on its dorsal aspect, and with the long knife an incision is made into the right ventricular cavity through the anterior ventricular wall in the direction of the pulmonary artery. With a pair of scissors this incision is prolonged up into the artery and down to the apex. The cavity of the ventricle is washed out gently, and the valves and endocardium examined.

The left atrium is exposed by joining the openings of the pulmonary veins, and the incision is continued into the atrial appendix. The endocardium and the atrial surface of the mitral value are inspected. An incision is made through the anterior wall of the left ventricle in the direction of the aorta. This incision passes through the pulmonary artery which lies in front and to the left of the aorta.

It will be noted that both the ventricles are opened in the direction of the great vessels leaving them.

The aorta is also opened. The cavity of the ventricle and the lining of the aorta are washed and inspected. The aortic valves are inspected, and the mitral valve can be opened from the cavity of the ventricle, the lower blade of the scissors being passed up into the left atrium between the two cusps of the mitral valve. The anterior cusp is divided. In this way a good view of the mitral valve and the endocardium of the left atrium is obtained. The tricuspid valve can be opened in the same way.

The coronary arteries are transected at close intervals (i.e. at intervals of approximately 3 to 4 mm) and preliminary assessments of the degrees of their patencies are made.

The examination of the heart is completed by making a few incisions through the thickness of the myocardium to look for pathological changes in the heart muscle.

The liver, the stomach, the spleen and the pancreas

The spleen is freed from its pedicle, weighed, washed and inspected. It is placed on the dissecting board and divided with a single incision of the long knife. The cut surface is inspected in a good light.

The pancreas is dissected free, divided in its length in the same way as the spleen, and the cut surface is inspected.

The stomach and the duodenum are dissected free from the liver. A pair of scissors is introduced at the ligatured end of the oesophagus, and the stomach is opened along its lesser curvature in a separate dish when a toxicological examination of the stomach and its contents is necessary. The nature of the stomach contents, their smell and other characteristics are noted. Specimens of the contents may be retained for examination, e.g. in cases of drowning in an unusual medium. The stomach is washed and its mucous and peritoneal surfaces carefully examined.

The gallbladder is dissected free from the under surface of the liver, opened and inspected. The liver is weighed and, after inspection of the surfaces, examined. Sections about one inch apart are made through the substance of the liver in a supero-inferior direction, the liver tissues not being divided completely so as to permit of a reconstruction of the site of any lesion that may be found. As the liver is divided, the cut surface is smoothed with the long knife and inspected in a good light.

The intestines

These are opened with a special pair of intestinal scissors. The gut is washed and inspected along its whole length.

The genitourinary organs

The kidneys and the bladder are placed on the dissecting table in the anatomical position, the aorta being posterior. With a pair of scissors introduced into the prostatic urethra, this is opened and the incision is carried through the prostate into the wall of the bladder, which is thus opened and inspected. The openings of the ureters are defined and the incision is carried up along each ureter to the pelvis of each kidney. In this way the ureters are examined. Each kidney is now dealt with.

Some of the perinephric fat is trimmed away from the lateral border of the kidney. At its hilum the tissues form a pedicle which can be grasped in the left hand so as to place the lateral border of the kidney in position for section. With the pedicle of the kidney thus held in the palm of the left hand, the heel of the long knife is placed at the upper pole of the kidney. With a single long incision carried well down towards the palm the kidney is halved, leaving a cleanly divided, even surface which is smoothed and inspected. With a toothed forceps the capsule of the kidney is stripped from the cut edge. The subcapsular surface of the kidney is inspected.

The rectum is dissected free from the bladder, opened and inspected.

In the female, after the bladder has been opened it is dissected free from the rest of the pelvic organs. The anterior vaginal wall is divided and the fornices are inspected. The vagina is opened from below upwards, exposing the cervix. The uterus is opened from the external os to the fundus, and the exposed interior is inspected. The ovaries and the fallopian tubes are inspected, and each ovary is divided and its cut surface examined.

SPECIAL DISSECTION OF THE PELVIC ORGANS IN THE FEMALE

The cave of Retzius is freed in the manner described at page 71 but the urethra and the upper vagina are not divided. The rest of the pelvic dissection is carried out as before.

The body is placed with its buttocks near the end of the dissecting table, and both lower limbs are widely abducted so as to give easy access to the field of dissection. An oval incision is made through the skin, beginning above the urethra and passing downwards on either side of the vulva to end behind the anus.

From the upper end of this incision in the region of the symphysis pubis the deeper tissues are dissected free, the knife first being carried under the symphysis pubis into the cave of Retzius above the urethra. The dissection is continued down along the border of the pubic ramus and the ischium close to the bone on either side, and through the ischiorectal fossae behind the anus on to the surface of the coccyx. In this way the distal genital tract, the rectum, and the anus are freed, and they are mobilized into the pelvic cavity from above, the genitourinary organs then being removed and dissected in the manner already described. In cases of suspected rape specimens of the pubic hair of the deceased should be removed and suitably labelled for subsequent identification. Smears taken from the secretions in the vagina or its fornices should be prepared on clean glass slides after the vagina has been opened. For signs of abortion in the dead, see page 374.

REMOVAL OF THE SPINAL CORD

In adults it is advisable to remove the spinal cord posteriorly. The body is placed in the prone position and a midline incision is made from the occipital protuberance to about the fourth lumbar vertebra if the whole spinal cord is to be removed. The skin and the underlying tissues are dissected away on either side of the spines of the vertebrae and the laminae are exposed. These are divided as close as possible to the transverse processes by means of an adjustable double-blade saw. It is easier to cut through the arches of the atlas and the axis with a pair of bone shears. A transverse incision is made at the lower end of the midline exposure to enable the dissector to grasp the lumbar end of the freed spinous processes with the bone forceps. The spinous processes can be lifted upwards in one piece.

The spinal cord surrounded by dura mater is now exposed and inspected. The dura is gripped with forceps and drawn aside gently to expose the extradural nerves, which are divided on either side. The dura and the lower nerve roots at the distal end of the spinal canal are divided transversely. The dura is picked up with the forceps so as to raise the cord gently, allowing the dissector to sever the remaining connections. The spinal cord and the dura mater are now divided as near the foramen magnum as possible and removed.

Dissection of the spinal cord

The cord in its coverings is stretched out on the dissecting board. The dura is opened by scissors and forceps in the midline, the cord being exposed and its membranes and outer surface inspected. The cord is sectioned by a series of transverse incisions about half an inch apart and the cut surfaces inspected. It is advisable to dip the knife in water before commencing this dissection, as the cord will otherwise stick to the blade.

SPECIAL EXAMINATIONS

Pathological examinations

In all cases of medico-legal importance, specimens for pathological examination may be submitted to central or regional laboratories.

Histological examination of tissues

Specimens of viscera or tissues for histological examination should be fixed in 10% formalin in saline, when the ordinary histological preparations are required. Sections of tissue for histological examination should not exceed 6–9 mm ($\frac{1}{4}$ to $\frac{3}{8}$ inch) in thickness.

Bacteriological examinations

All specimens for bacteriological examination, e.g. exudates, blood, excreta, etc. must be forwarded to the laboratory in sterile stoppered containers. All specimens must be collected under sterile conditions.

Blood cultures. Blood for blood culture must be obtained before the organs are disturbed. When the pericardial sac has been opened the anterior surface of the right ventricle is seared with a heated knife and the needle of a sterile syringe is passed into the ventricular cavity. Blood is withdrawn and placed immediately in the appropriate media which have been prepared beforehand.

If sufficient blood cannot be obtained from the ventricle, a sterile syringe may be passed through the seared anterior surface of the right atrium. When the atrium is used, it is necessary to steady it by clamping the right atrial appendix.

Modifications of this technique may be used to remove material from other organs such as the spleen, the liver, etc.

Meningeal smears. The area of meningitis is exposed with the usual sterile precautions. The subarachnoid space is opened with a sterile scalpel and a specimen taken from the space by means of a mounted sterile swab. Smears and cultures may be made from this specimen.

Splenic smears. The spleen is divided and a clean glass slide is placed in contact with the cut surface. In this way a suitable smear can be obtained for examination for such conditions as malaria.

Virological examinations

It may be necessary to submit specimens for examination for evidence of virus disease, e.g. rabies encephalitis. In such cases one half of the brain should be submitted for histological investigation and the other half should be sent for biological testing. The half of the brain for histological examination should be fixed in 10% formalin in saline.

If the other half of the brain can be delivered to the laboratory within 12 hours, no preservative should be added but the brain should be packed surrounded by ice. If the delivery of the brain is likely to take longer than 12 hours, it may be preserved in a 50% watery solution of pure neutral glycerol.

Biochemical examinations

Urine. Biochemical examinations of urine carried out within a few hours of death may be of value. The urine should be collected with a clean syringe by puncture of the bladder.

Blood. Biochemcial examinations of post-mortem blood for glucose urea, etc., are of limited value (pp 48 and 92). In cases of suspected drowning, blood collected from the right and left ventricles may be analysed for its sodium chloride or other electrolyte content. The interpretation of such analyses is dealt with at page 119. The collection of blood for analysis for ethyl alcohol is described at page 410.

Cerebrospinal fluid. Biochemical examinations of cerebrospinal fluid for glucose, urea and creatinine may be of value if the investigations are carried out on fluid collected within 12 hours of death (p. 49).

Vitreous humour

The care in the technique of collection is described by Coe.[4]

Specimens should be collected slowly with a syringe and a number-20 needle rather than with a vacuum tube. The strong negative pressure of the latter commonly pulls loose fragments of retina to contaminate the specimen. Such tissue fragments or blood distort chemical values significantly. Only crystal clear colourless fluid should be used. Centrifugation with use of the supernatant portion will prevent plugging of Technicon tubing. It is also important that all the fluid easily aspirated be withdrawn from the eye. This is due to the experimentally established fact that electrolytes and other solutes vary in concentration within different areas of the vitreous until diffusion equilibrium has been reached in the putrefactive phase. This unfortunately precludes serial sampling from a single eye to determine gradients of postmortem change.

Toxicological examinations

Instructions concerning the submission of specimens for toxicological examination are set out at pages 214–216.

EXHUMATIONS

The exhumation and examination of bodies may be ordered at any time after burial by magistrates or other designated administrative officers in terms of legal enactments operative in most countries of the world. Such orders are usually given in cases where a suspicion of foul play has been raised after the burial or where further medical evidence is required. Orders for exhumation may also be made in terms of Public Health Acts where a person is suspected of having died of an infectious or formidable epidemic disease.

Exhumation procedure

Before an exhumation can be carried out a written order must be obtained and this order must be produced to the person in charge of the burial place. In certain circumstances it may be possible to remove a body after exhumation to a mortuary for dissection. In our experience this has seldom been possible, particularly in country districts, and it has usually been necessary to conduct the post-mortem examination at the place of burial. We have found it most convenient to conduct these examinations in the early hours of the morning and preferably in the open. It is usually possible to improvise some form of dissecting table in the open, and we have found the use of a sheet of corrugated iron supported on trestles or boxes quite satisfactory for this purpose. The equipment which should be taken to an exhumation should include all the instruments necessary for conducting an ordinary autopsy with a toxicological box and additional jars in cases of suspected poisoning.

Great care must be taken in ensuring that the deceased is properly identified. The person in charge of the burial place should identify the grave in which the deceased has been buried and the undertaker should identify the coffin. The coffin may be recognized in other ways as well. If possible the deceased should be identified directly.

A complete autopsy should be carried out in the ordinary way. In cases of suspected poisoning the organs should be removed separately if they are recognizable, or all the contents of a body cavity may be removed in a single mass. The organs and tissues are placed directly in the prepared jars. Samples of the bones, hairs and nails should be taken in these cases, and it is also advisable to remove a portion of the burial shroud, portions of the coffin lining, and wood shavings, a part of the coffin, and samples of the soil above and below and on either side of the coffin. The parts removed for toxicological analysis must be carefully labelled.

Medical practitioners should exercise great care in carrying out an exhumation, particularly in the case of a person who is suspected of having died of an infectious disease.

REFERENCES

1 Krogman W M. The human skeleton in forensic medicine. Illinois: Thomas. 1962.
2 Prinsloo I, Gordon I. Post-mortem dissection artefacts of the neck and their differentiation from ante-mortem bruises. S Afr Med J 1951; 25: 358–361.
3 Gordon I, Shapiro H A, Taljaard J J F, Engelbrecht H E. Aspects of the hyoid–larynx complex in forensic pathology, Forensic Sc 1976; 7: 161–170.
4 Coe John I. Postmortem chemistry of blood, cerebrospinal fluid and vitreous humour. In: Wecht Cyril H. ed. Legal Medicine Annual 1976. New York: Appleton-Century-Crofts. 1977: pp 56, 81.

3

Rapid deaths from interference with oxygenation of the tissues*

For many years rapid deaths of medico-legal importance have been classified into three groups according to the supposed mechanisms of death, namely, coma, syncope, and asphyxia. Although these terms may describe terminal dominant symptoms, they do not provide an index of the mechanism of death, and the clinical conditions which they represent cannot be recognized at autopsy by any specific pathological changes. Many rapid deaths of medico-legal importance are fundamentally due to an interference with oxygenation of the tissues. For practical purposes such deaths may be classified by the manner in which the hypoxia (oxygen deficiency) or the anoxia (total lack of oxygen) is initiated.

Deaths due to an interference with oxygenation of the tissues result from hypoxia or anoxia. Hypoxic deaths can be initiated by hypoxic, anaemic, stagnant or histotoxic processes. Anoxic deaths can be initiated by anoxic or histotoxic processes. The terms hypoxia and anoxia are often used synonymously but, depending on the processes involved, we recognize the following forms of hypoxia and anoxia: hypoxic hypoxia, anaemic hypoxia, stagnant hypoxia, histotoxic hypoxia, anoxic anoxia and histotoxic anoxia.

GENERAL INTRODUCTION: THE GENERAL, NON-SPECIFIC APPEARANCES SEEN IN DEAD BODIES

No matter what starts the chain of events leading to the death of the deceased, the evidences of the fatal outcome seen in the body at a post-mortem examination will be determined by the fact that the breathing and the circulation of the blood have stopped.

If we exclude the signs of disease or injury, the external and internal signs of such a cessation of bodily function will depend largely on the amount of blood and its distribution in the organs and tissues at the time of death. These appearances are influenced by a variety of factors.

If death occurs instantly, the amount of blood in the various parts of the

---

* The material set out in this chapter is based upon the following papers: Gordon,[1] Gordon and Turner,[2] Shapiro,[3,4,5] Gordon and Mansfield[6] and Gordon.[7,21]

body will be the amount in the organs and tissues at the moment of death.

If death occurs relatively slowly, then because the failing heart is unable to pump the blood effectively around the circulation, there is a damming back of blood into the organs and tissues. In this way organs such as the liver and the lungs may become distended with the blood dammed back into their capillaries, producing in some cases an enlargement of the organ as well as a congestion of the parts with blood. This congestion is due to distension or overdistension of the capillaries with blood.

No ready means has yet been devised to measure this congested appearance of the organs quantitatively. Its description depends primarily on a subjective assessment which may well vary with different observers.

The significance of congestion, if it is present, is complicated further by the time interval after death when the observations are made.

It is unusual for a dead body to be examined immediately or very soon after death. The necessary formalities which must be complied with may take a day or two; or a weekend may intervene. As a result, medico-legal autopsies are seldom performed sooner that 24–48 hours after death. Our impressions of the internal appearances of dead bodies are therefore governed largely by factors operating during the early post-mortem interval.

As the blood in deaths from almost all causes (whether death is due to natural causes or not) rapidly becomes liquid and permanently unclottable within a very short time after death, the liquid blood will sink by force of gravity into the dependent parts (post-mortem lividity). This gravitation of blood into the dependent portions of the lungs may produce appearances which can be mistaken naked-eye for pneumonia.

The significance of congestion may be complicated further by other factors. There may be pallor of greater or less degree due to loss of blood, whether this occurred before or after death. The effects of shock on the circulation may also affect the external and internal appearances. Furthermore, when rigor mortis involves the muscles in the walls of the blood vessels, blood may be pushed from one part to another.

The final apppearance of the degree of congestion of the organs and tissues is therefore the resultant of a considerable number of variable factors.

The terminal congestion in the capillaries as the circulation fails, is associated with an inadequacy of the oxygen supply to the cells making up the walls of these capillaries. The integrity of these walls is thus impaired and, as a result, fluid from the fluid part of the blood contained in these capillaries may diffuse through the capillary wall into the neighbouring parts. This leads to oedema of the adjacent tissues.

This oedema (in greater or less degree) is thus often found in association with congestion of the parts. It may be very marked in organs such as the lungs. In cases of heart failure the lungs may become so flooded with fluid as to resemble the lungs in a case of drowning. The patient literally drowns in his own secretions.

There are several conditions other than drowning or heart failure which can flood the lungs with fluid in this way and these must be excluded before a conclusion can be reached about the significance of this observation.

As another result of the impairment of the integrity of the capillary wall, red blood cells may escape from the blood contained in the capillaries through the capillary wall, producing small bleeding points, pinpoint to pinhead in size. These are known as petechiae. They are really microscopic bruises.

Petechiae can form in many parts of the body, but they tend to form especially on the surfaces of certain internal organs. Together with congestion and oedema, petechiae constitute the third common sign seen internally in deaths from almost any cause.

Care must be taken in interpreting the significance of petechiae when they are observed (even in association with congestion and oedema) in the course of a post-mortem examination, because they can form after death, in areas of lividity and elsewhere, e.g. on the surface of the heart even in non-dependent areas.[6]

Congestion, oedema and petechial haemorrhages, in varying degrees, therefore comprise a group of basic pathological signs observed in bodies dead from almost any cause. Thus they do not have a specific significance indicating a particular type or mode of death and are best described (in Gordon's terminology) as *non-specific signs*. Their pathological significance is to be evaluated in relation to certain signs indicative of a particular way in which the train of events was set in motion leading to the death of the deceased. These are Gordon's *specific signs*, which will be described more fully in the following pages.

THE PARTICULAR OR SPECIFIC SIGNS IN THE DEAD

Gordon[1] distinguished between those particular signs on or in the body indicating the way in which the fatal chain of events was initiated (the so-called specific signs) and the general (non-specific) signs observed in all dead bodies, no matter in what way the fatal sequence was initiated.

The way in which the non-specific signs are produced has already been described. The specific signs are best illustrated by certain examples.

The skin of the neck in a case of throttling is likely to show the evidences of the application of force to that part by the fingers. There may therefore be abrasions (graze marks) produced by the finger nails and these may have a crescentic shape because of the way the neck was compressed by the throttling hand. The pattern of distribution of the abrasions may be consistent with having been produced by the forcible compression of the neck by the hand or hands of an assailant.

Lying beneath the skin, in the deeper tissues, there may be related areas of bruising in the soft parts, as a result of the compressing force applied through the fingers.

Furthermore, the force applied to the neck may have been sufficient to fracture certain bony or calcified structures in the front of the neck, e.g. the hyoid bone at the base of the tongue lying above the thyroid cartilage, or the thyroid cartilage itself may be fractured.

Thus the finger nail abrasions on the skin of the neck, the related underlying bruising of the soft parts and the fractures of the bony parts, singly or in combination, comprise a group of signs giving a specific indication of the way in which the sequence of events was initiated leading to the death of the deceased.

At the post-mortem examination there will, in addition, be found the non-specific signs common to deaths of almost all kinds, and not indicating throttling in particular.

In the same way, in cases of strangling or hanging, there will be the evidence of the ligature mark around the neck. The compression of the neck structures by the ligature will obstruct the return of blood to the heart from above the constriction, with the result that the blood will be dammed back into the veins (and eventually the capillaries), leading to the development of petechial haemorrhages above this obstruction. These petechiae may occur in the eyelids and the eyes. Thus a sign which in general is non-specific may in this case (when considered in relation to the specific sign of the ligature or the ligature mark) acquire a specific significance.

As a non-specific sign in cases of strangling, oedema of the lungs may be so marked as to resemble that seen in cases of drowning.

In deaths due to acute carbon monoxide poisoning, a bright cherry-red colour of the blood results from a relatively stable combination of the red blood pigment in the red blood cells with the carbon monoxide gas. This unusual colour of the appearance of the body, its organs and its tissues, will then constitute a specific sign, if other causes of such a colour are excluded.

In cases of drowning, the specific evidences will be provided by the nature of the fluid medium in the air passages and, in some cases, the stomach. In cases of choking there will be the foreign body in the throat. In corrosive poisoning there will be the staining around the lips and the mouth, resulting from corrosive acids or caustic alkalis.

CAUSES OF RAPID HYPOXIC DEATHS AND RAPID ANOXIC DEATHS

1. Deaths initiated by defective oxygenation of the blood in the lungs (hypoxic hypoxia) or by a total failure in oxygenation (anoxic anoxia):
   (a) From breathing in a vitiated atmosphere. These deaths are caused either:
   > By a displacement of oxygen from the atmosphere by inert gases, e.g. from exposure to the fumes in wells and vats, or
   > By exposure to gases in the atmosphere, e.g. from exposure to 'sewer gas'.

(b) From mechanical interference with the passage of air into or down the respiratory tract. Such obstruction may be caused either:

By closure of the external respiratory orifices, e.g. in smothering and overlaying, or

By obstruction of the air passages, e.g. in drowning, in choking by foreign body impaction, and in certain cases of throttling, strangulation, and hanging.

(c) From external compression on the chest and abdominal walls interfering with respiratory movements, e.g. falls of earth, traumatic 'asphyxia'.

(d) From a primary cessation of respiratory movements through paralysis of the respiratory centre, e.g. in certain cases of electrical injury and in certain forms of acute poisoning.

2. Deaths initiated by a reduced oxygen-carrying capacity of the blood (anaemic hypoxia):

This form of death occurs in cases of acute carbon monoxide poisoning, and acute massive haemorrhage.

3. Deaths due to impaired circulation resulting in a reduction of oxygen delivery per unit of time (stagnant hypoxia):

This form of death occurs in shock.

4. Deaths initiated by a depression of the oxidative processes in the tissues (histotoxic hypoxia or histotoxic anoxia):

This form of death is seen in acute cyanide poisoning.

MECHANISM OF FAILURE IN RAPID HYPOXIC DEATHS AND IN RAPID ANOXIC DEATHS

The mechanism of failure in rapid hypoxic and anoxic deaths cannot readily be determined by ordinary clinical methods, and such observations alone do not necessarily afford reliable evidence of the nature of the failure. With human beings it is usually impossible to obtain continuous records of the sequence of physiological events. Numerous animal experiments, however, have been undertaken to determine the main cardiorespiratory and biochemical changes which occur in various types of rapid hypoxic and anoxic deaths.

In order to obtain comprehensive information about the process of hypoxic and anoxic deaths, Swann[8] and Swann and Brucer[9] devised a series of experiments on unanaesthetized dogs. They investigated the following types of hypoxic and anoxic deaths: obstructive asphyxia; drowning in fresh water; sea water drowning; carbon monoxide poisoning; exsanguination and deaths caused by breathing gas mixtures low in oxygen, i.e. while breathing pure nitrogen, while breathing 2.43% oxygen in nitrogen, and while rebreathing through soda lime. In each experiment simultaneous observations were made of systolic and diastolic arterial blood pressures, venous pressure in the inferior vena cava, heart rate, heart sounds, electrocardiograms, intrathoracic pressure, pulmonary ventilation, respiratory rate, blood acidity, blood oxygen, blood carbon dioxide, blood lactic acid and haemoglobin, and plasma proteins.

These experiments showed that there were great individual differences in the times of survival of dogs subjected to various types of hypoxic or anoxic deaths. In fulminating anoxia caused by the inhalation of pure nitrogen, the respiratory cessation occurred after the cardiac cessation, but in the majority of the deaths the respiratory cessation occurred at approximately the same time as the cardiac cessation. The animals often showed low diastolic pressures, but the systolic pressures remained elevated until death was imminent. At the time of death, the systolic pressures declined sharply. Because of this sharp fall of systolic pressure, Swann believes that the final circulatory failure in hypoxic and anoxic deaths is determined by myocardial hypoxia or anoxia rather than by sudden peripheral vasodilatation.

In carbon monoxide poisoning and exsanguination the electrocardiographic changes showed special features of differentiation, but in all the other types of hypoxic and anoxic deaths, the electrocardiograms showed the same constant features. The terminal events in drowning were more complicated than in obstructive asphyxia because of the passage of electrolytes between the fluid in the alveoli and the blood plasma (p. 119).

Apart from the electrocardiographic changes in carbon monoxide poisoning and exsanguination and the special features in drowning, the pattern of cardiorespiratory and biochemical changes was essentially similar in all the forms of rapid hypoxic and anoxic deaths that were studied. Although these experiments were carried out on dogs, Swann[10] believes that man reacts in a similar manner.

THE PATHOLOGY OF RAPID HYPOXIC AND ANOXIC DEATHS

General pathological changes

During the process of death from rapid hypoxia or rapid anoxia, widespread tissue injury results from the lack of oxygen. It would appear that the capillaries are particularly susceptible to hypoxia and anoxia, and hypoxic or anoxic injury of the capillaries results in their dilatation. This is followed by stasis of blood in the dilated capillaries and in the venules, which accounts for the capillovenous engorgement which is a major feature of the general pathological findings in rapid hypoxic and anoxic deaths.

Injury to the capillary wall is often accompanied by petechial haemorrhages in the tissues. The haemorrhages may be found in the substance of viscera but they are most readily observed in the serous membranes, particularly in the visceral pleurae and the visceral pericardium. Although these petechial haemorrhages are not found invariably in rapid hypoxic and rapid anoxic deaths, they occur in the majority of such deaths.

Hypoxic or anoxic injury to the capillaries may also result in increased capillary permeability with transudation of plasma into the tissue spaces. In the early period after such injury, the transudation is followed by increased lymph drainage, and oedema does not develop as long as this drainage is adequate. Equilibrium can be maintained for a relatively short period only, and if the hypoxic or anoxic process continues, oedema of the tissues develops. Oedema of the lungs may be seen, but generalized oedema is not a prominent feature of the post-mortem findings.

Capillovenous congestion of the viscera, and petechial haemorrhages in the serous membranes, are non-specific general pathological changes which occur in all forms of rapid hypoxic and anoxic deaths. These changes are also seen in deaths from shock, and in many deaths from natural causes. Oedema of the viscera and effusions into serous cavities are commonly described in deaths from shock. The essential similarity in the post-mortem findings of rapid hypoxic and anoxic deaths and deaths from shock has been emphasized by Moon[11] and Moritz.[12]

Figure 3.1, which has been adapted from the work of Moon,[13] sets out the relationship between the various conditions causing rapid hypoxia and rapid anoxia and shock. The diagram illustrates how rapid hypoxia and rapid anoxia, initiated in various ways, give rise to the same vicious cycle of circulatory failure that occurs in shock.

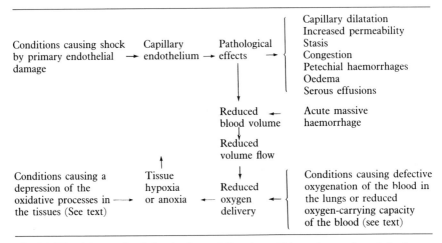

Fig. 3.1 The vicious cycle of the circulatory failure in rapid hypoxia, anoxia and shock as adapted from Moon.[13]

Biochemical and structural alterations

Parenchymatous degenerative changes develop in rapid hypoxic and rapid anoxic deaths, and although these changes may be sufficiently marked to be visible by light microscopy, they are non-specific in nature. In recent years attempts have been made to demonstrate specific biochemical and structural changes in cells and tissues in different forms of death. Histochemical techniques, tissue analytical biochemical methods and electron microscopy have been used for this purpose. Trowell[14] studied the changes produced in lymphocytes *in vitro* by various noxious agents. He found that four types of lesions (including an anoxic lesion) can result from the exposure of lymphocytes to various noxious agents, and that ultrastructural changes as observed by electron microscopy characterize the four principal lesions. In routine post-mortem examinations for forensic purposes, it is difficult to interpret electron microscopic findings because of the development of autolytic changes after somatic death and after cellular death. These autolytic changes may destroy or mask the subtle biochemical and ultrastructural morphological changes which are believed to be characteristic of particular mechanisms of cellular death as studied *in vitro* (Gordon).[7]

The sequential post-mortem changes in renal glomeruli have been studied by screening electron microscopy in five species of animals. Langlinais[15] distinguishes between changes resulting from circulatory arrest and those due to autolysis and claims that the studies demonstrate that evaluation by screening electron microscopy of tissue specimens from the kidney, is acceptable up to 60 minutes *post mortem*.

ASPHYXIA AS A PATHOLOGICAL ENTITY

The concept that asphyxia is a pathological entity which can be recognized by certain specific pathological changes, has led to considerable confusion in the literature on forensic medicine. Some authors use the term 'asphyxia' synonymously with 'hypoxia' and 'anoxia'. It is used by others to describe forms of death which are initiated by defective oxygenation of the blood in the lungs (hypoxic hypoxia or anoxic anoxia). There are others who restrict its use to that group of deaths which result from a mechanical interference with respiration. It is in the latter sense that the term is usually employed and understood in medico-legal practice.

It has been claimed on pathological grounds that visceral congestion, petechial haemorrhages, cyanosis, a condition of post-mortem fluidity of the blood and cardiac dilatation are pathognomonic signs of asphyxia. Certain biochemical changes have also been regarded as being characteristic of this condition.

Visceral congestion

Capillovenous congestion of the viscera occurs as a general pathological change in all forms of rapid hypoxic and rapid anoxic deaths, in deaths from shock, and in many deaths from natural causes.

Visceral congestion is usually well marked in deaths from mechanical interference with respiration. Swann and Brucer have stated that man probably survives for several minutes in deaths from mechanical interference with respiration, and the work of Moon suggests that the intensity of the congestive changes in this form of death depends upon the period of such survival rather than upon any special mechanism of death. The intensity of the congestive changes, however, does not serve to differentiate such deaths as similar changes are observed in many other forms of death. The appearances are complicated further by the effects of post-mortem lividity involving the viscera.

Petechial haemorrhages

Petechial haemorrhages in the visceral pleurae and visceral pericardium are often referred to as 'Tardieu spots', as they were originally described by Tardieu in a series of papers published during the last century. Tardieu consistently found these haemorrhages in deaths from 'suffocation' and regarded them as a *pathognomonic* sign of such deaths (Tardieu).[16] Ogston[17] recorded that soon after Tardieu published his original papers, his claim that petechial haemorrhages in the visceral pleurae and visceral pericardium were a specific pathological change was contested by Liman, the celebrated German medico-legal authority. The views of Liman receive substantial support at present, as pathologists have repeatedly described the occurrence of petechial haemorrhages in the serous membranes in many different forms of death. We have frequently observed such haemorrhages in deaths from shock, and in many deaths from natural causes, as well as in all the forms of rapid hypoxic and rapid anoxic deaths included in the classification set out in this chapter.

The non-specificity of petechial haemorrhages at autopsy has been conclusively established by the demonstration of the spontaneous development after death of subpericardial petechiae.[6] The naked-eye and histological appearances of subpericardial petechiae which developed after death are shown in Figs 3.2, 3.3, 3.4 and 3.5.

Cyanosis

Cyanosis depends upon an increase in the amount of reduced haemoglobin in the blood and may appear in any condition in which the proportion of oxyhaemoglobin in the blood is sufficiently diminished. 'Cyanosis' is a common post-mortem finding and is not confined to those deaths which are initiated by hypoxic hypoxia or which are caused by a mechanical interference with respiration (p. 40).

Post-mortem fluidity of the blood

When a post-mortem examination is undertaken shortly after death, the blood is usually fluid, and it undergoes spontaneous coagulation when

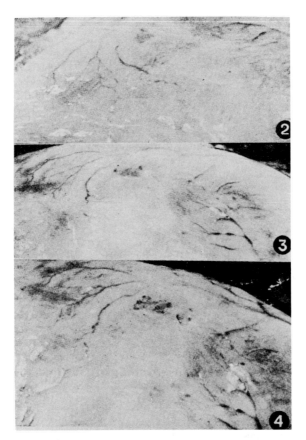

Fig. 3.2 Deceased male adult (aged 48 years). Cause of death, hypertension and arteriosclerosis. Post-mortem interval before commencement of autopsy, 4 hours. Pericardial sac opened at 9.52 a.m. Top: Photograph of anterior surface right ventricle taken at 9.54 a.m. Note *absence* of petechial haemorrhages.

Middle: Same case as illustrated in top. Photograph of anterior surface right ventricle taken at 10.03 a.m., i.e. 11 minutes after opening of pericardial sac. The photograph was taken from a slightly different angle but the region photographed can easily be identified as the same as in the upper third of the illustration. Note the development of petechial haemorrhages in the pericardium in the zone below the concave bend of the uppermost branching vessel.

Bottom: Same case as illustrated in upper and middle thirds of photograph. Photograph of anterior surface right ventricle taken at 10.13 a.m., i.e. 21 minutes after opening of pericardial sac. The photograph was taken from the same angle as in the middle illustration. Note the increase in the number of petechial haemorrhages which have appeared in the pericardium.

removed from the heart and vessels. If, however, the examination is under-taken a few hours after death, the blood may be clotted, or completely fluid and incoagulable, or partly clotted and partly fluid. In most deaths caused by mechanical interference with respiration, the blood is fluid and inco-agulable, but this condition of the blood is not confined to such deaths (p. 40).

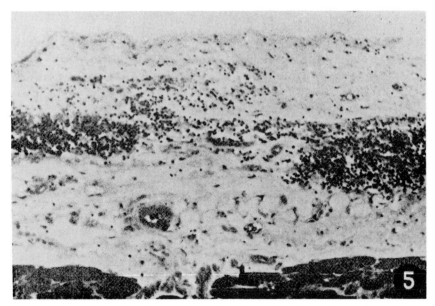

Fig. 3.3 Photomicrograph marked (5): A section of one of the haemorrhages shown in lower third of Fig. 3.2. Iron haematoxylin and cosin (× 150).

Mole[18] studied the factors which are responsible for post-mortem fluidity of the blood. He demonstrated the presence of a fibrinolysin in more than 90 per cent of samples of fluid and incoagulable blood. This lysin is active only while thrombi are being formed, and Mole considers that the lysin is adsorbed on to the thrombi and is released into solution when the fibrin is lysed. For this reason a given concentration of fibrinolysin is more likely to liquefy a clot when the process of coagulation is slow. Under certain conditions the fibrinolysin may be so active that fibrin is destroyed as rapidly as it is produced, and post-mortem thrombi never develop in the vessels. In other cases thrombi are formed but they undergo lysis.

In deaths from any cause, the condition of the blood at autopsy depends upon the concentration of fibrinolysin and the rate of intravascular coagulation after death. When the fibrinolysin is active and the rate of coagulation is slow, the blood is likely to be fluid. When the fibrinolysin is less active and the rate of coagulation is rapid, post-mortem clots are likely to form in the blood.

Mole has shown that in many deaths from a wide variety of causes, fibrinolysin is produced and the blood is found to be fluid at autopsy. These considerations have led him to emphasize that post-mortem fluidity of the blood is not characteristic of any special cause or mechanism of death.

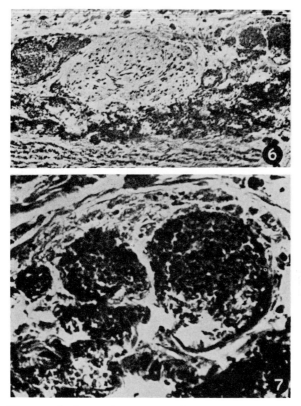

Fig. 3.4 Top: The general microscopic appearance of a petechial haemorrhage which developed spontaneously in the pericardium after death. Note the engorgement of the venules and the capillaries. A ruptured venule can be seen in the upper right hand zone of the photomicrograph. Orthotolidin, haematoxylin and eosin ($\times$ 160).

Bottom: Higher power view of ruptured venule above. Orthotolidin, haematoxylin and eosin ($\times$ 520).

Cardiac dilatation

Cardiac dilatation has been described as one of the characteristic signs of asphyxia. Cardiac dilatation is essentially a clinical concept and the use of the term in pathology for the purposes of morbid anatomical description is restricted. According to Anderson,[19] true cardiac dilatation can only be recognized at autopsy when it occurs in association with certain forms of cardiac hypertrophy.

In ascribing a special significance to cardiac dilatation in asphyxial deaths, it would appear that distension of the chambers of the heart has been regarded as evidence of cardiac dilatation. Distension of the atria and venticles is a common post-mortem phenomenon and may result from secondary muscular flaccidity. It has no significance as a specific pathological change.

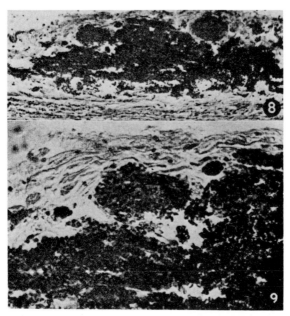

Fig. 3.5 Top: The general microscopic apppearance of a petechial haemorrhage which developed spontaneously in pericardium after death. Note the engorgement of the venules and the capillaries. A ruptured venule can be seen in the upper portion of the section to the left of the mid-line. Orthotolidin, haematoxylin and eosin (× 160).

Bottom: Higher power view of ruptured venule above. Orthotolidin, haemotoxylin and eosin (× 450).

Biochemical changes

The work of Swann and Brucer shows that estimations of the oxygen content, the carbon dioxide content, and the pH of agonal blood are of no value in differentiating obstructive asphyxial deaths from other forms of rapid hypoxic or rapid anoxic deaths. The claim that hyperglycaemia is characteristic of deaths from mechanical interference with respiration has been thoroughly investigated by Tonge and Wannan.[20] These authors have shown that an estimation of the post-mortem blood sugar is of no value in providing corroborative evidence of this condition. In a series of 145 cases, agonal hyperglycaemia was found in two only of 23 cases of asphyxial deaths. Except in cases of drowning, post-mortem chemical examinations are of no greater value than morphological studies in differentiating so-called asphyxial deaths from other forms of deaths.

Conclusion

As it has been shown that there are no qualitative differences in the general pathological changes in all deaths of medico-legal importance, asphyxia cannot be regarded as a distinct pathological entity which is recognizable on the basis of morbid anatomy. It is never justifiable therefore to certify that a deceased person has died of asphyxia if this opinion is based only upon a finding of visceral congestion, petechial haemorrhages, cyanosis, cardiac dilatation and a condition of post-mortem fluidity of the blood.

SUMMARY AND APPLICATION

In all forms of death the post-mortem findings may be divided into two groups. The first group comprises those of general pathological changes such as visceral congestion and petechial haemorrhages. These non-specific changes are always present in a greater or less degree in rapid hypoxic and rapid anoxic deaths as well as in deaths from shock and natural causes. The second group consists of the pathological changes which are dependent upon the type of death, e.g. the local injuries to the neck in throttling and strangulation, and the colour of the blood in acute carbon monoxide poisoning. Such changes are best described as special pathological changes.

In the description of post-mortem findings for medico-legal purposes, a clear distinction should be drawn between non-specific general pathological changes and special pathological changes which are dependent upon the type of death. This principle has been adopted in the succeeding chapters and all post-mortem findings have been considered under the following two headings:

1. Special pathological changes.
2. Non-specific general pathological changes.

REFERENCES

1 Gordon I. A clasification of deaths of medico-legal importance. Br Med J 1944; 2: 337–339.
2 Gordon I, Turner R. Deaths from rapid anoxia. Am Med Assoc Arch Path 1951; 52: 160–167.
3 Shapiro H A. Is asphyxia a pathological entity recognisable post mortem? J Forens Med 1953; 1: 65–67.
4 Shapiro H A. Medico-legal mythology—some popular forensic fallacies. J Forens Med 1954; 1: 144–169.
5 Shapiro H A. Tardieu spots in asphyxia. J Forens Med 1955; 2: 1–4.
6 Gordon I, Manfield R A, with the assistance of Duncan Taylor J E, et al. Subpleural, subpericardial and subendocardial haemorrhages: a study of their incidence at necropsy and of the spontaneous development, after death, of subpericardial petechiae. J Forens Med 1955; 2: 31–50.
7 Gordon I. The mechanism of death. J Forens Med 1967; 14: 125–130.
8 Swann H G. Studies in resuscitation. USAF Air Materiel Command Memorandum Report MCREXD Series 696–79G 1948.
9 Swann H G, Brucer M. The cardiorespiratory and biochemical events during rapid anoxic death. Tex Rep Biol Med 1949; 7: 511–636.
10 Swann H G. Personal communications, 1950.
11 Moon V H. Shock and related capillary phenomena. Oxford: Oxford University Press. 1938: p 211.

12 Moritz A R. The Pathology of Trauma. Philadelphia: Lea & Febiger. 1942: p 129.
13 Moon V H. Shock: its Dynamics, Occurrence and Management. Philadelphia: Lea & Febiger. 1942: p 208.
14 Trowell O A. Ultrastructural changes in lymphocytes exposed to noxious agents in vitro. Quart J Exp Physiol 1966; 51: 207–220.
15 Langlinais, Paulette B. Sequential postmortem changes of glomeruli. Arch Path Lab Med 1981; 105:482.
16 Tardieu A. Memoire sur la Mort par Suffocation. Ann d'Hyg Publ et Med Leg 1855 2e serie, t. iv. 371–441.
17 Ogston F. On punctiform ecchymoses in the interior of the body as a proof of death by suffocation. Br Med J 1868; 2:332.
18 Mole R H. Fibrinolysin and the fluidity of the blood post mortem. J Path Bact 1948; 60: 413–427.
19 Anderson W A D. Pathology. St. Louis: C V Mosby. 1948: p 533.
20 Tonge J I, Wannan J S. The post-mortem blood sugar. Med J Aust 1949; 1: 439–447.
21 Gordon I. The medico-legal aspects of rapid death initiated by hypoxia and anoxia. In: Wecht C H ed. Legal Medicine Annual, 1975. New York: Appleton-Century-Crofts. 1976: pp 29–47.

4

Deaths usually initiated by hypoxic hypoxia or anoxic anoxia

BREATHING IN A VITIATED ATMOSPHERE

Death from hypoxic hypoxia or anoxic anoxia may result from breathing in a vitiated atmosphere. A vitiated atmosphere is deficient in oxygen. This deficiency may be caused by a displacement of oxygen from the atmosphere by inert gases or by gases generated in the atmosphere.

Among the commoner gases found in vitiated atmospheres are carbon dioxide, carbon monoxide, methane, sulphuretted hydrogen and sulphur dioxide. A vitiated atmosphere usually contains more than one inert or toxic gas, e.g. 'sewer gas' contains carbon dioxide, sulphuretted hydrogen and methane.

Carbon dioxide is exhaled during respiration, and relatively high concentrations of this gas may accumulate in crowded, poorly ventilated places. In such circumstances persons may suffer from hypoxic or anoxic symptoms such as headache or drowsiness as the carbon dioxide displaces oxygen from the atmosphere, but it is exceptional for death to occur under these conditions.

Carbon dioxide, sulphur dioxide and carbon monoxide may be generated during the combustion of organic matter, e.g. after a mine explosion, and death is usually due to a combination of hypoxic or anoxic effects. The carbon dioxide displaces oxygen from the atmosphere; the sulphur dioxide, because of its strong reducing action, prevents haemoglobin from taking up oxygen, and the carbon monoxide displaces oxygen from its combination with the haemoglobin of the blood (p. 129). (However, there is evidence that acute carbon monoxide poisoning may induce histotoxic anoxia[1].)

Fatal toxic gas poisoning during fires is dealt with at page 137.

Carbon dioxide, methane and sulphuretted hydrogen are produced during the fermentation of organic matter, e.g. in sewers, deep wells, cellars, vats and silos. Death from exposure to a vitiated atmosphere in a sewer, deep well, etc., is usually due to the combined effects of several gases. Methane acts in the same manner as carbon dioxide by displacing oxygen from the atmosphere. Sulphuretted hydrogen is a strong reducing agent and although it does not combine with haemoglobin during life, it prevents the haemoglobin from taking up oxygen. After death, sulphuretted hydrogen reacts with the methaemoglobin in the blood to form the compound sulphmethaemoglobin.

Autopsy findings

Apart from the demonstration of carboxyhaemoglobin, sulphmethaemoglobin* or acid haematin in the blood in deaths from exposure to carbon monoxide, sulphuretted hydrogen or sulphur dioxide respectively, no special pathological changes are found at autopsy in deaths from breathing in vitiated atmospheres.

In all cases non-specific general pathological changes are found (Chapter 3). The intensity of the visceral congestive changes is usually well marked.

SUFFOCATION

Suffocation is an obstruction to the passage of air into the respiratory tract caused by a closing of the external respiratory orifices.

Suffocation includes the conditions of smothering and overlaying.

Occurrence

Accidental

Many infants who appear to be in good health are found dead in their cribs, cots or perambulators. Such deaths are sometimes ascribed to 'accidental mechanical suffocation' when it can be shown that the infant has turned into a prone position, and has apparently buried its face in a pillow or blankets. Werne and Garrow[2] investigated the deaths of 167 infants belonging to the group which is ordinarily certified as being due to 'accidental mechanical suffocation'. In 124 of the 167 cases, the cause of death could not be determined by naked-eye examination of the viscera and tissues, but complete histological studies revealed visceral lesions. Acute inflammatory changes of the respiratory tract were observed in most of these cases.

It has been shown in Chapter 3 that there is no means of differentiating so-called asphyxial deaths from other forms of death on the basis of general pathological changes such as visceral congestion and petechial haemorrhages.

Accidental suffocation of an infant by overlaying may occur in cases where the infant has to share the bed of its parent or parents.

This subject is dealt with in detail in the section on the 'sudden infant death syndrome' (pp 181–186).

---

* The demonstration of sulphmethaeamoglobin is not diagnostic of poisoning by sulphuretted hydrogen as the compound can be produced in the blood during putrefaction.

Suicidal

This type of suffocation is uncommon. In a case reported by Turner[3], a senior wireless operator on a merchant ship was found trussed up in his cabin with an oilskin sheet tied over his head (Fig. 4.1A). When the sheet was removed, a strap, which acted as a ligature, was found around his neck, and his arms were pinioned to his sides. His right hand was tied behind his back and a strap, which was termed the 'key strap' for convenience, was found grasped in his left hand (Figs 4.1B and 4.1C). The photographs show how the 'key strap' passed through the loop of another strap. It was found that when the 'key strap' was pulled, all the other straps were tightened and at the same time the oilskin became firmly bound to the body. The cause of death was given as suffocation and strangulation. The inquest proceedings suggested that the deceased had practised tying himself up in this unusual manner on several occasions before his death.

It has been suggested by some authorities who have referred to this case in reviews of previous editions of this book that this death was possibly one of so-called 'sexual asphyxia'. It is understood that 'sexual asphyxia' refers

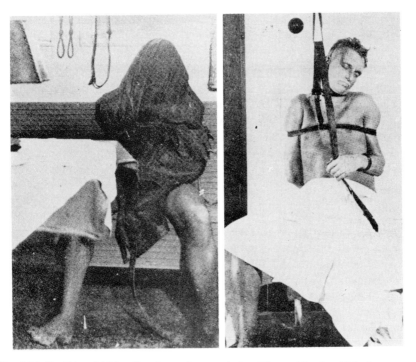

Fig. 4.1A Possible suicidal suffocation and strangulation. The position in which the deceased was found.

Fig. 4.1B Reconstruction of the position of the deceased after the removal of the oilskin (see text).

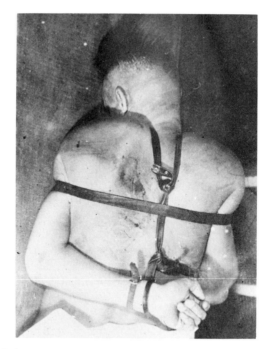

Fig. 4.1C Dorsal view.

to cases where the subjects obtain sexual gratification by adopting simple or complex techniques of self-induced hypoxia. The authors would agree that, although there was no evidence to this effect presented at the inquest the possibility of so-called 'sexual asphyxia' cannot be excluded. In such an event, the occurrence would have been more properly described as *accidental*.

Homicidal

Homicidal suffocation is relatively uncommon in adults, but it may occur in cases where the victim is too feeble to offer any resistance because of old age or illness. Homicidal suffocation is also seen where persons are over-powered while asleep or intoxicated. In one of our cases of homicidal suffocation a storekeeper was attacked by several assailants. A handkerchief was forced into his mouth, and a blanket was placed over his head and tied into position by a towel. Probably the best-known series of murders by suffocation were those committed by the notorious criminals, Burke and Hare, in Scotland in the early part of the nineteenth century.[4] The method of smothering employed by these men, which has become known as 'burking', consisted of a combination of compression of the chest with the forcible closure of the mouth and nostrils. In these murders the victims were usually attacked while asleep or while lying helpless through intoxication. One of the assailants used to throw himself over the chest of the victim while the other forcibly closed the victim's mouth and nostrils with his hands.

Suffocation or smothering is one of the commonest methods of infanticide. An infant may be smothered without the use of much force by such means as the placing of a pillow or bedclothes or the palm of the hand over the nostrils and mouth.

Mechanism of death

Death is usually due to hypoxic hypoxia or anoxic anoxia.

Autopsy findings

Special pathological changes

External wounds in the region of the mouth and nostrils. In homicidal suffocation abrasions and bruises are generally found in the region of the mouth and nostrils. These injuries are usually produced during struggling, but they may be absent in cases where the victim is unable to offer resistance or is rapidly over-powered, e.g. they may be absent in infants and young children and in aged and debilitated persons.

Non-specific general pathological changes

Non-specific general pathological changes as described in Chapter 3 are present. In most cases the intensity of the visceral congestive changes is marked. Numerous petechial haemorrhages are usually found in the pleurae and pericardium.

THROTTLING

Throttling or manual strangulation is the application of force to the neck of a person by pressure from the hands or forearm of another person.

Occurrence

Death from throttling is almost invariably homicidal, but instances of accidental throttling have been recorded. Homicidal throttling occurs in the course of assaults, and in cases of robbery and rape. Cases of accidental throttling have been recorded where firm pressure has been suddenly applied to the neck of a person during an embrace or in the course of 'horseplay'. Such deaths are probably caused by a reflex cardiac arrest which is brought about by compression of one or both of the carotid sinuses (p. 154).

Suicidal throttling has not been recorded.

Mechanism of death

Death from throttling may be due to one of following mechanisms:

1. Pressure on the sides of the neck may constrict the larynx and prevent the free passage of air down the respiratory tract. This results in hypoxic hypoxia which can lead to rapid death.

2. Compression of one or both of the carotid sinuses can result in reflex cardiac arrest and instantaneous death (p. 151).

3. Obstruction of the carotid arteries and internal jugular veins can result in cerebral hypoxia. Death may result if the cerebral hypoxia is maintained for a sufficient length of time.

Autopsy findings

Special pathological changes

External injuries. The nature and extent of the external injuries depend upon the method of throttling. An assailant may apply pressure to the neck with one hand, with both hands, or with his forearm. The assault may take place from the front, from the side, or from behind the victim. The pressure is most commonly applied to the upper part of the front of the neck. The soft tissues of the neck are not only compressed but they are forced upwards and backwards against the cervical vertebrae.

When the assailant uses one hand and the assault takes place from the front of the victim, the upper part of the neck immediately below the angles of the jaw is usually gripped. In such cases superficial bruises of the skin and crescentic abrasions caused by fingernail impressions may be observed on both sides of the neck. The bruises and abrasions may be more numerous on one side of the neck than on the other side.

Gonzales[5] states that a single abrasion on the right side of the neck and grouped abrasions on the left side of the neck are suggestive of a right-handed compression of the throat. The single abrasion is caused by pressure from the thumb and the grouped abrasions result from the pressure of the four fingers.

When an assailant using one hand changes his grip, or when he uses both his hands, multiple bruises and abrasions may be found over the front and sides of the neck (Figs 4.2A and 4.2B)

In certain circumstances there may be no external evidence of injury on

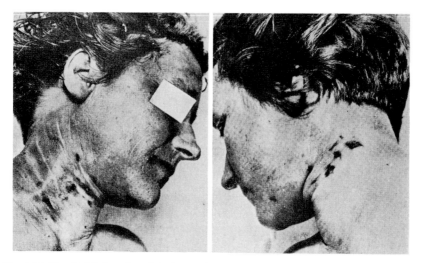

Fig. 4.2A Homicidal throttling. Injuries to the right side of the neck.

Fig. 4.2B Same case as Fig. **4.2A**. Injuries to the left side of the neck.

the neck. This occurred in one of our cases, described at page 57, where the accused placed a thick towel over the neck of his wife and throttled her through the towel.

When the assailant uses his forearm in throttling, the assault usually takes place from behind the victim. Pressure is exerted by the forearm against the arm of the assailant, and the larynx is compressed. In such cases external injuries are usually absent.

Injuries to the cervical tissues. Bruises may be found in the deeper layers of the skin, in the superficial fascia, in the deep fascia, in the sheaths of muscles, in the cervical muscles, and under the capsule and in the substance of the thyroid gland, and less commonly under the capsules and in the substance of the submandibular glands. Bruises may be observed in the retropharyngeal tissues and at the base of the tongue. Section of lymph nodes may show haemorrhages into their substance.

Injuries to the hyoid bone and the laryngeal cartilages. Fractures of the hyoid bone are commonly found in throttling. In order to demonstrate the presence of a fracture it is essential to expose the hyoid bone. A fracture appears as an irregular break in the continuity of the bone and is usually accompanied by haemorrhage at the site of fracture. The greater horn of the hyoid bone is united to the body of the bone by a plate of cartilage which ossifies at middle age. Romanes[6] states that the lesser horn is united to the body and the greater horn by a synovial joint which only disappears in old age. The cartilaginous separations between the greater horns and the body, and the joints between the lesser horns and the body should not be mistaken for fractures.

Fractures of the hyoid bone are not invariable in throttling, particularly in young persons. When fractures of the hyoid bone are found, it is highly suggestive of throttling as it is exceptional for the bone to be injured when other forms of blunt force are applied to the head and neck.

The laryngeal cartilages are less commonly injured than the hyoid bone, and it is unusual for these structures to be fractured before they have undergone ossification. Anson [7] states that:

> . . . certain parts of the laryngeal skeleton normally undergo calcification and ossification. Calcification begins at about 20 years of age in the thyroid and cricoid cartilages, and later in the arytenoid. The process begins a little later in the female than in the male, and does not extend so rapidly. The extent to which the cartilages are ossified and the time occupied in the process vary considerably. The elastic elements usually are not involved in the process. Calcification of the smaller cartilages, especially, is important clinically because such calcific areas may be mistaken for foreign bodies in roentgen examinations.

The foregoing statement is supported by the observations of Keen and Wainwright.[8]

In order to demonstrate the presence of fractures of the laryngeal cartilages it is essential to strip the larynx of its attached muscles and ligaments. Bruises of the laryngeal mucous membrane occur in throttling and may or may not be accompanied by fractures of the hyoid bone and laryngeal cartilages.

Camps and Hunt,[9] however, report the following case:

> We have also seen a fracture of the superior thyroid cornu in a man dying of ascending pyelonephritis in a hospital ward. There was no question of any ante-mortem violence, but the laying out of the body was admitted to have been done very roughly with hyperextension of the neck. Furthermore, there was a localised post-mortem extravasation of blood around the fracture. This would, in less certain circumstances, undoubtedly have been considered good evidence that the injury occurred before death, and illustrates the care required in interpreting such injuries.

These authors have also seen fractures of the hyoid bone as a post-mortem artefact.[9]

Obstruction to the venous return from the head and neck. Signs of mechanical obstruction to the venous return from the head and neck may be present. These signs include the following: Lividity of the face and lips; engorgement and petechial haemorrhages in the conjunctivae; and petechial haemorrhages in the skin of the face and neck.

Other injuries. Bruises and abrasions may be found on other parts of the body. In cases where the victim has been forced to the ground and has been held down, areas of bruising may be found in the following regions: in the scalp tissues over the back of the head; in the tissues overlying the spinous processes of the lower cervical and upper dorsal vertebrae; and in the tissues overlying the posterior surfaces of the shoulder blades. Bruising of the muscles of the anterior chest and abdominal walls may be found in those cases where the assailant has knelt upon the victim. When considerable force has been used, ribs may be fractured and contusions and ruptures of the abdominal viscera may occur.

Non-specific general pathological changes

Non-specific general pathological changes as described in Chapter 3 are present. In most cases the intensity of the visceral congestive changes is marked and numerous petechial haemorrhages are found in the pleurae and pericardium.

Additional points of medico-legal importance

The significance of fingernail abrasions of the skin

Characteristically grouped crescentic abrasions of the skin are quite rightly regarded as good evidence consistent with the manual application of force to the part. Shapiro et al[10] state that within their experience, medical experts have sought to draw inferences about the way in which the hand was applied to the neck in throttling, from the direction of the concavity of this type of abrasion. It has been assumed that, if the right hand of the assailant is applied to the neck of the victim from in front (i.e. with the assailant's right thumb on the right side of the victim's neck, and the remaining fingers of the assailant on the left side of the victim's neck) then the concavities of the crescentic abrasions will all face medially. This appears to be a plausible, common-sense view, but when tested, it was shown that the results were completely contrary. In a series of demonstrations, however, it has been shown that the concavities of crescentic markings often face laterally. In some cases a linear impression is obtained, but it is by no means usual for the concavity to follow the anatomical shape of the nail margin.

From an examination of this problem we have concluded that the shape of the finger nail largely determines the result. Nails with a straight border give unpredictable results; but as they become more pointed towards the centre of the free border, so do the apparently paradoxical results occur more frequently.

The unexpected direction of the concavity is determined by the anchoring of the skin of the victim by the central portion of the assailant's finger nail, thus displacing the skin so as to produce the reversed crescent. The sides of the free edge of the arch of the finger nail, in their contact with the skin, have no purchase and merely complete the sides of the concavity.

These observations indicate that it is extremely fallacious to infer the way in which an assailant's hand may have been applied to the part, from the direction of the concavities of crescentic abrasions.

Diagnosis of throttling in putrefied bodies

With the development of putrefaction and the associated progressive discoloration of the skin, it becomes increasingly difficult to detect external injuries in the neck. A similar difficulty arises in the diagnosis of bruises in the decomposed deeper cervical tissues. Although the discolorations produced in decomposing bruises are usually localized, similar areas of discoloration may be found when putrefaction affects localized ante-mortem intravascular collections of blood in the cervical tissues, or localized patches of post-mortem lividity. These difficulties have been considered in detail in connection with the case described at pages 50–53. It is particularly important to examine the hyoid bone for fractures in putrefied bodies, as such a finding is usually strongly suggestive of throttling (p. 102).

Post-mortem dissection artefacts of the neck and their differentiation from ante-mortem bruises

The handling of organs and the incision of vessels during routine post-mortem examinations often result in the extravasation of blood into the tissue spaces. These extravasations have been described as dissection artefacts, and their occurrence in cervical tissues is of special importance as they simulate ante-mortem bruises.

In dealing with the tissues of the neck in the routine post-mortem examination it is usual to reflect the skin by a subcutaneous dissection through the platysma muscle. This method of dissection ensures a clear exposure of the subcutaneous tissues and the ventral surfaces of the superficial muscles of the neck. It is not common practice to reflect individual cervical muscles from their attachments in order to expose the deeper structures of the neck. After the initial subcutaneous dissection, structures of the neck are usually removed *en masse* by downward traction from the floor of the mouth. The structures of the neck are then examined individually. In order to study the incidence and nature of dissection artefacts of the neck, Prinsloo and Gordon[11] followed this method of dissection in 18 cases. At the time of the initial dissections no extravasations of blood were observed in the subcutaneous tissues or in the fascia overlying the ventral surfaces of the superficial muscles. After the *en masse* removal of the structures, however, extravasations of blood were found in the deep connective tissues in 16 of the 18 cases. Although there was no evidence or suggestion of any ante-mortem cervical injury in these cases, there was no means of determining whether these extravasations were bruises or post-mortem artefacts. Accordingly, the method of dissection described at page 66 was devised to ensure that all the tissues of the neck were inspected *in situ* before removal. This method of dissection was carried out in 33 cases. Areas of extravasation of blood which were not seen at the time of the initial dissections, and were therefore produced after the dissections during the handling of the structures of the neck, were found in 20 of the 33 cases. In all instances the dissection artefacts simulated bruises. The dissection artefacts were found in the following situations: in the pretracheal connective tissues; in the investing fascial sheaths of the cervical muscles; in and around the carotid sheaths; in the capsule of the thyroid gland; and in the prevertebral or retropharyngeal connective tissues.

In view of the similarity in the naked-eye appearance between ante-mortem bruises and dissection artefacts, Prinsloo and Gordon examined selected bruises and dissection artefacts microscopically. Figures 4.3 and 4.4 show that on microscopic examination it is not possible to distinguish between dissection artefacts and ante-mortem bruises caused shortly before death.

Haemorrhage into the posterior crico-arytenoid muscles has been described in deaths from natural causes with no evidence of external trauma to the neck. This observation is important in avoiding an erroneous conclusion that these haemorrhages imply an application of force to this region of the neck.[12,13,14]

A large number of deaths which have to be investigated for forensic purposes occur in circumstances in which there is inadequate information relating to the events which have preceded the deaths. Many of these deaths are due to natural causes, and in the majority of this group, some lesion is found which is compatible with continued life, but which is also known to be associated with sudden death, e.g. coronary atheroma.

It is well recognized that external injuries and injuries to the hyoid bone and laryngeal cartilages may be absent in cases of homicidal throttling, and in such cases the demonstration of bruises in the deeper cervical tissues is essential for diagnosis. For this reason a difficult problem may arise when areas of extravasated blood are found in the cervical tissues in the course of a routine post-mortem examination which reveals some lesion which is compatible with sudden death from natural causes, but which is also compatible with continued life. If the extravasations of blood are bruises, then the possibility of the death having been caused by throttling must be considered, in spite of the presence of the pathological lesion. On the other hand unless an inspection of all the cervical tissues has been undertaken *in situ* it might be impossible to prove that the extravasations of blood are not dissection artefacts. The only certain method of ensuring that post-mortem artefacts are not mistaken for ante-mortem bruises is to examine all the structures of the neck *in situ* as a routine procedure in all deaths which have to be investigated for medico-legal purposes.

STRANGULATION

Strangulation is a constriction of the neck by a ligature, the constricting force being applied directly to the ligature.

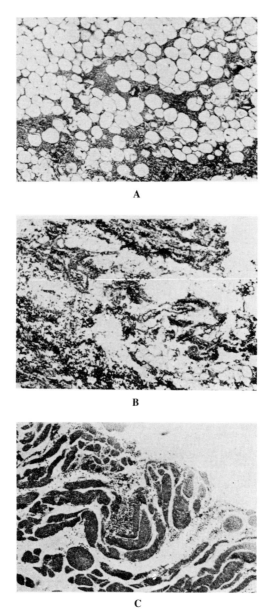

Fig. 4.3 A, Dissection artefact in the superficial fascia; B, Dissection artefact in the deep fascia. Note the extravasation of erythrocytes between the collagen fibres; C, Dissection artefact in muscle. Note the extravasation of erythrocytes over the surface of and between the muscle fibres (haematoxylin and eosin. × 290).

Occurrence

Accidental. This form of strangulation is uncommon but may occur under special conditions, e.g. intoxication. In one of our cases an intoxi-

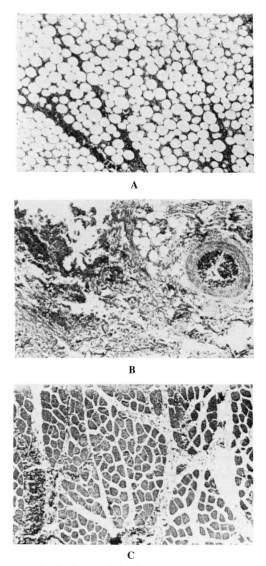

Fig. 4.4 A, Ante-mortem bruise in superficial fascia; B, Ante-mortem bruise in deep fascia; C, Ante-mortem bruise in muscle (haematoxylin and eosin. × 290).

cated person who was in the habit of sleeping next to his dog, climbed under a staircase. He then pushed his head through a loop in the dog's chain which was fastened to the lower step of the staircase. In this way he was accidentally strangled.

Suicidal. This form of strangulation is rare. A case of possible suicidal suffocation and strangulation has been described at page 97.

Homicidal. Homicidal strangulation is relatively common.

Mechanism of death

Death is usually caused by anoxic hypoxia but in certain cases it may be due to a reflex cardiac arrest which is induced by compression of the carotid sinus (p. 100).

Autopsy findings

Special pathological changes

The external ligature mark: General appearance. A single external ligature mark is usually present on the neck, but more than one mark may be found. These marks take the form of linear depressions in the skin, and their general appearance depends mainly upon the nature of the ligature material. Ligature marks are most distinct in cases where the ligature used is made of hard material such as coarse roping or wire. On the other hand, the marks may be indefinite in cases where the ligature used is made of soft-material. This condition was seen in one of our cases where a folded blanket was used as a ligature. It was also seen in one of our cases of infanticide where a stocking was used as a ligature.

Ligature marks are usually brown and dry at the time of examination, while abrasions and bruises of the surrounding skin are commonly found in relation to them. These abrasions and bruises are caused occasionally by the victim's finger nails in cases where an attempt has been made by the victim to release the ligature.

Situation. The ligature marks may be situated in any region of the neck, but they are usually found over the lower part of the larynx and the upper part of the trachea.

Direction. The marks are usually directed transversely across the neck.

Injuries to the tissues of the neck. Dissection of the neck usually reveals a moderate degree of bruising to the connective and muscular tissues, but such bruising is not an invariable finding.

In one of our cases the deceased was strangled with his own scarf. The scarf was found tied tightly around his neck. Although a broad depression was observed at the site of pressure of the scarf there were no abrasions or bruises of the surrounding skin. Disssection failed to reveal any bruising in the connective or muscular tissues of the neck and there was no injury to the hyoid bone or the laryngeal cartilages.

Injuries to the hyoid bone and the laryngeal cartilages. Fractures of the hyoid bone are unusual in strangulation. Fractures of the laryngeal cartilages occur, but they are relatively uncommon. Injuries to the mucous membrane of the larynx are less common in strangulation than throttling.

Obstruction of the venous return. Signs of mechanical obstruction to the venous return from the head and neck may be present. These signs have been described at page 83.

Non-specific general pathological changes

Non-specific general pathological changes as described in Chapter 3 are present. The intensity of the visceral congestive changes is usually well marked.

Additional points of medico-legal importance

Differentiation between homicidal strangulation and accidental strangulation by the umbilical cord in infants

In newly born infants it may be difficult to distinguish between homicidal strangulation and an accidental strangulation by the umbilical cord during the process of birth. This difficulty is increased when the cord is used as a ligature for homicidal purposes.

As a general rule, in the accidental form of strangulation by the umbilical cord there is relatively slight cervical tissue injury, while the lungs are usually incompletely expanded. In this connection, it should be noted that marked bruising of the cervical muscles may be produced during the ordinary course of labour. The presence of a complex type of knotting in the cord, e.g. the finding of a reef knot, suggests the homicidal form of strangulation.

Retention of ligature in cases of homicidal strangulation

In cases of strangulation the ligature should be kept for examination. If possible, the ligature should be taken off in such a way that the knot is retained intact. If the knot is situated over the front of the neck the ligature can be cut behind the neck and vice versa.

Case of homicidal strangulation

Some years ago, we dealt with an unusual case of alleged homicidal strangulation.

> A woman attended a beer-drinking party at a kraal. She was seen leaving the party during the night, and the following morning she was found dead about two miles from the kraal in a donga (a shallow gully or ravine). She was lying in a prone position with her mouth and nostrils buried in a pool of mud. There was evidence that she was under the influence of alcohol when she left the party, and it was concluded that she had fallen into the donga accidentally and had become suffocated in the mud.
>
> No injuries were observed on external examination of the body, and as foul

play was not suspected the deceased was buried without a post-mortem examination being held. Within a few days a young man made a voluntary statement to the police, in which he alleged that the deceased had been murdered. He stated that some months before her death the deceased had reported a headman to the police for committing adultery. The headman was prosecuted, and subsequently told several of his friends that he would avenge himself upon the deceased for this disclosure. The informant stated that on the night of her death he saw the deceased leave the kraal, and he noticed that she was followed by two men. He recognized one of the men as the headman, and he saw them both attack the woman. He said that they tied a folded blanket around her neck in such a way that they each held one of the ends. They then forced her into the donga, and took up positions on opposite banks. They pulled the deceased along by the blanket until she collapsed, and after she had fallen they removed the blanket from her neck and left her lying in the donga.

Upon this information an exhumation was ordered. The tissues of the neck were dissected and some evidence of bruising was observed, but the findings were obscured by putrefactive changes. No other cause of death could be found at the autopsy and strangulation was given as the probable cause of death, in spite of the absence of any external evidence of injury to the neck.

The failure to perform a post-mortem examination soon after death in this case provided a degree of uncertainty as to the cause of death, and seriously hampered the Crown in its prosecution. This case illustrates the need for holding complete autopsies as soon as possible in all reported sudden deaths.

HANGING

Hanging is a constriction of the neck by a ligature, the constricting force being applied indirectly to the ligature through the weight of the body.

In hanging, the body is usually wholly suspended with the feet above the ground, but hanging can occur with the body in a position of partial suspension. In the case shown in Figure 4.5, the deceased hanged himself in a sitting posture. It is possible that consciousness is lost rapidly in cases of this nature. It is of interest to note that the deceased wore a First World War badge on the lapel of his jacket. He committed suicide on the day of the outbreak of the Second World War.

Occurrence

Accidental

This form of hanging is uncommon, but cases have been recorded where children at play have hanged themselves, and where workmen in falling from scaffolding have been hanged by becoming entangled in ropes.

Suicidal

This is the commonest form of hanging.

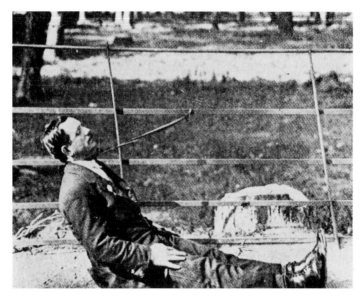

Fig. 4.5 Suicidal hanging

Homicidal

This form of hanging is rare.

Mechanism of death

Death can be due to hypoxic hypoxia or anoxic anoxia, the obstruction to the airway being caused by the upward displacement of the base of the tongue against the palate and the posterior pharyngeal wall. In certain cases, however, death may be due to a reflex cardiac arrest which is induced by compression of the carotid sinus (p. 154).

Fracture-dislocations of the cervical vertebrae may occur in certain types of hanging, e.g. in judicial hanging, and in cases of suicidal hanging where the deceased has jumped from a height and the fall has been arrested by a sudden jerk of the ligature.

Autopsy findings

Special pathological changes

Post-mortem lividity. In cases of complete suspension lividity is usually observed in the dependent lower limbs and in the hands. In males there may be considerable engorgement of the penis and testes.

The external ligature mark

General appearance. A single ligature mark is usually present on the neck.

The ligature, however, may be composed of a double strand or of several strands, and in these cases more than one mark will be observed on the neck.

A ligature mark is usually depressed below the skin surface, and it often corresponds in outline to the pattern of the ligature. In the early period after death the mark is pale in colour, but it later becomes brown and dry. Abrasions and bruises of the skin are occasionally seen in the bed of the depression, but there is usually no evidence of injury to the skin surrounding the ligature mark. Patches of lividity are often found immediately above the upper border of the mark.

Situation. The mark is usually situated over the upper part of the larynx but it may be lower in cases of partial suspension.

Direction. The direction of the ligature mark depends upon the type of ligature which has been used in the hanging.

Ligatures are usually tied in the form of fixed loops with single knots, but the knots may be multiple. In certain types of hanging a running noose ligature is used.

When a fixed loop is employed with a single knot in the midline either under the chin or at the back of the head, the mark is seen on both sides of the neck and is directed obliquely upwards towards the position of the knot over the front or back of the neck, as the case may be. When a fixed loop is used with the knot in the region of one ear, the mark differs on each side of the neck. On the side where the knot is situated the mark is directed obliquely upwards towards the knot, whereas it is directed transversely on the other side. When a running noose is employed the mark is seen on both sides of the neck, and is usually directed transversely across the front of the neck.

Injuries to the issues of the neck. Dissection of the neck usually reveals some degree of bruising of the connective and muscular tissues in relation to the ligature mark. These changes may be relatively slight in certain cases.

Injuries to the hyoid bone and the laryngeal cartilages. The hyoid bone may be fractured in hanging. Fractures of the laryngeal cartilages and injuries to the laryngeal mucous membrane are relatively uncommon.

Obstruction to the venous return. As in the cases of throttling and strangulation, signs of mechanical obstruction to the venous return from the head and neck may be present (p. 102).

Non-specific general pathological changes

Non-specific general pathological changes as described in Chapter 3 are present. The intensity of the visceral congestive changes is variable.

Additional points of medico-legal importance

Differentiation between suicidal hanging and the suspension of a body after death to simulate suicide

The problem of distinguishing between suicidal hanging and the suspension of a body after death to simulate suicide may arise. This differentiation is often difficult, as a well-defined ligature mark and bruising of the subcutaneous tissues may be produced after death.

In distinguishing between these two conditions:

1. It is important for the medical practitioner to arrange with the police in his district to inspect the place where the alleged hanging took place. At such an inspection the medical practitioner should determine whether the victim could have suspended himself in the manner in which he was found.

2. The autopsy should be complete, as some cause of death other than hanging is usually found in cases where a body has been suspended after death to simulate suicide. Difficulty may arise, however, in cases where bodies are suspended after homicidal strangulation or throttling.

3. A portion of the skin and deeper tissues in relation to the ligature mark should be examined histologically for evidence of tissue reaction. This investigation would only be of value in a case of hanging if the period of time that elapsed before death was sufficiently long for tissue reaction to develop (p. 244). The presence of tissue reaction in these circumstances would suggest that the deceased had been hanged. The absence of tissue reaction, however, does not exclude death by hanging.

4. If post-mortem lividity had become fixed before the suspension of the body, its distribution (e.g. dorsal) may negate the suggestion of ante-mortem suspension.

CHOKING BY FOREIGN-BODY IMPACTION

Death from choking may result from the impaction of foreign bodies in the pharynx, larynx, trachea, or bronchi.

Occurrence

Most deaths from choking are accidental. Children often place objects such as marbles or coins in their mouths and these objects may pass into the larynx or trachea during a sudden deep inspiration. Accidental deaths from choking are not uncommon in mental hospitals as persons with disordered or defective minds often cram large portions of food into their mouths (p. 156). Eller and Haugen[15] record that about 700 to 1000 deaths by 'choking on food' occur annually in the USA—as proved at autopsy. The National Safety Council of the United States has added 'inhalation of food' to its compilation of accidental deaths and estimates nearly 2500 such fatalities annually—more than those due to aircraft accidents, firearms, lightning and snakebite. 'Inhalation of food' is the sixth leading cause of accidental death in the USA.

The impaction of loose bodies such as surgical swabs in the larynx, trachea or bonchi while a patient is under the influence of a general anaesthetic may result in rapid death (p. 197). In cases of stupor, e.g. from acute alcoholic intoxication, death may be caused by the impaction of a denture in the pharynx or larynx.

Homicidal deaths by choking are uncommon, but cases may occur when the victims are aged or debilitated persons or are infants. In one of our cases of infanticide, a portion of cloth was forced into the upper end of the oesophagus of the infant and was found *in situ* at the autopsy. The mouth, palate and pharynx of an infant should always be carefully examined for injuries at autopsy in a case of this nature, as the foreign body is often removed by the assailant after death.

Mechanism of death

Large foreign bodies often become impacted in the pharynx and cover the laryngeal opening. By obstructing the airway completely such impacted bodies may cause death through hypoxic hypoxia or anoxic anoxia. Smaller foreign bodies which lodge in the larynx may not be large enough to obstruct the airway completely, but they may induce a laryngeal spasm. As a general rule laryngeal spasm passes off before the hypoxia becomes fatal. Sudden reflex neurogenic cardiovascular failure may occur in both forms of laryngeal obstruction. The cardiovascular failure is probably induced by reflex parasympathetic cardiac inhibition (p. 152).

If a foreign body passes through the larynx it may become impacted at the bifurcation of the trachea or it may lodge in a bronchus. When a foreign body impacted at the bifurcation of the trachea obstructs the free passage of air into the lungs, death may be caused by hypoxic hypoxia or anoxic anoxia, but irritation in this region is particularly liable to induce parasympathetic cardiac inhibition (p. 156).

Reflex cardiac inhibition may also occur when a foreign body is impacted in a bronchus. In one of our cases, a child, aged 3 years, 'choked' when eating a sausage. He appeared to recover but shortly afterwards, while resting, he suddenly became pale and died without showing any signs of respiratory distress. At the autopsy, there was a striking absence of visceral congestion and a portion of sausage was found in the right bronchus.

The impaction of a foreign body in the larynx, trachea or bronchi may give rise to severe reflex bronchiolar spasm. In one of our cases a youth participated in an obstacle race. Towards the end of the race each of the competitors had to eat an apple suspended from a string. While eating the apple the youth 'choked' and as he showed signs of respiratory distress he was taken to hospital. The signs of respiratory distress passed off before he reached the hospital and on examination no abnormality was observed on laryngoscopy or on radiological examination of the chest. He was discharged after a short period, but within an hour of leaving the hospital he rapidly developed signs of intense bronchospasm and died. No organic disease was detected at the autopsy, but several pieces of apple were found in the trachea.

The impaction of foreign bodies in the respiratory tract, especially in the bronchi, may result in delayed death from pneumonia, lung abscess or bronchiectasis.

DROWNING

Epidemiology

Drowning represents one of the three leading causes of death in the USA, accounting for over 7000 deaths each year.[16] The death rate has been estimated to be 2.5 per 100 000[17] but with the increase in popularity of boating and water sports, a larger population is at increasing risk.[16]

Complete immersion of the body is usual in drowning, in which case the drowning is a form of death in which there is defective oxygenation of the blood in the lungs, due to the presence of fluid in the respiratory tract, the fluid entering the air passages through the nose and the mouth. Although complete immersion is usual, drowning may occur when the nostrils and mouth only are covered by fluid. In the latter case, the possibility of an antecedent decreased level of consciousness must be considered, which includes loss of consciousness due to head injury, in epileptic subjects, from myocardial infarction, the ingestion of a narcotic substance, or, commonly, alcoholic intoxication.[18]

Occurrence

Drowning may be accidental, suicidal or homicidal. The vast majority are accidental.[18,19] Of these, nearly 80% are male.[16]

The relationship between alcohol consumption and accidental drowning is well documented.[18–21]

The most important effect of alcohol is its depressant effect on the central nervous system, impairing judgement and awareness, increasing the bravado, but producing a decreasing ability to react functionally and properly to an accidental situation.[18] Once immersion has occurred, the alcohol effect may further contribute in a more subtle fashion. Haight and Keatinge[22] showed that as alcohol depresses glucogenesis, alcohol consumption after exercise may produce a profound drop in the blood glucose level. This latter effect not only leads to weakness and confusion, but may also interfere with the normal body temperature regulating mechanisms.

Between 10[19] and 33%[18] of drownings are suicidal, with an approximately equal sex ratio.

Homicidal drowning is only occasionally reported and the victims are usually children.[19]

On the other hand, an attempt to disguise a homicidal crime by disposing of the body in water, is a more common occurrence.[23]

Types of drowning

Drowning can traditionally be classified morphologically into dry (atypical) and wet types, the distinction being based on the autopsy appearances of the lungs. A further distinction may be the clinical presentation of primary and secondary drowning.

Dry or atypical drowning

The incidence of this type of drowning is reported as comprising 10–15% of cases,[16] being most commonly encountered in children and adults under the influence of drugs (sedative hypnotics) or alcohol. Pleuckhahn[20] and Cairns et al[18] reported that these drowned persons did not appear to panic or struggle when submerged and fluid was not aspirated into the lower respiratory tract or stomach. Death thus appeared to be instantaneous, probably secondary to either vagally mediated cardiac arrest or laryngospasm, as a result of sudden entry of fluid into the nose and upper airways,[16,18] or during the submersion of an unconscious individual.

Wet drowning

In 1897, Brouardel conducted experiments on dogs as a result of which the process of wet drowning was divided into five stages. Essentially this type of drowning is related to the aspiration of the drowning fluid, leading to an hypoxic death. However, investigation of drownings occurring in fresh water and sea water, suggest that the mechanism of death involves more complex pathophysiological effects.

Drowning in fresh water

When a large volume of fresh water enters the lungs, rapid absorption of the water occurs into the pulmonary vascular system, due to the hypotonicity of fresh water. Haemodilution and hypervolaemia rapidly occurs with an associated massive haemolysis of red blood cells, leading to a rise in the level of potassium. In turn, levels of sodium chloride, calcium, proteins and haemoglobin are all reduced. The hypoxia and haemodilution are characteristically associated with ventricular fibrillation.[19] Further, the haemodilution has been shown to lead to a decrease in the blood alcohol concentration level by up to 33%.[16,23]

Drowning in sea water

The sodium chloride concentration of sea water is over 3%. Submersion in sea water results in a rapid diffusion of salts into the blood vascular system, with concommitant significant rise, particularly in the plasma concentration of sodium, chloride and magnesium. In order to establish osmotic equilibrium, fluid moves into the pulmonary alveoli. The end result is marked haemoconcentration and fulminant pulmonary oedema. Death supervenes within a few minutes, secondary to the hypotension and hypovolaemia. A marked bradycardia occurs, in contrast to ventricular fibrillation probably due to the raised plasma sodium level.[16,23]

In addition to the above morphological classification of drowning, i.e. wet and dry types, drowning may clinically be subdivided into primary and secondary types.

Primary drowning

Primary drowning occurs within minutes of submersion, with no resuscitation being instituted, or when death occurs too quickly to make resuscitation possible.

Many deaths secondary to cardiac arrest or ventricular fibrillation are of this type.

Secondary drowning

Secondary drowning occurs after resuscitation or treatment has made survival possible for a limited period, ranging from half an hour to several weeks. Death of this type is usually associated with metabolic acidosis, pulmonary oedema, chemical pneumonitis or severe infection.

Autopsy findings in non-putrid bodies

The difficulties which arise when attempts are made to relate speculative theories about the mechanism of death to post-mortem findings, had been considered in detail.[24]

The findings will vary, depending on whether dry or wet drowning has occurred.

General observation

It is essential to exclude from any description of anatomical signs as presumptive evidence of drowning, all signs of submersion or immersion, such as goose skin (or cutis anserina) and sodden and wrinkled feet and hands (in the case of the hands, the so-called 'washerwoman's' hands). After about two weeks, the skin loosens from the hands and feet. In 3–4 weeks the whole skin may loosen from the hands like a glove.[19] Although these signs have no evidential value in determining whether or not a person was breathing at the time of the submersion or immersion, Guhuraj[23] considers that the presence of cutis anserina, as well as retraction of the penis and scrotum and papilla mammae, suggest that the deceased was alive before the drowning event.

Since a submerged body tends to float face downwards, with the buttocks upwards and the legs and arms more or less hanging down in front of the body, any hypostasis which may be present, is usually present over the face, upper part of the chest, hands, lower arms, feet and calves. Movement of the body by the fluid will, of course, influence the development of the hypostasis, which may not be obvious in such circumstances.

The blood may become oxygenated secondary to water imbibition by the skin and the hypostasis may have a pink colour, suggestive of carbon monoxide intoxication.[19]

Special pathological changes in wet drowning

The respiratory tract. The characteristic signs of drowning are found in the respiratory tract. Frothy fluid which is often tinged with blood may be observed in the bronchi, trachea and larynx, and may appear about the mouth and nostrils. The entry of fluid into the lower respiratory tract stimulates the production of mucus. The mucus, water and possibly surfactant, may be whipped into a tenacious foam by violent respiratory efforts. The bubbles of the foam do not tend to collapse when touched. The lungs are usually voluminous. Pleural petechial haemorrhages may be present. Section of the lungs may reveal marked congestion, while large amounts of frothy fluid may be expressed from the cut surfaces. Fluid may be present in the pleural cavities.

The frothing of fluid in the respiratory tract is the most characteristic sign of drowning, but if artificial respiration has been performed, particularly by means of a respirator, the frothing and the amount of fluid in the air passages may be considerably reduced.

The trachea, bronchi and distal respiratory tract may contain substances such as sand or shell particles, which are ordinarily found in the medium in which the person drowned. Such substances in the distal respiratory tract, strongly suggest that the victim was alive at the time of drowning.[23]

The stomach and intestines. Fluid characteristic of the medium in which the drowning has taken place may be found in the stomach and intestines. This sign has a limited value, however, as fluid may enter the stomach and small intestine after death if the pressure of the fluid in the medium is sufficiently great.

The heart. Right ventricular dilatation[25] may be present secondary to the hypervolaemia, resulting in right ventricular strain and hypoxia, producing vasomotor increase in the pulmonary vascular resistance.

The middle ear and mastoid air cells. Haemorrhage into the middle ear as well as into the mastoid air cells may suggest that the victim was alive before drowning occurred.[26] However, these haemorrhages are also present in deaths not due to drowning and are also not constantly present in drowned cases.[27]

Non-specific general pathological changes

Non-specific general pathological changes as described in Chapter 3 are present. The intensity of the visceral congestive changes is usually well marked except in the voluminous lungs.

Autopsy findings in putrid bodies

The changes which are found in the tissues in putrefaction have been described in Chapter 1. Decomposition of a submerged body proceeds at a slower rate than on land. Running water may retard, and heavily polluted water may accelerate the process of decomposition. The water temperature, however, is the most important factor, and a water temperature of 5 to 6 °C may retard decomposition for several weeks. As decomposition reaches an advanced stage, marked gas production occurs, thus increasing the buoyancy of the body. If the body is not entangled, it will tend to float to the surface within 7 to 14 days.[19]

Although the lungs tend to putrefy more slowly than the other viscera, they ultimately undergo a process of softening and liquefaction, and this change is usually accompanied by an extravasation of blood-stained fluid into the air passages and pleural cavities. In addition, the gases which are evolved during putrefaction may pass into the fluid in the air passages and produce an appearance simulating the frothing which is found in drowning. For this reason it is usually impossible to determine whether a person has been drowned or not if the body is recovered in a state of advanced putrefaction. A presumption against drowning may be raised, however, if an injury which is incompatible with life is found on dissection of the body, provided that it can be shown that the injury could not have arisen after death.

Additional points of a medico-legal importance

Chemical methods for the determination of death by drowning

The various chemical methods which have been used for the determination of death of drowning have been reviewed by Moritz.[28] In most of these methods attempts have been made to detect chemical changes in the blood which depend upon an exchange of water and electrolytes between the inhaled fluid and the blood in the pulmonary capillaries. The best-known and most widely used of these methods is the method introduced by Gettler.[29] Gettler estimated the chloride content of the blood in the right and left ventricles in cases of drowning and compared his findings with a series of controls on persons who died of causes other than drowning. According to Gettler, the demonstration of a difference of at least 25 mg in the chloride content of the blood in the left and right sides of the heart provides evidence of drowning. In normal circumstances the chloride content of the blood is the same in both sides of the heart. When water enters the lung alveoli in large amounts the chlorides may diffuse between the inhaled fluid and the blood in the pulmonary capillaries. If the drowning has taken place in fresh water, the percentage of chlorides in the pulmonary capillaries is lowered, whereas the percentage is raised when drowning occurs in salt water. The reduction or increase in chlorides will therefore be more marked in the blood returning to the left atrium than in the blood entering the right atrium.

In analysing Gettler's method Moritz states that a reduction in blood chlorides is a common post-mortem phenomenon—the longer the interval between death and the examination the greater the reduction. Moreover, the reduction does not necessarily progress at the same rate in the two sides of the heart. Differences in the chloride content of the blood in the right and left sides of the heart may therefore develop in deaths from causes other than drowning. Because of the reduction in the blood chlorides after death, post-mortem changes are more likely to simulate the effects of drowning in fresh water than in salt water. Moritz states that if a body is examined within twelve hours of being recovered from fresh water, a disproportionate depression of the chlorides in the left side of the heart of 17 milli-equivalents or more per litre (i.e. 60.35 mg Cl per 100 ml) should probably be regarded as presumptive evidence of drowning.

Blood chloride estimations obtained twelve or more hours after death from drowning in fresh water are of little diagnostic value. On the other hand a failure to find a significant difference in the chloride content on the two sides of the heart would not exclude drowning if the body has been recovered from fresh water.

Chloride determinations have greater diagnostic value in cases of suspected drowning in sea water. In 80% of the cases of drowning in sea water reviewed by Moritz abnormally high chloride values were obtained. In most of these cases the chloride level was not only higher in the left side of the heart, but the differences between the two sides were greater than had been observed in the control series. Moritz states that 'a preponderance of chlorides in blood from the left side of the heart of 17 milli-equivalents or more per litre (i.e. 60.35 mg Cl per 100 ml) constitutes presumptive evidence of drowning in salt water.'

If in suitable cases it is decided to submit samples of blood for chloride determination the samples should be taken separately from the right and left ventricles into dry tubes. About 10 ml of blood should be obtained from each ventricle, and whenever possible an estimate of the sodium chloride content of the medium should also be undertaken. Schwär[30] has drawn attention to factors other than the length of the post-mortem interval which can influence the results of chemical determinations, e.g. there may be a continuation of the fluid/electrolyte flow in the pulmonary vessels after respiratory movement has ceased.

Magnesium concentration determinations, from the right and left ventricle of the heart, pose problems similar to those of chloride concentration estimations. However, Coutselinis and Boukis[31] documented increased levels in magnesium concentration in the cerebropspinal fluid in cases of sea water drowning.

A relatively new and potentially useful investigation is the estimation of serum strontium as a diagnostic criterion of the type of drowning water. Abdallah et al[32] reported on the value of serum strontium levels in rabbits before and after death by drowning. They reported the presence of raised serum strontium levels which were significantly influenced by the type of water in which the drowning occurred. These workers further showed that the increase in serum strontium levels was reciprocally related to the volume of the water aspirated. It would thus appear that determination of serum strontium levels may be a practical technical method for differentiation between death due to drowning and post-mortem immersion of a victim. Further, differentiation between drowning occurring in sea or fresh water is possible. With the exception of serum strontium in bones, the difference in its concentration in the various soft tissues and organs is negligible. Of importance, serum strontium levels in the body fluids are insignificantly affected by resuscitation, haemolysis or early putrefaction. In addition, pathophysiological behaviour of serum strontium is similar in man and animals.

Plasma specific gravity estimations are helpful if undertaken within 12–24 hours of death.[30] Later investigations are complicated by the effects of haemolysis and putrefactive changes.

The significance of diatoms in the diagnosis of death by drowning

Diatoms and fluid media. Thomas, Van Hecke and Timperman[33] state that 'it is now generally accepted that, during drowning in water containing microscopic plankton (diatoms, algae, plant fibres, etc.) the latter penetrate in small quantity into the lung capillaries, reach the left heart and are thus dispersed throughout the body by the arterial circulation.' Certain of the diatoms have acid-resistant silica shells. Thomas and his co-workers claim that if such diatoms can be demonstrated in tissues which can only be reached by the systemic circulation, e.g. the bone marrow, a strong presumption is raised that the deceased was breathing at the time of immersion in a fluid medium. The bone-marrow of long bones such as the femur, the tibia and the humerus is examined. In collecting the bones for examination, particular care is taken to avoid a risk of contamination from the outside by diatoms present on the skin and clothing on the body. The following technique is adopted by Thomas and his co-workers:

> One or more long bones are extracted from the body. All soft tissues attached are cut off and the bone scrubbed thoroughly. Halfway along the shaft, for a distance of a couple of centimetres, a layer of bone is cut out to a depth of about 2 mm., by means of a machine tool. Alternatively one can also perform this operation in two different places nearer the epiphyses. This procedure effectively prevents contamination of the bone-marrow. The shaft is then sawn through at the sites marked out by the machine tool. The bone marrow can now be collected by means of a gynaecological curette of adequate size. Experience teaches that from 15 g. to 40 g. of marrow can thus be recovered. The marrow is placed in a Kjeldahl flask in which it is chemically digested by adding small quantities of nitric acid at a time. Sulphuric acid is contra-indicated because it produces precipitates which completely obscure the microscopic picture. Heating is best done with an ordinary Bunsen burner. The operation lasts 1-2 hours and yields a transparent yellow fluid with a supernatant disc of fat. The yellow fluid is next centrifuged. The deposit (usually hardly visible to the naked eye) is poured on to a slide and examined, while still wet, under a coverglass.

Valuable surveys of the use of the diatom method in the presumptive diagnosis of drowning have been set out by Timperman.[34,35]

If it is established that in man diatoms are not absorbed from the normal alimentary tract, then the demonstration of diatoms in the systemic circulation, viscera, bone marrow etc., would be good evidence of the inhalation of a medium containing diatoms. In these circumstances, it will be necessary to establish the absence of disease of the alimentary tract as a result of which diatoms may have entered the circulation through the gut.

A further difficulty is that it is not known for how long diatoms remain, e.g. in bone marrow, once they have been lodged there. Thomas suggests that they may persist for years.

In cases other than drowning the involuntary or accidental inhalation of even a small amount of a fluid medium containing diatoms may lead to the persistence of the diatoms in the bone-marrow, etc., for an unspecified time in years.

Although there are many methods possible for identification of plankton, recently described methods[36,37] include centrifugation of 'drowning lung tissue' in a colloidal silica gradient. Using this method, zooplankton as well as phytoplankton can be successfully isolated. A further method for diatom detection is that of an ultrasonic irradiation procedure using a tissue stabilizer. This method is less time consuming than other methods. In cases of decomposed bodies, demonstration of diatoms is possible since, by virtue of their silica skeleton, diatom decomposition tends not to occur.

Diatoms and atmospheric air. As Spitz and Schneider[38] claim that atmospheric air may contain diatoms, inhalation of such a medium containing diatoms will also lead to the absorption of diatoms through the lungs and their deposit in bone marrow etc. For these reasons the demonstration of diatoms in the systemic circulation, viscera, tissues, etc. is not incontrovertible evidence of drowning. The proper inference to be drawn from such an observation is that it presents evidence of the inhalation of a medium containing diatoms whether the medium is water or air.

Diatoms and the effects of hydrostatic pressure on bodies recovered from the sea bed. Nanikawa and Kotoku[39] describe their autopsy fidings in a body recovered from the sea bed at a depth of 120 metres. Their findings suggested that the body was that of an adult male who probably died of natural causes and was buried at sea. Diatoms found in the lungs were considered to have reached the lungs after death.

This finding is in accord with other observations.[40,41] Tomonaga[42] showed that at a water pressure below 130 m, water enters systemic organs and diatoms can be detected in these organs.

Karkola and Neittaanmäki[43] claim that pulmonary alveolar macrophages, diatoms and crystalline dirt particles migrate into left heart blood in drowning. They consider that their results show promise for the development of a new forensic diagnostic method.

The relationship between diatoms and a diagnosis of death by drowning, has given rise to a large body of literature with pros and cons taking part in a 'war of diatoms'.

Perper and Wecht,[44] in their conclusion on diatom identification and the diagnosis of drowning, consider that accurate diatom counts can, in most cases, easily discriminate between drowning and non-drowning cases,[45,46] especially when other methods are impractical, e.g. following resuscitation attempts, post-mortem mutilation or decomposition; the authors conclude by considering the diatom method to be the most reliable drowning test.

Peabody,[47] however, considers that no final conclusion can be drawn from the presence of diatoms in various body organs.

Injuries on drowned persons

Wounds may be found on external examination of drowned persons. Such wounds may be produced before, at the time of, or after immersion. Before immersion they may be of accidental, suicidal or homicidal origin. At the time of immersion they may be produced by the deceased striking hard objects such as rocks or stones. After immersion a body may be washed up against hard objects in the water or be attacked by fishes and crustaceans.

It is often difficult to distinguish between these types of injury. Ante-mortem wounds can only be differentiated from post-mortem wounds if the ante-mortem injury has preceded the drowning by at least one hour or longer. In such cases histological evidence of tissue reaction may be found in the wounds. The absence of tissue reaction, however, would not exclude an ante-mortem origin for the wound (p. 242).

The problem of determining whether a person was alive or dead at the time of immersion

Death may occur from reflex shock or natural causes during immersion, while a body may be disposed of after death to conceal a murder. The signs of drowning will be absent in these cases, but difficulties may arise if the body has been recovered in a state of advanced putrefaction.

Reflex shock is seen most commonly in old or debilitated subjects or in cases of immersion in very cold water. It is never possible to establish that death was due to reflex shock, but a presumption may be raised in certain circumstances if all other possibilities can be excluded.

Death from natural causes during bathing is uncommon. In these cases some lesion which could have caused death rapidly is usually demonstrable at autopsy.

Dead bodies are sometimes disposed of in the sea, rivers, or wells to conceal murder. In these cases, apart from the absence of the signs of drowning, the injury responsible for the death can usually be demonstrated, provided that putrefaction is not too far advanced. The type of problem which arises in these circumstances may be illustrated by the findings in one of our cases:

One evening a farm worker was overheard quarrelling with his wife in a small hut which they occupied on the farm. When the farmer went to call the worker on the following morning, he found that both the man and his wife had left with all their belongings. Ten days later the farmer noticed a grain bag floating in his dam. The bag contained the body of the woman. Her head was projecting from the open end of the bag and the rest of the body was firmly compressed in the bag. The deceased's hands and feet were wrinkled and sodden. Externally the skin was distended and green in colour. Areas of desquamation of the skin were seen over the chest, the neck and face, but no external wounds could be found. A series of vertical, parallel incisions approximately 13 mm apart were made through the skin of the face, neck, chest and abdomen, and the underlying tissues were examined in strips. In this way several areas of reddish-brown discoloration were found in the subcutaneous tissues. These areas of discoloration were examined microscopically and found to consist of foci of blood extravasation having the appearance of bruises.

Examination of the internal organs revealed several small bruises in the intestines and a moderately extensive subarachnoid haemorrhage over the lateral surface of the left cerebrum. No fluid or frothy material was observed in the larynx, trachea or bronchi. The lungs were not distended and no haemorrhages were observed in the pleurae. On section, the lungs were a uniform dark-red colour and only a small amount of blood-stained fluid could be expressed from their cut surfaces.

Although the tissues of the body showed moderate putrefactive change, this change was not sufficiently advanced to have obscured the pathological changes ordinarily associated with drowning. The number, situation and the extent of the bruises suggested that they were probably ante-mortem in origin. Furthermore, the subarachnoid haemorrhage did not appear to have been caused by any disease process. On the basis of these findings it was stated that the deceased was dead at the time of her immersion and the probable cause of death was given as subarachnoid haemorrhage caused by trauma with associated injuries to other parts of the body.

The accused was arrested five months after the crime. He admitted that he had assaulted his wife, but he stated that he had not intended to kill her. When, after the assault, he found that she was dead, he became frightened, and after placing the body in a bag he disposed of it in the dam. He then left the farm. The accused was found guilty of murder with extenuating circumstances.

In certain circumstances a person may be rapidly overpowered and be thrown into water while he is alive and breathing, and under these conditions signs of drowning will be found at autopsy. It is therefore essential that all bodies that are recovered from fluid media should be carefully examined to exclude foul play, whether the deceased has been drowned or not.

Microscopical examination of the lungs and other organs in instances of death associated with immersion, has revealed no findings of sufficient specificity to allow the diagnosis to be made with certainty. If, however, the gross post-mortem findings, the microscopical appearance of the organs, the evaluation of diatom distribution and the circumstances leading to death are considered, the diagnosis of death due to immersion should be able to be made with a reasonable degree of certainty.

Electronmicroscopy has been employed, both to gain an insight into the pathophysiology of drowning and to improve the specificity of diagnosis. Fresh and sea water has been introduced experimentally into the trachea of rats, and the fine ultrastructural changes have been recorded. There is, however, at present no comparable human model.[48–50]

If the body is infected with fleas or lice at the time of submersion, an estimation of the time of submersion may be more accurately made, since fleas can survive up to 24 hours and lice can survive for 12–48 hours after submersion.

REFERENCES

1 Becker L C. Augmentation of myocardial ischaemia by low level carbon monoxide exposure in dogs. Arch Environ Hlth 1979; 34:274.
2 Werne J, Garrow I. Sudden deaths of infants allegedly due to mechanical suffocation. Am J Publ Hlth 1947; 37: 675–687.
3 Turner R. Personal communication, 1940.
4 Roughead W. The Trial of Burke and Hare. London: Hodge. 1921.
5 Gonzales T A. Manual strangulation. Arch Path 1933; 15: 55–66.
6 Romanes G J. Cunningham's Textbook of Anatomy. Oxford: Oxford University Press. 1972: p 128.
7 Anson B J. Morris' Human Anatomy. New York: McGraw-Hill. 1966: p 1414.

8 Keen J A, Wainwright J. Ossification of the thyroid, cricoid and arytenoid cartilages. S Afr J Lab Clin Med 1958; 4: 83–108.

9 Camps F E, Hunt A C. Pressure on the neck. J Forens Med 1959; 6:127, 129.

10 Shapiro H A, Gluckman J, Gordon I. The significance of finger nail abrasions of the skin. J Forens Med 1962; 9: 17–19.

11 Prinsloo I, Gordon I. Post-mortem dissection artefacts of the neck and their differentiation from ante-mortem bruises. S Afr Med J 1951; 25: 358–361.

12 Camps F E, Hunt A. Pressure on the neck. J Forens Med 1959; 6: 116–136.

13 Tamáski L. Kehlkopfmuskkelblutungen bei plötzlich verstorbenen. Zacchia 1961; XXIV: Serie 2a Fasc 4.

14 Paparo G P, Siegel H. On the significance of posterior crico-arytenoid muscle haemorrhage. Forens Sci 1976; 7: 61–65.

15 Eller W C, Haugen R K. Food asphyxiation—restaurant rescue. New Engl J Med 1973; 289: 81–82.

16 Fisher R S. Immersion injury and drowning. In: Isselbacher K. J. ed. Harrison's Principles of Internal Medicine 10th ed. Tokyo: McGraw Hill. 1983: pp 754–755.

17 Spyker D A. Submersion injury. Epidemiology, prevention and management. Paed Clin N Am 1985; 32(1): 113–125.

18 Cairns F J, et al. Deaths from drowning. N Z Med J 1984; 97: 65–67.

19 Gierten J C. Drowning. In: Forensic Medicine, Vol. III. London: W B. Saunders. 1977: pp 1317–1333.

20 Plueckhahn V D. Alcohol and accidental drowning. Med J Aust 1984; 141: 22–25.

21 Dietz P E, Baker S P. Drowning—epedemiology and prevention. Am J Public Hlth 1974; 64: 303–312.

22 Haight J S J, Keatinge W R. Failure of thermoregulation in the cold during hypoglycaemia induced by exercise and ethanol. J Physiol 1973; 22: 87–97.

23 Guhuraj P V. Forensic Medicine. India, Longman. 1982: pp 177–184.

24 Gordon I. The anatomical signs of drowning. A critical evaluation. Forens Sci 1972; I: 389–395.

25 Rezek P R, Millard M. The heart, dissection and anatomy. In: Klemperet P. ed. Autopsy pathology. Springfield, Illinois: Thomas. 1963: p 250.

26 Niles N R. Haemorrhage in the middle ear and mastoid in drowning. Am J Clin Pathol 1963; 40:281.

27 Fatteh A. The diagnosis of drowning. In: Wecht C H. ed. Handbook of Forensic Pathology. Philadelphia: Lippincott. 1973: p 159.

28 Moritz A R. Chemical methods for the determination of death by drowning. Phys Rev 1944; 24: 70–88.

29 Gettler A O. A method for the determination of death by drowning. J Amer Med Assoc 1921; 77: 1650–1652.

30 Schwär T G. Drowning—its chemical diagnosis. A review. Forens Sci 1972; 1: 411–417.

31 Coutselinis A, Boukis D. The estimation of magnesium concentration in cerebro-spinal fluid as a method of drowning diagnosis in sea water. Forensic Sci 1976; 7: 109–111.

32 Abdallah A M, Hassan S A, Kabil M A, Ghanim A E. Serum strontium estimation as a diagnostic criterion of the type of drowning water. Forens Sci Int 1985; 28: 47–52.

33 Thomas F, Van Hecke W, Timperman J. The detection of diatoms in the bone marrow as evidence of death by drowning. J Forens Med 1961; 8: 142–144.

34 Timperman J. Medico-legal problems in death by drowning. J Forens Med 1969; 16: 45–75.

35 Timperman J. The diagnosis of drowning. A review Forens Sci 1972; 1: 397–409.

36 Terazawa K, Takatori T. Isolation of intact plankton from drowning lung tissue by centrifugation in a colloidal silica gradient. Forens Sci Int 1980; 16: 63–66.

37 Fukui Y, Hata M, Takahashi S, Matsubara K. New method for detecting diatoms in human organs. Forens Sci Int 1980; 16: 67–74.

38 Spitz W U, Schneider V. The significance of diatoms in the diagnosis of death by drowning. J Forens Sci 1964; 9: 11–18.

39 Nanikawa R, Kotoku S. Medico-legal observations on a dead body drawn up from the sea bed with special reference to ethanol and diatoms. Forens Sci 1974; 3: 225–232.

40 Mueller B. Gerichtlike medizin. Berlin: Springer Verlag. 1953.

41 Shinzawa Y. On the invasion of water into the dead bodies in water. Nagasaki Med J 1957; 32: 256–270 (Japanese).

42 Tomonaga T. On some questions in the practice of diatom method as the evidence of drowning and on the corpse under high water pressure. Jap J Leg Med 1963; 17: 188–189 (Japanese).

43 Karkola K, Neittaanmäki H. Diagnosis of drowning by investigation of left heart blood. Forens Sci Int 1981; 18: 149–153.

44 Perper J A, Wecht C H. Microscopic diagnosis in forensic pathology. Illinois: Charles C. Thomas. 1980: Chap 7.

45 Koseki T. Fundamental examinations of experimental materials and control animals on the diagnosis of death from drowning by the diatom method. Acta Med Biol 1968; 15: 207–219.

46 Burger E. Zur Frage des Beweiswertes fur das Auffinden von Diatomeen im Grossen Kreislauf. Dtsch Z Gericht Med 1968; 64: 21–28.

47 Peabody A J. Diatoms and drowning—A review. Med Sci Law 1980; 20: 254–261.

48 Reidbord H E, Spitz W U. Ultrastructural alteration in rat lungs: Changes after intratrachael perfusion with freshwater and seawater. Arch Pathol 1966; 8: 103–111.

49 Reidbord H E. An electron microscopic study of the alveolar-capillary wall following intratrachael administration of saline and water. Am J Pathol 1967; 50: 275–289.

50 Nopanitaya W, Gambill T G, Brinkhous K M. Fresh water drowning. Pulmonary ultrastructure and systemic fibrinolysis. Arch Pathol 1974; 98: 361–366.

5

Deaths usually initiated by anaemic hypoxia, histotoxic hypoxia or histotoxic anoxia

ACUTE CARBON MONOXIDE POISONING

Occurrence

Accidental. Accidental carbon monoxide poisoning occurs:

1. From an exposure to household gas—by the careless handling of gas apparatus, or from the use of faulty lighting installations, stoves, geysers, etc. Poisoning may also arise from the inhalation of household gas which has percolated through walls and floors from leaking gas mains or pipes. This form of poisoning is particularly dangerous as the constituents of household gas such as the sulphur compounds, which impart a pungent odour to the gas, may be removed in the process of percolation. In these circumstances, dangerous amounts of carbon monoxide may accumulate without warning.

2. From the use of flueless braziers in poorly ventilated rooms or buildings.

3. From an exposure to the exhaust gas of petrol engines. This type of poisoning occurs occasionally when the engine of a motor car is allowed to run in a closed garage.

4. From an exposure to the gas in mines following upon underground fires or explosions.

5. From an exposure to the gas during fires.

Suicidal. This type of poisoning arises most commonly from an exposure to household gas. It may also occur from the use of flueless braziers or from exposure to the exhaust gas of motor vehicles.

Homicidal. This form of poisoning is rare.

A case of attempted murder by carbon monoxide poisoning is recorded:

> The accused and a woman, at the latter's suggestion, decided to commit suicide by introducing exhaust gas into a closed motor car in which they were sitting. The accused made the necessary arrangements for introducing the fumes into the car, and started up the engine.
>
> They both lost consciousness in the car, but they were later removed to hospital where they eventually recovered. At the subsequent trial the accused was convicted of an attempt to murder his companion. This conviction was confirmed by the Judges of the Appellate Division.

Mechanism of death

Death is due to anaemic hypoxia*. In this form of poisoning carbon monoxide displaces oxygen from its combination with haemoglobin, and forms a relatively stable compound known as carboxyhaemoglobin. The affinity of haemoglobin for carbon monoxide is about 300 times as great as its affinity for oxygen. When blood is exposed to an atmosphere containing both gases in equal concentration, 300 parts of the carbon monoxide are absorbed by the haemoglobin for each part of oxygen.

In carbon monoxide poisoning, therefore, the haemoglobin becomes rapidly saturated with carbon monoxide and the oxygen-carrying capacity of the blood is reduced. According to Wokes,[1] carbon monoxide poisoning may result after a few minutes' exposure to air containing 1 in 500 of carbon monoxide, while a concentration of 1 in 5000 may cause symptoms after 5 to 6 hours' exposure.

The carbon monoxide concentration in the blood at which death occurs varies greatly. Gettler and Freimuth[2] state that most deaths occur at a blood concentration of between 60 and 75% but values as low as 33.6% and as high as 83.1% have been recorded in fatal cases of acute carbon monoxide poisoning.

Autopsy findings

Special pathological changes

Colour of the blood. The characteristic finding is a cherry-red colour of the blood. This colour is observed externally in the lips and skin and is particularly well marked in the patches of lividity. In addition, the colour is observed on dissection in the blood of the larger vessels of the heart and in the tissues and viscera throughout the body.

Changes in the central nervous system. A detailed analysis of the changes which have been described in the literature as occurring in the brain, the spinal cord and the peripheral nerves in delayed deaths from carbon monoxide poisoning has been given by von Oettingen.[3] Among the changes described in the brain are the following: haemorrhages in the meninges, cortex, and white matter; selective cellular necrobiosis of ganglion cells in the cortex; and bilateral softening of the lenticular nuclei with a predilection for involvement of the gobus pallidus regions.

Non-specific general pathological changes

Non-specific general pathological changes as described in Chapter 3 are present. The intensity of the visceral congestive changes is usually well marked.

---

* There is evidence that acute carbon monoxide poisoning may also induce histotoxic anoxia.[4]

Toxicological analysis

Carboxyhaemoglobin may be detected in the blood by spectroscopic examination or by chemical analysis. Each method may be used for qualitative or quantitative purposes.

Such analyses must be undertaken by suitably qualified chemists or toxicologists. Medical practitioners should submit 10 ml of venous blood for a quantitative analysis for the presence of carboxyhaemoglobin.

Additional points of medico-legal importance

The value of estimations of carboxyhaemoglobin in deciding whether a person was alive or dead when a fire reached him

The average carbon monoxide blood concentration of normal persons living in urban areas has been found to be about 1% with a maximum of 6% in certain occupations, e.g. taxi drivers, garage workers, etc. Gettler and Freimuth[2] have shown that carbon monoxide is not absorbed by a body after death. These facts are of value in deciding whether a person who is found in the ruins of a fire was alive or dead when the fire reached him.

Persons who die before the fumes of the fire reach them have a blood concentration which is within the normal limits, while persons who die during an exposure to the fumes have a concentration which exceeds 10%.

Irreversible changes in the central nervous system and delayed death in carbon monoxide poisoning

The chemical reaction which results in the formation of carboxyhaemoglobin is reversible, but the release of carbon monoxide from its compound is a slow process. The hypoxic effects of carbon monoxide poisoning are therefore maintained for some period after the removal of a victim from a contaminated area.

The total period of the hypoxia may be sufficiently long for the development of irreversible changes in the central nervous system and delayed deaths from this cause may occur. In one of our cases three men went to sleep and left a flueless coal brazier burning in their room throughout the night. On the following morning one of them was found dead, while the other two were deeply unconscious. These two men subsequently died without recovering consciousness 12 and 48 hours respectively after their removal from the place of exposure.

Dissociation of oxygen from oxyhaemoglobin in acute carbon monoxide poisoning

Carbon monoxide interferes with the dissociation of oxygen from the oxyhaemoglobin which remains in the blood in this form of poisoning. The condition of a person with his blood half-saturated with carbon monoxide is more serious, therefore, than the condition of a person suffering from anaemia with 50% haemoglobin.

The deleterious effect of carbon monoxide on the dissociation of oxyhaemoglobin may be counteracted by carbon dioxide. This fact explains the characteristic collapse which occurs in carbon monoxide poisoning, when the victim is taken into the open air, as the concentration of carbon dioxide is considerably less in the air than in the contaminated atmosphere. For the same reason carbon dioxide should always be given with oxygen in the treatment of this form of poisoning.

Similarity of symptoms in acute carbon monoxide poisoning and acute alcoholic poisoning

Medical practitioners should always consider the possibility of acute carbon monoxide poisoning when conducting medical examinations on persons who are alleged to have been drunk while in charge of motor vehicles. The symptoms of acute carbon monoxide poisoning may resemble those of acute alcoholic poisoning. If there is reason to think that a person may be suffering from carbon monoxide poisoning about 10 ml of venous blood should be submitted for analysis for carboxyhaemoglobin.

ACUTE POISONING BY HYDROCYANIC ACID AND CYANIDE COMPOUNDS

This form of poisoning may result from the inhalation of the fumes of the acid or from the ingestion of the acid or its chemical compounds.

The compounds which give rise to poisoning most commonly are potassium and sodium cyanide, but the ingestion of other compounds such as silver cyanide and mercury or zinc cyanide may lead to death.

Occurrence

Accidental. Hydrocyanic acid is used extensively for fumigation purposes and accidental inhalation poisoning may arise from this cause. Fatalities may result from persons entering houses and buildings after fumigation before the fumes of the acid have been adequately dispersed.

Suicidal. This is the commonest type of poisoning, and usually results from the ingestion of cyanides by persons who have access to such compounds, e.g. chemists, doctors, photographers, gilders, electroplaters and gold-mine workers.

Homicidal. This form of poisoning is rare but cases of homicidal poisoning by the introduction of cyanides into foodstuffs have been recorded.

Mechanism of death

In this form of poisoning there is an interference with the intracellular oxidative processes in the tissues, and death is due to histotoxic hypoxia or histotoxic anoxia.

The lethal dose of hydrocyanic acid by inhalation varies greatly, and depends upon the concentration of the gas in the atmosphere and the period of exposure. A concentration of 0.2 to 0.3 mg per litre of air may lead to instantaneous death, while lesser amounts would be fatal if inhaled over a sufficiently long period of time. Hydrocyanic acid may be fatal in amounts of 0.05 g when taken by mouth, while the lethal dose of potassium cyanide is generally given as 0.25 g (pp 217–219).

Large doses of the acid or its compounds are usually taken in cases of suicidal poisoning and death occurs within a few minutes. When the amount taken is smaller death may be delayed for several hours.

Death is relatively more rapid in inhalation poisoning than in poisoning by ingestion.

Autopsy findings

Special pathological changes

Colour of the blood. The characteristic finding is a bright pink colour of the blood. Oxygen is not removed from the capillaries in the tissues and all the vessels of the body, including the veins, contain arterial blood. The colour is observed externally in the lips and skin and is well marked in the patches of lividity. The mucous membranes of the body, including the gastric mucosa, are pink in colour, and this colour is also observed in the organs and tissues.

The odour of bitter almonds. A characteristic odour of bitter almonds may be detected on dissection of the body. In cases of suspected cyanide poisoning the cranial cavity should be opened first as the odour is usually well marked in the brain tissues.

Non-specific general pathological changes

Non-specific general pathological changes as described in Chapter 3 are present. In most cases the intensity of the visceral congestive changes is slight.

Toxicological analysis

Hydrocyanic acid is an extremely volatile substance, and medical practitioners should submit specimens for analysis in well-stoppered test tubes or jars as soon after the autopsy as possible. All specimens for analysis should be sent, without delay, to a suitably qualified chemist or toxicologist.

REFERENCES

1 Wokes F. A textbook of applied biochemistry. London: Bailliere, Tindall & Cox. 1937: p 324.
2 Gettler A O, Freimuth H C. The carbon monoxide content of the blood under various conditions. Am J Clin Path 1940; 10: 603–616.
3 Von Oettingen. Carbon monoxide: its hazards and the mechanism of its action. Washington: United States Government Printing Office: Publ Hlth Bull 1944; No 290: p 137.
4 Becker L C. Augmentation of myocardial ischaemia by low level carbon monoxide exposure in dogs. Arch Environ Hlth 1979; 34:274.

6

Deaths from burns, exposure to high and low environmental temperatures, and electrical injuries

DEATHS FROM BURNS

Burns are produced by the application of flame, or hot liquids or gases, or solid heated substances to the surface of the body. Similar lesions of the skin are caused by the action of certain chemicals and through contact with electrically charged conductors.

Occurrence

Deaths from burns are usually accidental but they may be of suicidal or homicidal origin.

Accidental deaths from burns are seen most frequently in infants, children, and aged persons. Accidental deaths from burns occur when persons who are under the influence of drugs or alcohol are unable to escape when a fire breaks out. Inebriated persons often start fires by careless acts. In one of our cases the badly charred remains of a woman were found on a bed. Three empty brandy bottles and two packets of cigarettes were found on a chair beside the bed. The evidence at the inquest disclosed that the deceased had been drinking heavily before her death and it was probable that the bed clothes caught alight while she was smoking in bed.

Suicidal burning is relatively uncommon.

Homicidal burning is unusual but is seen in cases where paraffin or some other inflammable material is thrown over the victim and his clothing then set alight. Bodies may be burned after death in order to conceal homicidal injuries, and for this reason complete autopsies should always be performed upon bodies which are removed from burned-out buildings, cars, etc.

Mechanism of death

The highest death rate from burns occurs within the first 24 hours. These deaths are usually attributed to shock and toxaemia. Toxaemia persists up to 72–96 hours and probably accounts for those deaths which occur within this period. Sepsis is the most important factor in deaths which occur 4 to 5 days or longer after burning. It is doubtful whether the liver changes

134

which occur in burns are sufficient to cause death (p. 136).

Deaths may also arise indirectly through bronchopneumonia, especially in infants, while haemorrhage from acute erosions of the duodenum and other parts of the intestinal tract is an occasional cause of delayed death after burning. Fatal renal damage may also occur.

Autopsy findings in early deaths from burns

Special pathological changes

External lesions. Burns are found on external examination of the body. The situation, extent, and nature of the burns should be described. The extent of burning varies greatly in fatal cases, and although a relatively large surface of the body is usually involved, death may result from lesions which are limited in extent, particularly in infants. There is also considerable variation in the depth of fatal burns.

Burns are usually described as burns of first, second, third, fourth, fifth, or sixth degree according to a classification originally introduced by Dupuytren. A first-degree burn consists of an erythema of the skin without vesication. A second-degree burn results in injury to the superficial and deep layers of the epidermis and is characterized by the formation of vesicles in the burned skin. A third-degree burn results in the destruction of the full thickness of the epidermis and the epithelial glands and hair follicles. In fourth-degree burns there is complete destruction of the dermis extending into subcutaneous tissues. Muscles are involved in fifth-degree burns and in sixth-degree burns there is complete carbonization of the burned part with charring of bones.

Wilson[1] states that Dupuytren's classification is of limited practical value as it is very difficult, on naked-eye examination, to determine the exact depth of burning. He has suggested that burns should be classified into the following three types:

Type I. Epidermal burns. In this type of burn the lesion is confined to the epidermis and takes the form of an erythema with or without superficial vesication.

Type II. Dermo-epidermal burns. In this type of burn the epidermis and dermis are separated and the dermis is involved in the destructive process.

Type III. Deep burns. In this type of burn the skin is totally destroyed and underlying structures are exposed. In some deep burns, islands of intact dermis may be found in the wounds.

Apart from its value in clinical surgery, Wilson's classification is useful for the purpose of describing morbid anatomical findings in post-mortem reports.

Heat rigor. Heat rigor may be observed in the muscles. This phenomenon is seen particularly in cases where there has been deep charring of the body (p. 33 and Fig. 1.15).

Liver necrosis. For many years a centrilobular necrosis of the liver has been observed in fatal burns. This form of necrosis was originally attributed to the acute toxaemia which accompanies burns, but in recent years experimental and clinical evidence has shown that these lesions are caused by the coagulating agents used in treatment rather than by the burns themselves.

In an experimental study Hartman and Romence[2] found that although minor degenerative lesions occur in the livers of burned animals which had not received coagulation therapy, the incidence of liver damage was greatly increased when tannic acid, silver nitrate, and ferric chloride were used as dressings for burns. Rae and Wilkinson[3] showed that tannic acid is especially liable to produce liver damage.

Non-specific general pathological changes

Non-specific general pathological changes as described in Chapter 3 are present. In most cases the intensity of the visceral congestive changes is marked. Petechial haemorrhages are commonly found in the pleurae, pericardium and endocardium.

Additional points of medico-legal importance

Was a person found in the ruins of a fire alive or dead when the fire reached him?

A person who dies after the fumes of a fire have reached him usually has a carbon monoxide blood concentration which exceeds 10% (p. 130), and carbon particles are found in his air passages.

These two signs are absent when a person dies before the fumes of a fire reached him. They are absent, therefore, in cases of murder when a body has been burned after death.

The presence of the signs, however, does not necessarily indicate that death was due to burning alone. The signs only establish that a deceased person was breathing at the time that the fire reached him. They are present, therefore, when a person is burned while he is unconscious following upon some injury. In the British case of Rex *v.* Rouse, to which reference has already been made (p. 34), carbon particles were found in the air passages of the deceased while the blood contained a moderate amount of carboxyhaemoglobin. On the basis of these findings, it was stated that the deceased was alive for a short period after the fire started.

If the concentration of carboxyhaemoglobin is sufficiently high, the characteristic cherry-red colour of the blood will be observed. Stein[4] has noted that under the influence of heat the cherry red colour of carboxyhaemoglobin changes to a brownish colour. The change begins at about 65 °C and the rate at which the change occurs depends upon the concentration of the solution, the pH of the medium in which it is contained, and the duration of heating. On spectroscopic examination heating results in a disappearance of the bands, but on adding sodium dithionite the characteristic bands of globin haemochromogen can be seen. These changes with denatured carboxyhaemoglobin are, however, not as readily demonstrable as with oxyhaemoglobin solutions. Kilroe-Smith and Shapiro[5] found that this characteristic colour of human blood containing carboxyhaemoglobin disappears to the naked eye when the blood is heated in a test tube to about 80 °C.

The proposition stands that if carboxyhaemoglobin, in excess of the amount which might normally be present (p. 130) or if the characteristic cherry-red colour of the blood is observed in a body recovered from a fire, this is good evidence that the deceased was alive before the fire reached him. The failure to observe in a dead body removed from a fire, the characteristic cherry-red colour of carboxyhaemoglobin does not warrant the inference that the body was dead before the fire reached it.

An estimation of the ethyl alcohol content of the blood of the deceased may be of indirect value in suggesting that the deceased might have been under the influence of alcohol, and might therefore have been unable to escape at the time that the fire occurred.

The cause of death in fires

Deaths in fires are usually due to burning, but they may be caused by acute carbon monoxide poisoning or other forms of toxic gas poisoning. Dutra[6] states that dangerous quantities of nitrogen dioxide and nitrogen tetroxide are liberated by the burning of nitrogen-containing materials such as nitrocellulose film and artificial leatherette. The burning of wool or silk liberates ammonia and hydrogen cyanide. Hydrogen sulphide and oxides of sulphur are yielded during the burning of wool and other sulphur-containing substances. Acrolein, which is a highly irritating compound, is liberated by the thermal decomposition of neutral fats or materials containing glycerine. The combustion of polyvinyl chloride produces carbon monoxide and other noxious substances.

In certain instances death may be due to injury from falling masonry or other structures. In addition, it is stated that death can arise from 'reflex shock' from fear, but this is very difficult to prove.

Differentiation between ante-mortem and post-mortem burns

It may be possible on naked-eye examination to state that a burn is ante-mortem in origin if it shows evidence of an advanced inflammatory reaction. For instance, if a vesicle caused by a burn contains pus it may be assumed that the burn was produced before death. In most cases, however, naked-eye appearances cannot be relied upon, and the only method of distinguishing between an ante-mortem and a post-mortem burn is a histological examination for evidence of tissue reaction. Marked cellular exudation and reactive changes in the tissue cells in relation to a burn may be regarded as evidence that it was produced before death. The absence of tissue reaction, however, does not necessarily indicate that a burn was produced after death, as the death may have occurred so rapidly after the burning that there was insufficient time for the development of tissue reaction.

Vesicles caused by burning are usually produced before death, but they can arise after death. It has been held that an ante-mortem vesicle can be distinguished from a post-mortem vesicle by the appearance of a red line of demarcation between the vesicle and the rest of the skin, by the presence of albumin and chlorides in the fluid of the vesicle, and by a reddening and swelling of papillae in the floor of the vesicle. These criteria of distinction are of little practical value as a red line of demarcation is not an invariable accompaniment of an ante-mortem vesicle, while albumin and chlorides have been demonstrated in post-mortem vesicles, especially in obese and oedematous persons. Furthermore, as the prominence of the papillae in the floor of a vesicle depends partly upon the depth of the vesicle, it is difficult to assess the significance of such swelling on naked-eye examination alone. The only reliable method of distinguishing between an ante-mortem and a post-mortem vesicle is to excise the vesicle and its related tissues and examine the structure histologically for evidence of tissue reaction.

Post-mortem artefacts caused by heat resembling ante-mortem injuries

External wounds. When bodies are exposed to very high temperatures the tissues may rupture, and splits resembling incised or lacerated wounds may appear in the skin. These artefacts can usually be differentiated from ante-mortem wounds by the absence of haemorrhage into the related tissues.

Fractures of the skull and intracranial haemorrhages. Fractures of the skull and intracranial haemorrhages are often found in charred bodies. There are three possible cause for such injuries:

1. They may be produced by ante-mortem violence.

2. They may result from the action of heat on the skull and its contents.

3. They may be caused after death by injuries from falling masonry or other structures. It is important to be able to distinguish between these injuries.

In cases of murder bodies may be deliberately burned in order to conceal an ante-mortem head injury. In most of these cases the bodies are burned after death. In some cases the victim may be burned while he is unconscious and the burning usually takes place within a short period of the infliction of the head injury (Rex. *v.* Rouse, p. 34). In certain cases, however, the victim may survive the head injury for an hour or longer before he is burned, and in these circumstances microscopic evidence of tissue reaction may be found in the bone at the margins of the fracture and in the membranes overlying the haemorrhages. In most cases the period of survival between the head injury and the burning is insufficient for the development of tissue reaction, and the distinction between ante-mortem fractures of the skull and ante-mortem intracranial haemorrhages, and fractures and haemorrhages produced by heat and post-mortem injuries, must be based on macroscopic examinations.

Moritz[7] states that there are two types of thermal fractures of the skull. In one type the fracture results from a rapid increase in intracranial pressure and the fragments are displaced outwards. In the other type the fracture appears to be due to a rapid desiccation of the bone with contraction and only involves the outer table of the skull. In this type there is no displacement and the lines of fracture are frequently stellate. Moritz states that in both types of fracture there is likely to be secondary mechanical disturbance of bone. This may be caused by falling debris or rough handling of the body and, if the bone is brittle enough, depressed fractures can result. It is apparent from the description given by Moritz that it can be extremely difficult to distinguish between a thermal fracture of the skull and an ante-mortem fracture due to violence, but such a differentiation may be possible. Ante-mortem fractures in cases of homicide often appear as localized depressions of the skull. Close examination of such fractures or fragments of bone will often show a shelving inwards of the outer table of the bone along the edges of the fracture. This shelving of the outer table is characteristic of a depressed fracture.

Although ante-mortem fractures of the skull are usually accompanied by adjacent extradural haemorrhages and contusion and laceration of the brain, if the brain is extensively charred it may be impossible to recognize areas of contusion in the tissue.

Sampson[8] has shown that post-mortem extradural haemorrhages can be caused by heat alone, and may be unaccompanied by fractures of the skull. Such haemorrhages may be localized and may closely simulate ante-mortem extradural haemorrhages (Fig. 6.1).

The facts set out in this section show that in a charred body it may be impossible, even in the presence of a localized extradural haemorrhage, to establish that a head injury has been caused by ante-mortem violence unless an uncharred portion of the brain shows areas of contusion and laceration.

Examination of clothing for combustible substances

The clothing of a person who has been remvoed from a burned-out structure should be examined for combustible substances. In the case of Rex v. Rouse, to which reference has been made, petrol was demonstrated on a portion of unburned clothing removed from the left groin. Such a finding may have considerable value in a charge of murder when it is alleged that the deceased was burned after death.

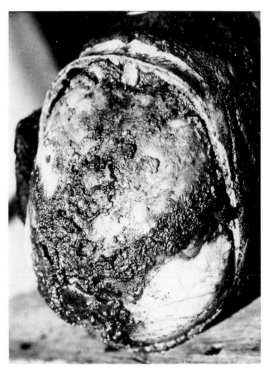

Fig. 6.1 Post-mortem extradural haemorrhage caused by heat. The calvarium has been removed and the intact dura mater covering the cerebrum is seen beneath the collection of clotted blood distributed over the external surface of the dura mater. (Prof. L. S. Smith's case.)

DEATHS FROM EXPOSURE TO HIGH AND LOW ENVIRONMENTAL TEMPERATURES

The body core temperature of a normal resting adult is controlled at a relatively stable level. Early morning rectal temperature is generally within 0.5 °C of 37 °C. There is a circadian rhythm such that the rectal temperature tends to be 0.5 °C to 1 °C higher in the evening than in the early morning.

If the rectal temperature rises to above 40 °C or falls to below about 35 °C, there is a risk of tissue damage and ultimately death. The deviations of body temperature may take three forms, namely:

1. Heat gain can exceed heat loss, with rise in body temperature—hyperthermia;
2. Heat loss can exceed heat gain and body temperature will fall — hypothermia; and
3. Control mechanisms maintaining normal body temperature may fail and the body temperature will rise or fall—abnormally labile body temperature.

DEATHS FROM EXPOSURE TO HIGH ENVIRONMENTAL TEMPERATURES OCCURRENCE

In a detailed review, Anderson et al[9] list three categories of heat illness:

1. Heat oedema, heat syncope or heat cramps—non-fatal;
2. Heat exhaustion—rarely fatal;
3. Heatstroke—classical and exertional types.

Heatstroke results from hyperpyrexia following exposure to excessive heat. Deaths from heatstroke include situations such as those which can occur during military training; with exercise in a hot environment (football, marathon runners); during summer in hot regions; in mining operations, e.g. when workers are not acclimatized; in elderly persons; and under the influence of medicines, particularly in therapy with substances which can inhibit sweating.[10]

Clinical findings

Heatstroke is the most severe form of heat-induced disease and body tissue is seriously damaged as a result of the high body temperature. The risk of heatstroke increases markedly when the rectal temperature exceeds 40 °C. At 43 °C, brain and liver functions are seriously impaired.

Autopsy findings

The degree of pathological changes are conditioned by the degree of heat pyrexia and the time duration before death. The thermal damage to tissue affects many organs.

Hart et al[11] presented data to indicate that there are differences both in the clinical course and the autopsy findings in classical as opposed to exertional cases of heatstroke. The differences include diffuse intravascular coagulation, rhabdomyolysis and acute renal failure being rarely found in the classical cases but being commonly present in exertional heatstroke deaths. Kew et al[12] in a series of 40 cases of exertional heatstroke, documented an incidence of 10% with evidence of acute renal failure.

Kew et al[13] reported that liver biopsies in mine workers who developed heatstroke demonstrated the presence of damage due to the hyperthermia per se, together with the complicating factors of hypoxia, ischaemia and disseminated intravascular coagulation. The authors postulated that in several cases of liver damage, the liver failure itself could have contributed to a fatal outcome.

Rubel and Ishak[14] documented the histopathological changes in the liver of 50 cases of fatal exertional heatstroke. In five cases, where acute death occurred, they demonstrated the presence of parenchymal congestion and fatty change, but no fibrin thrombi were present. In other patients, who survived up to 8 days following hospitalization, fatty change was a common feature, as were degenerated hepatocytes resembling Councilman bodies. There was minimal evidence of extensive hepatic necrosis or evidence of regeneration of hepatic parenchymal cells. In those who survived more than 12 hours, more than half the cases showed the presence of bile stasis, frequently associated with an acute cholangitis and bile ductular proliferation.

Chao et al[15] detailed the autopsy findings in 10 acute heatstroke deaths that occurred after running or after route marches in high environmental temperatures. At autopsy, features of diffuse intravascular coagulation were prominent.

Anderson et al[9] in a detailed review on heatstrole, confirmed and extended these findings, highlighting two further aspects. First, the problem of antecedent disease. The risk for transmural myocardial infarction occurring during heatstroke appeared to be greatest for patients with underlying coronary artery disease. Further, elderly victims or patients with cerebrovascular disease were more prone to the formation of cerebral oedema with associated parenchymal petechial haemorrhages as well as marked Purkinje cell damage. Secondly, autopsy findings could be predicted with reference to the time that had elapsed between the occurrence of heatstroke and death—which occurred after several hours to 10 days. Thus, a whole spectrum of autopsy findings may occur in relation to survival time. Further, the presence of pulmonary oedema could reflect over-zealous fluid replacement therapy.

Kew et al[16] documented changes in the heart in 26 unselected patients with heatstroke. Their study was based on the clinical findings, serum isoenzyme and electrocardiographic changes and, where possible, pathological examination of the heart. Evidence of cardiac damage was found in 17 of the 26 patients and 69% had a significant increase in the percentage of LDH 1. Electrocardiographic tracings were abnormal in 58% of the cases. Two of the patients died and histopathological examination of the heart showed the presence of interstitial oedema and myofibre degeneration.

Kim et al[17] undertook a detailed study of skeletal muscle changes in three cases of fatal heatstroke. Their findings were similar to those occurring in other forms of rhabdomyolysis and included swollen and irregular fibres, with zones of defective staining and loss of striations. There was also focal extravasation of red blood cells into the endomysium as well as phagocytosis and regeneration of myofibres.

Shibolet et al[18] presented a detailed report on the clinical presentation and mechanism of the production of heatstroke in 36 cases occurring in healthy young males, engaged in strenuous physical activity. Many of their findings have been confirmed in the above survey.

Lethal sunburn is quite distinct from heatstroke and may be considered to be a metabolic type of poisoning, resulting from the release of kinins and other toxins from the damaged skin.

DEATHS FROM EXPOSURE TO LOW ENVIRONMENTAL TEMPERATURES

Hypothermia is usually defined as a condition in which the body core temperature is below 35 °C.

Occurrence

Deaths from exposure to cold (air or water), occur in many countries, particularly in the colder latitudes and altitudes, and during winter. Death is seldom due to the cold *per se*, and exhaustion, fatigue, lack of food, disease, injuries, drug and/or alcoholic intoxication are usually major contributors to the cause of such exposure-related hypothermic deaths. Immersion hypothermia, since body heat is lost at a rate three times faster than in cold, dry air at the same temperature, is a potent and rapid cause of fatalities.

Mechanism of death

Clark and Edholm[19] indicate that exposure to cold results in a progressive decrease in metabolic processes in all organs, a lowered oxygen dissociation of oxyhaemoglobin and oxymyoglobin as well as diminished blood flow through tissues. With reference to the nervous system, this leads to unconsciousness and mechanisms for temperature regulation become progressively inoperative.

Hypothermia protects the central nervous system from the effects of ischaemia, and is an important cause of apparent death.

The effects of low temperature on the heart are particularly important, the heart rate and cardiac output falling progressively as the temperature falls. Atrial fibrillation is common and at temperatures below 28 °C there is a high risk of ventricular fibrillation, which is often the terminal event. Cases reported by Keatinge[20] demonstrate such cardiac disorders.

Autopsy findings

In accidental hypothermia, the process of death lasts 3–12 hours in cold, dry air and snow conditions; in water it can be as short as 5 minutes. As a consequence, few specific or morphological changes may be seen at autopsy. Studies of catecholamine and other stress hormone levels may be informative. These parameters are stable in blood after death, and the level of the increased concentration of catecholamines may reflect the duration and individual reaction.[21] Tests for blood ethanol and drugs are mandatory. Ethanol or psychotropic drugs are reported to be present in up to 70% of deaths. Subjects under the influence of drugs or ethanol[22] probably die more rapidly.

Hirvonen[23] in a series of 22 cases of fatal accidents or suicidal hypothermia, suggested that the best diagnostic signs at autopsy included a purple skin and oedema involving the face, hands and feet; internally the most conspicuous finding may be that of gastric erosions or haemorrhages. Although the heart was macroscopically normal in Hirvonen's cases, microscopical examination revealed the presence of small foci of myocardial degeneration.

A bright red colour of the blood has been described as being characteristic of deaths from cold. Decreased dissociation of the oxyhaemoglobin and the reduced capacity of the tissues to utilize oxygen may partly account for this observation. However, refrigeration after death can also produce a bright red colour of the blood. Hypoxia leads to increased capillary permeability and it would appear that in deaths from cold the transudation of plasma in certain regions is so great that plugs of tightly packed red blood corpuscles are left in the vessels. Kreyberg[24] has observed that stasis of this nature is often accompanied by haemorrhages into the tissues. The stasis, with arrest of blood flow, also affords an explanation for the occurrence of visceral infarcts described at autopsy.

Non-cardiogenic pulmonary oedema is common.[25]

There is no single sign at autopsy which enables one to make a definitive diagnosis of death due to hypothermia. However, the circumstances, the macroscopical, microscopical and biochemical changes in the cadaver, all help to justify the diagnosis with reasonable certainty.

DEATHS FROM ELECTROCUTION

There are two forms of death from electrocution, namely, deaths caused through contact with electrical conductors and deaths caused by lightning stroke. The pathological changes in these forms of death are essentially similar.

Occurrence

Most deaths from contact with electrical conductors are accidental and are caused by contacts with broken or non-insulated wires in faulty domestic or industrial appliances. Suicidal and homicidal deaths of this nature are rare.

Deaths from lightning stroke are invariably accidental.

Mechanism of death

Death is usually instantaneous but it may be delayed for several hours. According to Barrera,[26] the rapid form of death is due either to cardiac failure or to respiratory failure. Barrera claims that in practically all instances the respiratory failure could be overcome by sufficiently prolonged artificial respiration, but the cardiac failure appears to be due to a sudden cardiac arrest. This cardiac arrest has been ascribed to ventricular fibrillation, but Alexander[27] believes that the more likely cause is an intense stimulation of the vagal nerve centres in the medulla oblongata.

In cases where death is delayed, unconsciousness is the most common symptom, and occurs even in cases where the brain itself has not been in the direct path of the current or discharge. Unconsciousness is often accompanied by signs of circulatory and respiratory failure and in cases where specific lesions are not demonstrable in the central nervous system it is probable that the unconsciousness is caused by hypoxia or anoxia which is secondary to the cardiac and respiratory failure.

According to Moritz[28] the occurrence of electrical injuries caused by contact with electrical conductors depends upon (1) the kind of current; (2) the amount of current; (3) the path of the current; and (4) the duration of the current flow.

1. Alternating currents are more effective in producing lesions than direct currents and some alternating frequencies are more dangerous than others. Moritz states that the 60-cycle alternating current which is commonly used in domestic and industrial supplies is particularly prone to injure the medullary centres and the heart.

2. The amount of current that will flow through or over the body may be determined by the formula $C = V/R$, in which C is the current in amperes, V is the potential, and R is the resistance of the body in ohms. If the voltage is high or if the resistance is low, the flow of current through the body is proportionately great.

3. Moritz states that death is more likely to occur if the brain stem or heart are in the direct path of the current.

4. In general, the severity of an electrical injury is directly proportional to the duration of the current flow.

Most deaths due to contact with electrical conductors result from exposure to high-tension currents, but ordinary domestic currents of low tension (e.g. 110 volts) may cause death if there is a favourable contact between the skin and the external conductor and if either the brain stem or the heart lies in the path of the current. On the other hand, high-tension currents (e.g. 1200 to 2000 volts) may not prove fatal if the contact is poor or if the exposure is momentary.

Autopsy findings

Special pathological changes

External lesions caused through contact with conductors. External lesions are usually observed at the sites of entry and exit of the current. These lesions may be absent when there is extensive contact between the skin and the external conductor, e.g. external lesions were absent in one of our cases where a girl was accidentally electrocuted in a bath.

In certain cases multiple lesions are found in the region of flexures, where the current has passed across joints instead of around them.

The external lesions at the site of entry closely resemble ordinary burns. Jenny[29] has shown that the skin offers most of the resistance to the passage of an electric current through the body and that part of the electrical energy is transformed into heat in the skin. He states that lesions of the skin caused by electrical injury cannot be differentiated from ordinary burns on histological examination. As a general rule, the extent and degree of tissue injury at the site of entry is directly proportional to the tension or voltage of the current.

Thomsen et al[30] state that the morphology of electrical lesions differs markedly from that of heat lesions. They found this difference both by light and electron microscopy and claim that electricity has a specific action on epidermal cells.

Lesions resembling burns are usually seen at the site of exit of the current. In certain cases the skin at the site of exit may be split in the form of punctured or lacerated wounds.

External lesions caused by lightning-stroke. In deaths from lightning-stroke external lesions are usually found, but they may be absent. Spencer[31] describes the external lesions as 'burns' and classifies them into three types: linear 'burns', arborescent 'burns' and surface burns.

1. Linear 'burns'. These 'burns' are linear in shape and vary from 6–25 mm in width and from 2.5–30 cm or more in length. As moist skin offers less resistance than dry skin, linear burns are often found in the moist creases and folds of the skin.

2. Arborescent or filigree 'burns'. These 'burns' are characterized by the formation of superficial thin, irregular, and tortuous markings on the skin. These markings have a general pattern resembling the branches of a tree and are therefore described as arborescent markings.

3. Surface burns. These lesions are true burns and occur beneath metallic objects worn or carried by the deceased. The heat which causes these burns may be sufficiently great to fuse or magnetize the metal. The clothing of persons who are struck by lightning may be torn and burned. In some cases the clothes are completely stripped off the body and boots or shoes are burst open. Surface burns may be found in relation to the burned portions of clothing.

Injuries to muscles and bones. In most instances of fatal electrocution the external lesions do not extend deeper than the tissues which lie immediately subjacent to the skin. In some cases, however, the lesions may extend through the subcutaneous tissues and involve muscles and bone. Jenny has described lesions of the muscles which simulate the changes which occur in the crush syndrome (p. 334). Injury to bone may result in the elevation of periosteum, the destruction of the superficial layers of the bone (e.g. the external table of the skull), or fractures.

Lesions of the central nervous system. A detailed description of the neuropathological changes in fatal electrocution has been given by Critchley.[32]
These changes are: focal petechial haemorrhages in the brain and spinal
cord, especially in the medulla and grey matter of the anterior horns; chro-
matolysis involving particularly the pyramidal cells, the nerve cells of the
medullary nuclei and of the anterior horns, and the Purkinje cells of the
cerebellum; wide dilatations of the perivascular spaces which measure from
25 to 250 μm in diameter, and are most numerous in the brain stem and
cervical cord; and fragmentation of the axons and changes in the myelin
sheaths of peripheral nerves. Hassin[33] has described certain microscopic
disruptive lesions in the brains of criminals who sustained high-tension electrical injuries in legal electrocutions. These lesions affected the brain
parenchyma and the arteries. Irregular tears and fissures appeared in the
brain tissue and adjacent cortical layers were separated from one another.
The separation was particularly conspicuous between the pia mater and the
subpial lamina zonalis of the cerebral cortex, and between the Purkinje cell
layer and the granular layer of the cerebellum. In some cases the walls of
arteries were completely ruptured. In other cases there was fragmentation
of the internal elastic membranes of arteries.

The wide dilatations of the perivascular spaces described by Critchley and
the disruptive lesions noted by Hassin are not confined to electrical injuries
caused by contact with high-tension conductors. They are commonly found
in the high-tension electrical injuries of lightning-stroke. Pritchard[34] states
that these lesions cannot be accounted for by the heating and electrolytic
effects of the current. He suggests that electrostatic forces are more likely
to produce the lesions. Pritchard explains the development of electrostatic
forces in the following manner:

If a person makes an effective contact with a conductor at high potential
or if he is struck by lightning, his body becomes suddenly highly charged
with electricity. Electrostatic forces will develop on any charged body
because of the mechanical repulsion which is exerted between all similarly
charged particles. Accordingly the accumulation of an electric charge on the
surface of the human body produces a force which acts outwards upon the
surface because each element of the surface is repelled from all other
elements. The distending or expanding force on the surface has the same
effect as a proportionate reduction in the atmospheric pressure acting upon
the body. The force passes inwards as a wave of decompression. As the
tissues yield in proportion to their rigidity and cohesion there is a distortion
of spaces within soft structures and a separation of parts that have relatively
little cohesion. Pritchard believes that the characteristic dilatation of perivascular spaces and the localized gaps and tears which appear in the brain
after high-tension electrical injuries are due to these electrostatic effects.

Associated injuries from mechanical trauma. The electrostatic forces
described by Pritchard are responsible for the gross mechanical effects on

the body and its clothing which occur in high-tension electrical injuries. When a person comes in contact with a high-tension electrical conductor or is struck by lightning he may be flung violently to the ground. If he is standing near to other objects which are similarly affected, e.g. trees, in lightning-stroke, he may be hurled several yards away from them. In lightning-stroke the sudden violent displacement from one another of persons or objects that are struck is due to the development of mutually repulsive forces between them.

Injuries from mechanical trauma, involving especially the skull and its contents, must be distinguished from the lesions produced by the electrical trauma.

Non-specific general pathological changes

Non- specific general pathological changes as described in Chapter 3 are present. In most cases the intensity of the visceral congestive changes is slight. Widespread petechial haemorrhages may be found in the serous membranes.

REFERENCES

1 Wilson J V. The pathology of traumatic injury, Edinburgh: Livingstone. 1946: p 26.
2 Hartman F W, Romence H L. Liver necrosis in burns. Ann Surg 1943; 118: 402–416.
3 Rae S L, Wilkinson A W. Liver function after burns in childhood. Lancet 1944; 1: 332–334.
4 Stein H B. Unpublished observations, 1973.
5 Kilroe-Smith T A, Shapiro H A. Unpublished observations, 1973.
6 Dutra F R. Medico-legal examination of bodies recovered from burned buildings. Am J Clin Pathol 1949; 19: 599–607.
7 Moritz A R. Personal communication, 1946.
8 Sampson B F. Intracranial haemorrhages after death by burning. Clin Proc 1946; 5: 189–194.
9 Anderson R J, Reed G, Knochel J. Heatstroke. Adv Intern Med 1983; 28: 115–140.
10 Khogoli M, Weiner J S. Heatstroke: report on 18 cases. Lancet 1980; 2: 276–278.
11 Hart G R, Anderson R J, Crumpler C P, Shulkin A, Reed G, Knochel J P. Epidemic classical heatstroke. Medicine 1982; 61: 189–197.
12 Kew M C, Abrahams C, Seftel H C. Chronic interstitial nephritis as a consequence of heatstroke. Quart J med 1970; 39: 189–199.
13. Kew M C, Minick O T, Bahu R M, Stein R J, Kent G. Ultrastructural changes in the liver in heatstroke. Am J Pathol 1978; 90: 609–618.
14 Rubel L R, Ishak K G. The liver in fatal exertional heatstroke. Liver 1983; 3: 249–260.
15 Chao T C, Sinniah R, Pakiam J E. Acute heat stroke deaths. Pathology 1981; 13: 145–156.
16 Kew M C, Tucker R B K, Bersohn I, Seftel H C. The heart in heatstroke. Am Ht J 1969; 77: 324–335.
17 Kim R C, Collins G H, Cho C, Ichikawa K, Givelber H. Heatstroke: Report of three fatal cases with emphasis on findings in skeletal muscle. Arch Pathol Lab Med 1980; 104: 345–349.
18 Shibolet S, Coll R, Gilot T, Sohar E. Heatstroke: Its clinical picture and mechanism in 36 cases. Quart J Med 1976; 144: 525–548.
19 Clark R P, Edholm O G. Man and his thermal environment. London: Edward Arnold, 1985.

20 Keatinge W R. Sudden death in cold water and ventricular arrhythmia. J Forens Sci 1981; 26: 451–461.

21 Hirvonen J, Huttenen P. Increased urinary concentrations of catecholamines in hypothermic deaths. J Forens Sci 1982; 27: 264–271.

22 Weyman A E, et al. Accidental hypothermia in an alcoholic population. Am J Med 1974; 56: 13–21.

23 Hirvonen J. Necropsy findings in fatal hypothermia cases. Forens Sci 1976; 8: 155–164.

24 Kreyberg L. Tissue damage due to cold. Lancet 1946; i. 338–340.

25 O'Keefe K M. Non-cardiogenic pulmonary oedema from accidental hypothermia. Colo Med 1980; 77: 106–107.

26 Barrera S E. Electrical injuries and fatal electrocution: effect on nervous system. In: Glasser   ed. Medical Physics, Chicago: Year Book Publishers, 1944: p 341.

27 Alexander L. Clinical and neuropathological aspects of electrical injuries. J Industr Hyg 1938; 20: 191–243.

28 Moritz A R. Physical agents in the causation of injury and disease. In: Anderson W A D. ed. Pathology, 3rd edn St. Louis: Mosby, 1957 pp 135–138.

29 Jenny F. Thermal injuries due to electrical accidents. Schweiz med Wschr 1947; 77: 780–782.

30 Thomsen H K, Danielsen L, Nielsen O, Aalund O, Nielson K G, Karlsmark T, Genefke I K. Early epidermal changes in heat- and electrically injured pig skin. I. A light microscopic study; II. An electron microscopic study. Forens Sci Int 1981; 17: 133, 145.

31 Spencer H A. Lightning: Lightning-stroke and its treatment. London: Baillière, Tindall & Cox, 1932.

32 Critchley M. Neurological effects of lightning and of electricity. Lancet 1934; 1: 68–72.

33 Hassin G R. Changes in the brain in legal electrocution. Arch Neurol Psychiat 1933; 30: 1046–1060.

34 Pritchard E A B. Changes in the central nervous system due to electrocution. Lancet 1934; 1: 1163–1167.

7

Deaths from acute neurogenic cardiovascular failure. The adult respiratory distress syndrome

The nervous control of cardiovascular function is carried out by the autonomic nervous system which consists of two mutually antagonistic divisions—the sympathetico-adrenal and the parasympathetic divisions. The functions of these two divisions, as they affect the circulation, may be summarized as follows: the sympathetico-adrenal division stimulates the cardiovascular system to meet the body's demands in physical and emotional stress and its effects are most fully developed in states of emergency. The parasympathetic division exerts a tonic and inhibitory control on the cardiovascular system. Its influence is conservative and restorative. Acting together these divisions provide a balanced control and allow of integrated changes in the system to meet the ever-varying needs of the body.

Cardiovascular function may be reflexly affected through the autonomic nervous system:

1. By emotion;
2. By variations in pressure in the carotid sinuses;
3. By changes in the gaseous concentrations in the blood; and
4. By the excitation of peripheral afferent somatic or visceral nerves.

Reflex excitation of this nature may cause either sympathetico-adrenal stimulation of the circulation or parasympathetic inhibition of the circulation. There is much individual variation in the sensitivity of the cardiovascular system to reflex nervous excitation. In some persons there appears to be a constitutional imbalance of the autonomic system, with heightened sympathetic or parasympathetic tone.

CAUSES OF REFLEX CIRCULATORY CHANGES

Emotion

Sudden psychic shock is liable to cause parasympathetic inhibitory effects, while emotional disturbances such as fear, especially when accompanied by painful sensations, may cause sympathetico-adrenal stimulation.

Emotional influences, by facilitation, may also sensitize the autonomic nervous system so that the effects of reflex peripheral nervous excitation are more readily produced.

Variation in pressure in the carotid sinuses

Variations in the pressure inside the carotid sinuses may produce profound reflex changes in the circulation. An increase in the tension of these sinuses, due to pressure applied over them, may cause strong parasympathetic stimulation.

Excitation of peripheral nerves

The peripheral nerves convey both pressor and depressor afferent fibres. Stimulation of the pressor fibres causes generalized vasoconstriction with a rise in blood pressure. Stimulation of the depressor fibres causes generalized vasodilatation with a fall in blood pressure.

The afferent nerve fibres possess different thresholds to exciting stimuli, so that weak stimuli cause depressor effects and stronger stimuli cause pressor effects.* Painful stimuli are associated with pressor effects. The anal, vaginal and spermatic cord regions of the body appear to have many parasympathetic fibres so that stimulation of these regions may cause profound parasympathetic effects. Stimuli from the viscera, caused by pulling upon attachments or by distension of hollow muscular organs, may cause depressor (parasympathetic) stimulation.

Other influences

Physical exertion, cerebral anaemia and hypoglycaemia cause sympathetico-adrenal stimulation. A similar effect is produced by a low oxygen tension or a high carbon dioxide tension in the blood. The sympathetico-adrenal stimulation is caused both by direct action on the medullary centres and by reflex action through the chemoreceptors of the aortic and carotid bodies.

EFFECTS OF REFLEX AUTONOMIC STIMULATION

Sympathetico-adrenal stimulation of the circulation normally results in acceleration and augmentation of the pulse, increase in myocardial contractility and irritability, and generalized vasoconstriction and venoconstriction with a rise in blood pressure. Parasympathetic stimulation normally results in

---

* It would appear that the nerve fibres which convey pressor stimuli are the same fibres which convey the sensations of pain and extremes of temperature, while the fibres which convey depressor stimuli also convey the sensations of touch and temperature.

inhibitory circulatory effects, such as slowing of the pulse, depression of myocardial contractility and conductivity and generalized vasodilatation (particularly of the venous and of the splanchnic bed), with a fall in blood pressure.

Sympathetico-adrenal stimulation or parasympathetic stimulation may lead to sudden, fatal circulatory failure. Deaths caused by such mechanisms present characteristic clinical features and are associated with non-specific autopsy findings. Such deaths are often of special medico-legal importance.

DEATHS FROM SYMPATHETICO-ADRENAL STIMULATION

Pathogenesis

An important effect of sympathetico-adrenal stimulation is the increase of myocardial irritability. This is shown by the occurrence of ventricular extrasystoles. Ventricular fibrillation, which is known to give rise to rapid death, may be regarded as an extreme expression of myocardial irritability. There is reason to believe that stimuli which in a normal heart may cause extrasystoles, may cause ventricular fibrillation when the heart is hyperirritable.[1–3]

Dock[4] reported that accidental deaths have occurred in man following upon the intravenous injection of epinephrine, while Nathanson[5] conducted experiments which suggest that ventricular fibrillation may be induced by epinephrine injections in persons suffering from coronary artery sclerosis. Nathanson[5] demonstrated that in persons over 40 years of age numerous ventricular extrasystoles from multiple foci may be rapidly and readily provoked by the intravenous injection of small doses of epinephrine. He considers that such extrasystoles could readily progress to fibrillation and that, in persons with coronary artery disease, sudden death may be precipitated by reflex nervous stimulation.*

Ventricular premature extrasystoles are a sign of electrical irritability and they may cause ventricular fibrillation by two mechanisms:

1. The ventricular premature extrasystoles may repeat themselves and progress to ventricular tachycardia and fibrillation.

2. The R-upon-T phenomenon.[7,8,9] If a ventricular premature systole falls during the 'vulnerable' period of ventricular repolarization it can cause a 'fragmented' ventricular response and lead to ventricular fibrillation. Catecholamines, hypoxia and acidosis make the ventricle more sensitive to this phenomenon.

Raab[10] stated that one of the easiest and quickest ways in which to cause

---

* It has been shown that myocardial anoxia caused by experimental coronary artery occlusion induces ventricular fibrillation. Leary[6] suggested that spasm of the coronary arteries, reflexly provoked by peripheral nervous stimualtion, may precipitate fatal angina pectoris. Stimulation of the sympathetic division of the autonomic nervous system, however, causes coronary dilatation and it is doubtful whether reflex sympathetic stimulation causes sudden death by this mechanism.

fatal circulatory failure in an animal is to give the animal an injection of epinephrine. He mentions that accidental deaths in man following upon such injections have been recorded. He points out that sudden deaths without adequate morphological findings to account for the death have occurred in circumstances strongly suggestive of coincidence with sympathetic neurocirculatory disturbances. Raab claims that in fatal cases of this nature he has isolated excess amounts of epinephrine-like catechols from the heart, and he considers that the accumulation of the hormonal discharges from the adrenal gland or peripheral nerve terminals may cause sudden deaths by provoking ventricular fibrillation.

It would appear that there is strong evidence to indicate that any reflex nervous stimulation which may cause extrasystoles in a normal heart can produce ventricular fibrillation in a heart rendered irritable by drugs, or by disease processes such as coronary arteriosclerosis.

Deaths from fibrillation in persons with normal hearts may result from electrical shock, poisoning with digitalis or accidental intravenous injection of epinephrine. Although it is doubtful whether persons with normal cardiovascular systems can die from simple peripheral reflex stimulation or from physical effort or emotion,[11] exceptions to this cannot be excluded.[12]

Hypotension which may result from pain or fear, from loss of effective circulating blood volume, drugs or reflex action will cause hypoxia. Hypoxia from a low cardiac output or respiratory indequacy will render the ventricular cells more sensitive to catecholamine release and lead to ventricular fibrillation.

Clinical features

Ventricular fibrillation causes rapid cardiac failure. The onset of ventricular fibrillation may be preceded by the occurrence of coupled beats or short bursts of extrasystoles. In certain circumstances, however, the final arrhythmia may be introduced by a single premature beat.

From the onset of the arrhythmia, inco-ordinate and imperfect contractions of the heart rapidly lead to circulatory failure. Death from cardiac inhibition occurs instantaneously, but circulatory failure due to ventricular fibrillation usually takes several minutes to develop. Rare cases have been recorded in which the fibrillation was paroxysmal in nature and of such short duration that the subject recovered.[13]

The clinical features are those of a hyperacute congestive cardiac failure. The onset of symptoms is sudden. There may be severe anginal pain. Dyspnoea is a marked feature and cyanosis develops rapidly. Pulmonary oedema is a prominent feature and may be so severe that blood-stained froth may exude from the mouth and nostrils. Death may occur in a few seconds or a few minutes. There may be a history of previous anginal attacks or of chronic cardiac disease with or without congestive failure, but frequently such disease is latent and unsuspected during life and deceased may have appeared to have been in good health.

Pathological changes

Some pre-existing cardiac disease is usually demonstrable at autopsy. There may be coronary artery sclerosis, cardiac hypertrophy or fibrosis and/or fatty changes of the myocardium, chronic valvular disease (particularly of the aortic valves), or syphilitic atresia of the coronary orifices. There may be signs of earlier chronic congestive failure, such as chronic passive congestion of organs and dependent oedema. Pulmonary congestion and oedema are present and may be marked. Care must be exercised, however, to differentiate froth in the air passage due to marked pulmonary oedema from the froth that may be produced in the respiratory tract due to early putrefaction. Petechial haemorrhages in the pleurae are common, and may be very numerous.

PARASYMPATHETIC CIRCULATORY INHIBITION

Pathogenesis

Syncope

It is believed that syncope or fainting is due to a vasovagal attack resulting from reflex parasympathetic stimulation. Cotton and Lewis[14] showed that vasovagal attacks could be prevented by the intravenous injection of atropine.

The stimuli which provoke such syncopal attacks have been described at pages 150–151.

Syncope is caused by reflex bradycardia or asystole, or by reflex splanchnic vasodilatation. There appears to be a combinaton of these cardiac and vascular effects in some cases. As a result of the acute reflex circulatory changes, a sudden fall in the blood pressure occurs which causes cerebral ischaemia with a very rapid loss of consciousness. There are often preceding signs, such as undue sweating, nausea and vertigo, but there may be no such warning. The subject loses consciousness rapidly. There is marked pallor but cyanosis does not develop. There is no respiratory distress. Complete recovery usually follows. The attacks may occur in healthy persons.

Fainting attacks may often be provoked by pressure over the carotid sinuses. In their studies on the carotid sinus in health and disease. Weiss and Baker[15] showed that there is a great variation in individual susceptibility to vasovagal attacks. In hypersensitive persons the slightest pressure over the carotid sinus may provoke an attack.

Engel et al[16] on their clinical, electroencephalographic and electrocardiographic studies on vasodepressor and carotid sinus syncope, demonstrated that fainting attacks could be provoked in sensitive persons by such stimuli as venipuncture, distension of the rectum, colon or vagina, hyperventilation or pressure over the carotid sinus. They noted that such attacks could be aborted by painful stimuli which caused opposing sympathetic stimulatory reflex effects, and that the emotional state of the subject was an important factor in sensitizing him to attacks.

In the majority of cases the inhibitory cardiac stimulus is momentary and the heart's action is soon restored. If the stimulus should persist, however, and asystole continue, the ventricles soon 'escape' and take up their own rhythm independently of the atria and restore the circulation. This 'escape' is not due to fatigue of the vagus or to stimulation of the muscle by distension of the ventricles, but is due to the stimulation of a sympathetic reflex.[47] The stimulus for this reflex is the rising pressure in the distended veins which empty into the right side of the heart.

Fatal syncope

Although Lewis[12] doubted whether vasovagal attacks ever proved fatal, a large number of cases has been recorded of sudden and unexpected deaths from reflex cardiac syncope.

The deaths in these cases occurred in circumstances which would readily account for fainting from reflex autonomic nervous stimulation. According to the available reports the deceased persons developed typical syncopal attacks and died with great rapidity. The extreme rapidity with which these attacks occurred was typical of some reflex nervous mechanism. The sudden loss of consciousness with pallor and without cyanosis, dyspnoea or convulsions appears to be more consistent with the development of sudden cardiac asystole than ventricular fibrillation. At the autopsies no organic disease, particularly of the cardiovascular system, was found to account for these deaths.

Gardner,[18] in a number of cases, noted general post-mortem appearances which he considered to be striking and characteristic. These appearances were: an absence of so-called 'asphyxial' signs (hypoxic signs), collapse and emptiness of the great veins, emptiness of the right chambers of the heart, absence of congestion of the lungs, and pallor of the skin. We have noted similar findings in cases of this type.

It would appear that in all these cases reflex vagal asystole of the heart occurred, and that this asystole was not followed by an 'escape' of the ventricles. This suggests a failure of the nervous reflex mechanism for restoration of the heart beat.

Starling[19] stated that 'if cardiac asystole is reflexly produced by vagal stimulation and the arterial system is dilated so that the mean systemic pressure is low, or when "asphyxial" gasps of the animal are prevented by anaesthesia or by section of the spinal cord, the heart may fail to recover from inhibition produced even by transient stimulation of the vagus.' A possible explanation of these deaths may be that when cardiac asystole is associated with splanchnic dilatation, the pressure in the great veins may fall below that required to stimulate the 'escape' mechanism for restoration of the heart beat.

In reflex deaths occurring under general anaesthesia, the failure of the 'escape' mechanism to operate may be due to the differential effects which narcotics may have on the autonomic nervous system, whereby at some stage in anaesthesia the parasympathetic division may still be active while the sympathetic division is depressed and inactive.

Circumstances in which syncopal deaths may occur

The application of a constrictive force to the neck

There is evidence to show that when a constrictive force is applied to the neck, as in hanging or strangulation, death may occur with great rapidity. In such cases the deaths cannot be regarded as being due to hypoxic hypoxia. In these cases there is often a striking absence of visceral congestion. Death would appear to be due to parasympathetic inhibition of circulatory function caused by a rising pressure in the carotid sinuses as a result of the direct pressure over them, or by occlusion of the arteries above the sinuses by the ligature. If the ligature is situated below the sinuses but in a position in which the carotid arteries can be occluded, death may be due to ventricular fibrillation from reflex sympathetico-adrenal stimulation.

A number of sudden deaths has been reported in which pressure has been only momentarily applied to the neck. Simpson[20] reported the death of a young girl who collapsed suddenly when a soldier playfully pinched her neck while they were dancing. At autopsy no organic disease was demonstrated and death was attributed to vagal inhibition. When such a death follows upon an embrace, the circumstances may suggest rape and murder, but the possibility of unintentional accident should not be overlooked.

Foreign bodies in the respiratory tract

Sudden reflex death may occur following the impaction of food in the larynx or the unexpected inhalation of fluid into the upper respiratory tract. In these forms of death the striking feature at autopsy is the relative absence of visceral congestion, and it would appear that the deaths may arise through parasympathetic inhibition.*

Puncture of the pleural cavity and other minor operations

A number of deaths has been recorded following the puncture of a pleural cavity, usually for the induction of a pneumothorax. Capps,[21] in a review

---

* Persons with disordered or defective minds often cram large portions of food into their mouths, and as a result may choke to death. Such accidental deaths are not uncommon in mental hospitals. Simpson[20] has pointed out that deaths of this nature may not be due to 'asphyxiation' but may be caused by reflex vagal inhibition of the heart due to the sudden impaction of food in the glottis. We have seen cases of a similar nature. As these deaths may occur with extreme rapidity, there may be no time to carry out any effective emergency treatment. For this reason, care should be exercised before members of the hospital staff are criticized by the suggestion that an early relief of the obstruction would have saved the patient's life.

of the literature, concluded that deaths of this nature are usually due to reflex cardiac inhibition.

Similar deaths have been reported following upon other minor operations, such as the passing of a urethral sound.

Apprehension on the part of the patient appears to be an important factor facilitating such fatal reflexes. Appropriate premedication may be desirable for the purpose of calming a nervous patient. In minor operations the routine use of local anaesthesia for the purpose of blocking the afferent reflex nervous paths appears to be most important in obviating these rare accidents.

Blunt force

Unexpected blows to the larynx, chest, abdomen and genital organs have on rare occasions caused sudden deaths from reflex cardiac failure and not from organic injury. The rapidity with which such deaths occur, the absence of visceral congestion, and the absence of any marked traumatic lesion at autopsy suggest the possibility of reflex inhibition.

Distension of hollow organs

Reflex cardiac inhibition may be caused by the sudden distension of hollow muscular organs, e.g. during attempts at criminal abortion when instruments are passed through the cervix or fluids are injected into the uterus (p. 370). Gastric dilation secondary to air sufflation may produce a similar effect.

Acute myocardial infarction

This may be associated with ischaemia or 'ischaemic denervation' of the sinoatrial node and sinus bradycardia or complete heart block. The bradycardia may then induce hypotension, further decrease in coronary blood flow and death.[22]

Ageing of the impulse-forming and conducting systems of the heart

Sinus bradycardia and partial or complete A-V block are degenerative diseases associated with advancing age. Parasympathetic stimulation in these circumstances further depresses the heart rate and may induce a Stokes-Adams attack which may be fatal.

DIAGNOSIS OF DEATH FROM ACUTE NEUROGENIC CARDIOVASCULAR FAILURE

When an apparently healthy person dies suddenly and unexpectedly and no adequate cause for the death is found at autopsy, the possibility of the death having been caused by acute neurogenic cardiovascular failure must be considered.

The most important factor in establishing a diagnosis of acute neurogenic cardiovascular failure is the carrying out of a careful and detailed autopsy to exclude any other cause for sudden death. This examination should include histological studies of suitable sections of the myocardium. If other causes for sudden death are excluded, and if definite evidence is available to indicate clearly that the death occurred with dramatic suddenness and followed promptly upon the occurrence of an appropriate nervous stimulus, a diagnosis of neurogenic cardiovascular failure may be inferred with reasonable certainty. Often, however, it may be suspected but may not be definitely known that an appropriate nervous stimulus occurred immediately before death, or it may be known that such a stimulus occurred but it may not be possible to establish that death followed promptly after the application of the stimulus. In such cases, although it may be suspected that death was caused by acute neurogenic cardiovascular failure, this cannot be proved and the cause of death must remain in doubt.

If some pre-existing, though clinically latent, cardiac lesion is found at autopsy, if the fatal symptoms were consistent with acute congestive cardiac failure (with acute dyspnoea and cyanosis which may be of very short duration), and if acute congestive visceral changes are present, it may be inferred that the probable final mechanism of death was a ventricular fibrillation precipitated by reflex sympathetico-adrenal stimulation. If the heart is found to be normal at autopsy, if the fatal clinical signs were those of syncope (with pallor and loss of consciousness without dyspnoea), and if visceral congestion is absent, it may be inferred that the probable final mechanism of death was cardiac inhibition induced by parasympathetic stimulation.* Often, however, although the suddenness of the death and the promptness with which it followed the occurrence of an appropriate simulus may justify a diagnosis of acute neurogenic cardiovascular failure, the absence of detailed information of the terminal clinical signs and the indefinite nature of the visceral congestive changes may leave the diagnosis of the exact mechanism of the death in doubt.

---

* The effects of congestion are seen most readily in the lungs, and from the description which has been given of the mechanism of death in acute neurogenic cardiovascular failure, it might appear that the two types of failure could be differentiated at autopsy by the fact that pulmonary congestion is absent in deaths from cardiac inhibition and is relatively prominent in deaths from ventricular fibrillation. In most cases, however, autopsies are not undertaken until various post-mortem changes have developed. Sheehan[23] claims that post-mortem changes such as hypostasis and rigor mortis (affecting the heart and blood vessels) can produce an artificial congestion and oedema of the lungs. The onset of putrefaction may also facilitate the redistribution of blood and fluids in the vessels and tissues. Because of the development of these post-mortem changes the state of congestion of the lungs at autopsy does not afford a means of differentiating between deaths from cardiac inhibition and ventricular fibrillation.

ADULT RESPIRATORY DISTRESS SYNDROME (ARDS)—THE LUNG AS TARGET ORGAN

Definition

Petty[24] defines the adult respiratory distress syndrome (ARDS) as a sudden clinical, pathophysiological state characterized by severe dyspnoea, hypoxaemia, diffuse bilateral pulmonary infiltrations and 'stiff' lungs, following massive acute lung injury, usually in persons with no prior major lung disease.

Historical considerations

Blennerhassett[25] describes the historical considerations which led to the definition of the acute respiratory distress syndrome as follows:

> Development of respiratory failure following direct trauma to the lung (blast lung) has long been recognized. The acceptance that lung pathology may be a consequence of serious extrapulmonary trauma and/or shock took much longer to gain acceptance. The usual rationalization in the past of fatal pulmonary edema in shock states, and in particular, that developing in the patient undergoing vigorous resuscitative measures hours or days after the primary event, was that the edema was due to overhydration from transfusion; this fallacious argument still dies hard in some pathology departments. Gradually forthcoming however, and particularly in studies emanating from Viet Nam, was the concept of lung damage accompanying non-pulmonary trauma. Such terms as traumatic wet lung, shock lung, Da Nang lung, post-traumatic pulmonary insufficiency, respiratory insufficiency syndrome, congestive atelectasis and a number of others were commonly used. It remained for Ashbaugh et al to describe in 1967 progressive pulmonary insufficiency developing in 12 patients, 7 with multiple trauma, 1 with acute pancreatitis and 4 with multiple or obscure causes for shock. They coined the term adult respiratory distress syndrome (ARDS) to describe the clinical entity. The aptness of the bringing together of these causes of the clinical syndrome and unifying the concept under the ARDS title has been repeatedly confirmed and justified.

ARDS results from either direct damage to the lung, e.g. the aspiration of liquid gastric contents, or indirectly following shock from any cause. In spite of the wide variety of causes, the resultant pathological changes are similar. The descriptive term, diffuse alveolar damage (DAD) is used for these changes which commence with injury to capillary endothelial cells and Type I pneumocytes. Katzenstein and Askin[26] have tabulated the causes of diffuse alveolar damage (DAD) as follows:

Causes of diffuse alveolar damage

Infectious agents
  Viruses
  Mycoplasma
  Other (especially in immunocompromised patients)

Inhalants
   Oxygen
   Nitrogen dioxide
   Sulphur dioxide
   Smoke
   Other noxious gases and fumes

Ingestants
   Chemotherapeutic agents
      azathioprine
      carmustine (BCNU)
      bleomycin
      busulfan
      chlorambucil
      cytosine arabinoside
      cytoxan
      melphalan
      methotrexate
      mitomycin
   Other drugs
      colchicine
      gold
      hexamethonium
      hydrochlorothiazide
      nitrofurantoin
      placidyl
      practolol
   Heroin
   Kerosene
   Paraquat

Shock
   Traumatic
   Hemorrhagic
   Septic
   Neurogenic
   Cardiogenic

Radiation

Miscellaneous
   Acute pancreatitis
   Cardiopulmonary bypass

Air embolism
Near-drowning
Uraemia
High altitude
Heat
Molar pregnancy
Systemic lupus erythematosus
Postlymphangiography

Unknown causes

The pathology of diffuse alveolar damage

Naked eye changes. At autopsy the lungs are firm, airless and plum-coloured, and may have a liver-like appearance. The weight of each lung is usually in excess of 1000 grams.

Histological changes. The histological appearances depend upon the duration of the illness and have been divided into two overlapping stages—an early *exudative stage* within the first week of injury, and a *proliferative (or organising) stage* which occurs after one or two weeks.

1. *Exudative stage.* Initially there is interstitial and intra-alveolar oedema, and variable intra-alveolar haemorrhage. After several days, characteristic eosinophilic hyaline membranes replace necrotic alveolar epithelium and Type II pneumocytes begin to proliferate. A chronic inflammatory infiltrate is present in the interstitium.

2. *Proliferative stage.* This is characterized by fibroblastic proliferation in the interstitium as well as focal organization of alveolar exudate and further proliferation of Type II pneumocytes. The end result is fibrosis.

The initial injury is thought to occur in capillary endothelial cells with leakage of fluid into the interstitium and later into the alveolar spaces. Destruction of Type I pneumocytes results in the formation of hyaline membranes which consist of necrotic cellular debris and fibrin. Exudative and proliferative changes may occur together either due to the persistence of the initial cause or to superadded causes. For example, an initial cause such as traumatic shock may be complicated by secondary infection as well as the need to administer high concentrations of oxygen for adequate ventilation, both of which may contribute to further alveolar damage.

The mortality in diffuse alveolar damage (DAD) is approximately 50%, and death may occur in either stage. Recovery may be complete or with varying degrees of impaired pulmonary function.

REFERENCES

1 Levy A G. The exciting causes of ventricular fibrillation in animals under chloroform anaesthesia. Heart 1913; 4: 319–378.
2 Levy A G. The action of nicotine on the heart under chloroform. Heart 1926; 12: 387–389.
3 Brow G R, Long C L H, Beattie J. Irregularities of th heart under chloroform anaesthesia: their dependence on the sympathetic nervous system. J Am Med Assoc 1930; 95: 715–717.
4 Dock W. Transitory ventricular fibrillation as a cause of syncope and its prevention by quinidine sulphate. Am Heart J 1929; 4: 709–714.
5 Nathanson M N. Pathology and pharmacology of cardiac syncope and sudden death. Arch Intern Med 1936; 58: 685–702.
6 Leary T. Coronary spasm as a possible factor in producing sudden death. Am Heart J 1935; 10: 338–334.
7 Wiggers C J, Wegria R. Ventricular fibrillation due to single localised induction and condenser shocks applied during the vulnerable phase of ventricular systole. Am J Physiol 1940; 128: 500–505.
8 Han J, Garcia de Jalon P, Moe J K. Fibrillation threshold of premature ventricular responses. Circ Res 1965; 18: 18–25.
9 Lown B, Fakhro A M, Hood W B, Thorn G W. The coronary care unit—new perspectives and directives. J Am Med Assoc 1967; 199: 156–165.
10 Raab W. Sudden death of a young athlete, with an excessive concentration of epinephrine-like substances in the heart muscle. Arch Pathol 1943; 36: 388–392.
11 Kaysii A I. Death from inhibition and its relation to shock. Br Med J 1948; 21: 131–134.
12 Lewis T. Diseases of the Heart. London: McMillan. 1933: pp 103 and 104.
13 Schwartz S P, Jezer A. Transient ventricular fibrillation: the clinical and electrocardiographic manifestations of the syncopal seizures in a patient with auriculoventricular dissociation. Arch Intern Med 1932; 50: 450–469.
14 Cotton T F, Lewis T. Observations upon fainting attacks due to inhibitory cardiac impulses. Heart 1918; 7:23.
15 Weiss S, Baker J P. Carotid sinus reflex in health and disease: its role in causation of fainting and convulsions. Medicine 1933; 12: 297–354.
16 Engel G L, Romano J, McLin T R. Vasodepressor and carotid sinus syncope: clinical, electroencephalographic and electrocardiographic observations. Arch intern Med 1944; 74: 100–119.
17 Nahum L J, Hoff E C. The influence of the cardiac sympathetics and adrenin on the phenomena of ventricular escape. Am J Physiol 1935; 113:101.
18 Gardner E. Mechanism of certain forms of sudden death in medico-legal practice. Med leg criminol Rev 1942; 10: 120–133.
19 Starling E H. Human physiology, 7th ed. Philadelphia: Lea & Febiger. 1936: pp 734–738.
20 Simpson K. Deaths from vagal inhibition. Lancet 1949; 256: 558–560.
21 Capps J A. Air embolism versus pleural reflex as the cause of pleural shock. J Am Med Assoc 1937; 109: 852–854.
22 James J N. Pathogenesis of arrhythmia in acute myocardial infarction. Am J Cardiol 1969; 24: 791–799.
23 Sheehan H L. The pathology of shock in obstetrics. Transactions of the International Congress of Obstetricians and Gynaecologists. Dublin: Parkside Press. 1949: p 152.
24 Petty T L. Adult respiratory distress syndrome: Definition and historical perspective. Clin Chest Med 1982; 3: 3–7.
25 Blennerhassett J B. Shock lung and diffuse alveolar damage. Pathological and pathogenetic considerations. Pathology 1985; 17: 239–247.

26 Katzenstein A-L A, Askin F B. Diffuse alveolar damage. Surgical pathology of non-neoplastic lung disease vol 13 in the series Major problems in pathology. Philadelphia: W.B. Saunders.1982: pp 9–42.

8

The medical investigation of the cause of death: sudden, and unexpected deaths in adults, children and infants: sudden infant death syndrome

An important and often one of the most difficult tasks of a medical practitioner or pathologist is the investigation of the cause of death. Deaths which require medico-legal investigation may be divided into two main groups:

1. Deaths which are known or which are suspected to have been caused by non-natural causes, e.g. deaths from violence, criminal neglect, or poisoning.

2. Deaths which are not suspected to have been caused by non-natural causes but which are reported to a coroner (a medical examiner, a magistrate or a responsible judicial or administrative officer) because a satisfactory certificate stating that death was due to natural causes has not been issued by a medical practitioner. Such certificates may not have been issued for one of the following reasons:

(a) The deceased was not attended by a medical practitioner.

(i) The death may have occurred so rapidly and so unexpectedly that no medical practitioner could be summoned in time; or

(ii) The deceased may have been ill for some time before death, but a registered medical practitioner did not attend the deceased because of a failure on the part of relatives or others to realize the seriousness of the illness; through the non-availability of a medical practitioner; through poverty; or because of superstitious beliefs.

(b) The deceased was attended by a medical practitioner who, although he may not have suspected that the death was due to non-natural causes, may have been unable to say with certainty that it was due to natural causes.

In most jurisdictions, the coroner or a corresponding officer instructs the medical practitioner to investigate the cause of death. In most instances, the responsible administrative officer does not specify how the investigation is to be carried out, nor, as a rule, does he state that a dissection of the body must be undertaken. In most jurisdictions a medical practitioner or a pathologist is authorized to examine the internal organs of the body (i.e. to perform an autopsy) if the medical practitioner considers that such an examination is necessary. The decision to dissect a body rests entirely with the medical practitioner. In some cases, the circumstances of the death, the clinical history, and the external appearance of the body may lead the medical practitioner to form a firm opinion as to the cause of death, and he may decide not to carry out an autopsy. This however, is a procedure which must be used with proper discretion. Unless there is clear evidence from reliable sources to indicate that death was due to natural causes, it is the opinion of the authors that an autopsy should be performed even though there are no known circumstances to suggest that the death was due to other than natural causes. A detailed autopsy should always be held, not only when it is suspected that death was due to non-natural causes but also when it is definitely known from the history or from the external appearances of the body that death was due to non-natural causes. This is necessary because the exact nature of the fatal injuries, the presence and nature of other injuries, and the physical state of the deceased at the time of his death are all factors which may prove to be of medico-legal importance. Although much of the information obtained at an autopsy may ultimately prove to be of no medico-legal value, it may be impossible to determine whether any particular finding is significant or not at the time at which the investigation is carried out. Information of importance may be unobtainable at a later stage, because of putrefaction, but even in putrefied bodies it is seldom possible to be certain that legally important information may not be found on dissection of the body. The failure to carry out a detailed autopsy at the time of investigation of the cause of death may prejudice the course of justice, and the responsibility for such an omission rests entirely with the medical practitioner concerned. It is therefore strongly recommended— unless there is other clear and reliable evidence to indicate with reasonable certainty that the death was due to natural causes—that when a medical practitioner is required to investigate the cause of death, he should always carry out a full and detailed dissection of the body.

CLASSIFICATION OF THE CAUSES OF DEATH

The causes of death may be grouped according to the autopsy findings as follows:

1. Deaths due to natural causes:
   Group 1, where a lesion is found at autopsy which is incompatible with life.
   Group 2, where a lesion is found at autopsy, which is known to cause death, but which is also known to be compatible with continued life.
2. Deaths due to non-natural causes:
   Group 3, where a lesion is found at autopsy which is incompatible with life.
   Group 4, where a lesion is found at autopsy which may have caused

death, or which may have precipitated death, but which is also known to be compatible with continued life.

3. Deaths due to obscure causes:
Group 5, where no lesion is found at autopsy or if a lesion is found it is of a minimal or indefinite nature.

Deaths due to natural causes

Group 1

In some deaths from natural causes the autopsy reveals a lesion which is incompatible with life because of its nature, site, or extent, e.g. the rupture of an aortic aneurysm or a massive intracerebral haemorrhage involving the brain stem.

Group 2

In a large proportion of deaths from natural causes some lesion is found at autopsy which may have caused death but which is also compatible with continued life, e.g. arteriosclerosis of the coronary arteries. In these cases the failure to detect any other cause of death is presumptive evidence that the lesion was responsible for the death but it is not conclusive proof. The clinical history is often of value in determining the probable cause of death in such circumstances. In the case of coronary arteriosclerosis, if the deceased had several attacks of angina pectoris before his death it is reasonable to assume that the lesion was the cause of his death. In certain circumstances, however, the clinical history may raise the possibility of some other cause of death. For instance, if the deceased suffered from gastrointestinal symptoms with vomiting and diarrhoea, or if he had a series of convulsions before his death, the possibility of irritant poisoning or poisoning by substances such as strychnine would have to be excluded before the death could be attributed to the coronary arteriosclerosis.

The clinical history is of major importance in the investigation of deaths which are classifiable in this group. The medical practitioner must not only find a lesion which is accepted as a possible cause of death but he must be satisfied that the clinical history is consistent with the cause given. If the clinical history is of an unusual nature, the possibilities suggested by the history should be excluded before the death is attributed to the lesion.

Deaths due to non-natural causes

Group 3

At autopsy, certain injuries may be found which are incompatible with life in any person, e.g. injuries such as decapitation, or avulsion of the heart from the large blood vessels. Provided that it can be established that they were caused before death, it may be definitely asserted that such injuries were the cause of death.

Group 4

In some deaths injuries may be found at autopsy which, because of their nature, site, or extent may not appear to be sufficient to account for death in a healthy person. An injury of such a nature, however, may be the cause of death as it may have produced death by some complication which arose directly from the injury but which is not readily demonstrable by any post-mortem changes. At autopsy it is often impossible to assess the degree of shock or the extent of haemorrhage which may have followed a particular injury. In such cases a failure to find any other adequate cause of death and a knowledge of the circumstances in which the injury occurred and of the symptoms shown by the deceased, may enable the medical practitioner to ascribe death to the injury with reasonable certainty.

In other circumstances although an injury may not appear to be an adequate cause for death, the autopsy may reveal some natural disease process which is known to cause death, e.g. coronary arteriosclerosis. In some of these cases the circumstances of the death and the symptoms shown by the deceased at the time of the collapse may suggest that his death was precipitated by the injury through reflex sympathetico-adrenal stimulation (p. 152).

Deaths due to obscure causes

Group 5

In certain deaths where the post-mortem examination fails to reveal any macroscopic lesion which will satisfactorily account for death, the death may be due to some obscure natural or non-natural cause. As the majority of chemical poisons produce no recognizable or characteristic lesions in the tissues, the possibility that death may have been caused by poisoning arises in these cases. These deaths, however, are frequently due to natural causes, but they may be due to certain types of injury, or complications of injury, or to poisoning. The nature of these deaths may often be determined by further investigations.

THE INVESTIGATION OF DEATHS DUE TO OBSCURE CAUSES

The investigation of a death due to obscure causes in which no lesion which will satisfactorily account for death is found at autopsy, may be clinical or laboratory. Clinical investigation, for the most part, is based on interviews with persons who observed the deceased before he died. The object of such interviews is to obtain as detailed an account as possible of the signs and symptoms shown by the deceased before his death. Information as to his occupation, habits, and previous residence may be of value in the case of deaths due to natural causes, while the police may supply information concerning factors which may relate the death to a non-natural cause. Laboratory investigations may be bacteriological, virological, biochemical, or histopathological (pp. 76–77) or toxicological (pp. 214–216).

Until the investigations are completed in deaths of obscure origin, it is often advisable to retain the stomach and its contents, the liver, and both kidneys, in case a toxicological analysis should prove necessary.

In this section an account is given of some of the more important obscure or uncommon causes of death. In many of the conditions described, either the clinical history, the circumstances of the death, or the autopsy findings may indicate the probable cause of death and suggest the laboratory investigations which should be undertaken to confirm the diagnosis. For this reason, in addition to the description of autopsy findings, we have summarized the most important clinical features of some conditions and have outlined laboratory methods which may prove of value in diagnosis.

Obscure causes of death from natural causes

Some of the conditions described in this subsection are serious infectious diseases which are endemic in some countries, e.g. plague and typhus. Descriptions of these diseases have been included because (in terms of a country's health legislative requirements) medical practitioners may have to confirm, by post-mortem examination, a suspicion that a death has been caused by an infectious disease.*

---

* When there is reason to believe that the deceased may have died from an infectious disease (more especially if the suspected disease is a formidable epidemic disease such as plague) suitable precautions should be taken by the medical practitioner conducting the autopsy to protect himself and his assistants against the danger of infection. In order to kill fleas or lice that may be present on the body and the clothing, the clothed body and the vicinity in which it has been found, should be sprayed with a liquid insecticide. If the body is in a room the whole room should be sprayed.

The medical practitioner and his assistants should wear protective aprons, gowns, rubber gloves, and top-boots. Trouser ends should be tucked into the boots and should be well dusted with insecticide powder. During the autopsy special care should be taken to avoid injuring the hands and fingers with instruments or spicules of bone. If the practitioner or one of his assistants is injured, the wound should receive immediate attention. Bleeding should be encouraged by pressure at the margins of the wound and the depths of the wound should be thoroughly washed under running water before appropriate antiseptic treatment is applied. It is also advisable to consider the administration of suitable antibiotics or chemotherapeutic agents as a prophylactic measure. When the autopsy has been completed the body and the surrounding vicinity should be washed or sprayed with appropriate disinfectant solutions. Particular care should be taken in handling specimens which have been retained for laboratory investigation. All instruments should be sterilized. Soiled protective clothing and gloves should be soaked in disinfectant solutions, but in certain circumstances it may be advisable to destroy such articles.

Acute infections

Death due to an infection is usually preceded by symptoms such as fever. However, the infectious process may progress rapidly, or the initial symptoms may go unrecognized or unheeded, so that the individual may die without a diagnosis having been made.

It is important that a specific microbiological diagnosis be made in such cases, as it may be a contagious disease to which other members of the commuity may have been exposed. Therefore, appropriate microbiological investigations, in particular bacterial and viral cultures, should be performed on autopsy material such as blood, pus, bone-marrow and other relevant tissues or fluids. Attempts should be made to prevent contamination of such specimens during their collection.

In this section, infections are considered in terms of organ systems and infectious agents.

Upper respiratory tract infections

In this group of diseases, death is due to airway obstruction with consequent hypoxaemia. The major infections in this category are acute epiglottitis, [1–3.] croup [3–6] and diphtheria.[7,8]

Epiglottitis is usually caused by *Haemophilus influenzae* type b[9,10] and is characterized pathologically by oedema of the epiglottis, aryepiglottic folds, ventricular bands and the arythenoids and clinically producing abrupt and complete airway obstruction. The disease is almost exclusively one of young children, although adult cases have been described associated with significant mortality.

Croup (acute laryngotracheobronchitis)[3–6] is characterized by mucosal oedema and inflammation, mainly in the subglottic region. It is usually caused by parainfluenza virus or other respiratory viruses.

Diphtheria,[7,8] a rare but epidemiologically important cause of upper airway obstruction, is due to diphtheria toxin produced by certain strains of *Corynebacterium diphtheriae* and characterized by membrane formation, which may extend from the pharynx into the larynx. Other causes of death in this condition include cardiac arrhythmias,[11] adrenal insufficiency and peripheral motor nerve paralysis.[12]

In individuals, especially children, apparently dying of upper airway obstruction, the possibility of foreign body inhalation should always be considered.

Lower respiratory tract infections[13]

Bronchiolitis.[14–16] This is a disease of young infants, usually caused by respiratory syncytial virus.[17] It is characterized clinically by tachypnoea, wheezing and evidence of air-trapping. Death, when it occurs, is due to respiratory failure. Pathologically there is bronchial and bronchiolar epithelial cell necrosis, interstitial pneumonia, patchy atelectasis and emphysema.

Asthma. Although not primarily an infection, this disease is often precipitated by infections due to respiratory viruses or *Mycoplasma pneumoniae.*[18,19,20,21]

Pneumonia. This is a common infection in both children and adults.[22–24] It may progress rapidly, resulting in respiratory failure and death. In young children, viruses such as respiratory syncytial virus,[25] adenovirus and measles virus,[26] and bacteria including *Streptococcus pneumoniae* (pneumococcus), *H. influenzae* and *Staphylococcus aureus* are the most important causes of pneumonia. In older children and young adults *Strep. pneumoniae* is the most important cause of severe pneumonia, whereas in the elderly, as well as hospitalized patients, Gram-negative bacilli,[27,28] *Strep. pneumoniae*[21] and *Staph. aureus*[29] are the important causes of pneumonia. These can be cultured by routine methods.

Legionnaires' disease,[21, 30–33] is a recently recognized form of severe pneumonia occurring mostly in the elderly, in smokers and in immunocompromised individuals. The causative organism, *Legionella pneumophila*, can be detected by immunofluorescence of lung tissue or bronchial secretions or by culture on spedial media.

Another recently emerging pathogen, causing pneumonia in immunocompromised patients, particularly those with acquired immune deficiency syndrome (AIDS), is *Pneumocystis carinii*.[34,35] These patients can be identified by specific staining of bronchial washings or preferably sections of lung tissue.

Whooping cough (Pertussis). This is an infection of the respiratory tract caused by *Bordetella pertussis*,[36–38] which can be cultured on special media. Clinically the condition is characterized by paroxysmal cough followed by a crowing inspiratory sound. In young infants it may present with apnoea. Death is due to hypoxaemia or encephalopathy. Pathologically, epithelial cell necrosis, accumulation of secretions in the airways and hypoxic changes are present.

Diarrhoea

This is one of the commonest infectious diseases of human beings, and one of the greatest causes of infant mortality worldwide. Death is due to dehydration, which is usually clinically obvious. The recognized causative organisms and methods of demonstrating their presence are shown in Table 8.1. Shigella infections may occasionally be fatal as a result of a toxic encephalopathy or the haemolytic–uraemic syndrome.

Heart

Cardiac infections which may result in a rapidly fatal course include acute endocarditis, myocarditis and purulent pericarditis.

Table 8.1 Micro-organisms causing diarrhoea, and methods used to demonstrate their presence (After Berkowitz and Klugman as set out in the Acknowledgements)

Micro-organism	Method (applied to faeces)
Viruses	
27 32 nm viruses, e.g. Norwalk agent[39,40] and	Electron-microscopy Antigen detection
Rotavirus[41–45]	Electron-microscopy
Bacteria	
Escherichia coli[46–49] various mechanisms	Culture; sophisticated methods necessary to demonstrate pathogenicity
Salmonella spp.	Culture
Shigella spp.	Culture
Yersinia enterocolitica[50,51]	Culture, using cold enrichment
Campylobacter jejuni[52–56]	Culture, special media at 42°C
Vibrio cholerae[57]	Culture
Clostridium difficile[58–62]	Culture, demonstration of toxin
Protozoa	
Giardia lamblia[63]	Microscopy
Entamoeba histolytica[64,65]	Microscopy
Cryptosporidium spp.[66]	Microscopy; acid-fast staining

Acute infectious endocarditis.[67] This is usually due to *Staph. aureus*, but may be due to other bacteria such as pneumococcus. Intravenous drug abusers are at a particularly high risk of acquiring this infection, as well as endocarditis due to *Candida albicans*. Pathologically there is inflammation, vegetative formation and destruction of cardiac valves, and the organism may be cultured from blood or from the vegetation.

Myocarditis. Although this may complicate many infections, it is usually viral in origin.[68] Death is due to cardiac arrhythmias or cardiac failure. It is particularly important to make an aetiological diagnosis in newborns, as myocarditis due to Coxsackie virus has occurred in outbreaks in maternity hospitals.

Purulent pericarditis. This diagnosis is frequently missed clinically, and death may occur as a result of cardiac tamponade.

Infections of the central nervous system

These conditions may be missed ante-mortem, as the individual's level of consciousness is often impaired, making the obtaining of a history difficult. The most important infection of the nervous system is acute bacterial meningitis.[69,70] This usually follows haematogenous spread of organisms to the meninges, but may follow compound fractures of the skull. The common causative organisms are *H. influenzae*, *Strep. penumoniae* and *Neisseria meningitidis* in young children; *Strep. pneumoniae* and *N. meningitidis* in older children; and *Strep. pneumoniae*, Gram-negative bacilli and *Listeria monocytogenes*[71] in the elderly. Microbiological investigations are very important, as the pathological features are not specific for each infectious agent. Both *H. influenzae* and *N. meningitidis* are contagious, so that household contacts of such cases should be made aware of their exposure and given chemoprophylaxis.

Other forms of intracranial suppuration. Brain abscess, subdural and extradural collections of pus are often secondary to infections of the middle ear cavity or paranasal sinuses. Their microbiology is usually mixed, with streptococci and anaerobic bacteria being the most common organisms isolated.

Viral encephalitis. Several different viruses may cause encephalitis. Herpes simplex virus is the commonest cause of sporadic encephalitis. In herpes encephalitis there is marked cerebral oedema, especially of the temporal lobes.[72] This infection may be confirmed by the presence of eosinophilic intranuclear inclusions histologically, by the demonstration of specific antigen, or by isolation of the virus from brain tissue. Many other viruses such as the enteroviruses and Epstein–Barr virus can cause encephalitis. Epidemic encephalitis in certain parts of the world is caused by arborviruses such as Eastern and Western equine encephalitis. The diagnosis is usually made serologically.

Rabies. This should always be considered in cases dying of apparent encephalitis.[73] Confirming this diagnosis is important as post-exposure prophylaxis may be indicated in other individuals exposed to the rabid animal. The diagnosis is established by demonstrating the viral antigen or by the presence of Negri bodies in brain parenchyma or by culture of the virus. This should be done in an appropriately equipped laboratory, which may be the local veterinary laboratory.

Poliomyelitis[74,75] This is an enterovirus infection in which involvement of the motor nuclei of the spinal cord and brain-stem sometimes occurs. A generalized encephalitis may also occur. Death is usually due to involvement of the brain-stem or of the respiratory muscle innervation. The diagnosis is made by culture of the virus from central nervous system tissue, from nasopharyngeal secretions or faeces, or by serological means.

Guillain–Barré syndrome.[76,77] This is a post-infectious condition due to demyelination of peripheral nerve roots. It may resemble poliomyelitis clinically, but the motor involvement is usually more diffuse and symmetrical than in poliomyelitis. It may progress very rapidly and result in respiratory failure within a few hours of onset.

Tetanus.[78] This disease, caused by a potent exotoxin produced by *Clostridium tetani*, introduced into wounds, or into the umbilicus of newborns, is characterized by severe muscle spasms. Death is due to hypoxaemia or to autonomic disturbances. The diagnosis is made clinically. The pathology is not specific. The microbiological diagnosis can be made by strict anaerobic culture of the organism from wound material, but this is rarely accomplished.

Slow (virus) infections. There is increasing evidence that pre-senile dementia, encephalopathy and death may be due to so-called slow viruses. An infectious aetiology of Creutzfeldt-Jakob disease[79,80] has been established and infection of the central nervous system by the AIDS virus can also cause encephalopathy. The identification of these agents in brain tissue requires highly specialized isolation techniques not routinely available.

Generalized infections

These may not be associated with characteristic symptoms nor with symptoms referable to specific organ systems. The pathology may also be non-specific. Making a specific diagnosis, therefore, often depends on the history which provides information about the epidemiological setting in which the infection was acquired, and on microbiological investigations. In addition to using blood, pus, cerebrospinal fluid, urine and viscera as sources of material for microbiological investigation, skin lesions and bone marrow should also be used. Of particular importance in the history are features suggesting possible exposure to specific micro-organisms, or possible factors predisposing the patient to certain infections. These include travel within the previous year, animal and bird exposure, arthropod exposure, occupational exposure, food and water sources, blood transfusions, sexual exposure, and factors compromising the individual's immune system.

Generalized viral infections

Disseminated herpes simplex infection.[81] This is an uncommon infection occurring mostly in immunocompromised patients and in children with severe protein-energy malnutrition. The clinical course is usually characterized by fulminating liver failure associated with a bleeding tendency. The pathology, which is particularly marked in the liver and adrenal glands, is characterized by cell necrosis, the presence of eosinophilic intranuclear inclusions and multinucleate giant cells.

Haemorrhagic fevers. Several viruses, each occurring in certain geographic locations, cause disseminated infections during which a haemorrhagic state may occur. These infections include yellow fever,[82] Lassa fever,[83] Marburg virus disease,[84] Ebola fever,[85] Congo-Crimean haemorrhagic fever, all of which occur in Africa, Argentinian[86] and Bolivian haemorrhagic fever[87] in South America, and Dengue and Congo-Crimean haemorrhagic fever in Southern Asia and the Caribbean Basin. Most of these infections are associated with biochemical and histological evidence of hepatitis. Diagnosis is made serologically or by isolation of the virus in specially equipped laboratories. Although these infections are considered somewhat 'exotic', the ease of modern travel has made their appearance possible anywhere in the world.

Viral hepatitis. Fatal cases of hepatitis are usually due to hepatitis B virus or non-A non-B infections.[88-90] Hepatitis B can be confirmed by demonstration of hepatitis B surface antigen in serum or hepatitis B surface and core antigens in the liver. Making a specific diagnosis of hepatitis B is important in that close contacts, especially sexual contacts, should be offered hepatitis B hyperimmune globulin.

Rickettsial infections[91]

These are a group of infections caused by different species of rickettsial organisms and transmitted by different arthropods. They include epidemic (louse-borne) typhus, murine (flea-borne) typhus, and tick-borne spotted fevers such as Rocky Mountain spotted fever and African tick-bite fever. The causative organisms infect endothelial cells, resulting in capillary thrombosis and perivascular inflammation. The main target organs are the brain, heart and skin, and clinically patients present with fever, headache and a maculo-papular rash. The diagnosis is usually made serologically, but the organism can be isolated by innoculation of blood into animals.

Bacterial infections

Death from generalized bacterial infections is usually due to organ dysfunction as a result of extensive inflammation, from toxaemia (exotoxaemia or endotoxaemia) and from activation of various chemical cascades, such as the coagulation, kinin, plasminogen and complement cascades. The symptoms and signs are usually non-specific, so that microbiological investigations are essential for making an aetiological diagnosis. The epidemiological history, as discussed above, may be helpful. The apparent source of the bacteraemia, e.g. a lymph-node in plague or tularaemia, may give a clue as to the causative organism, as may metastatic foci of infection, e.g. the skin in meningococcaemia. The pathology is usually non-specific, but may show features of shock or of metastatic foci of infection.

Parasitic infections

Of the many different parasites affecting man, the most important are the malarial parasites. Millions of fatalities occur worldwide annually, mostly in endemic areas. Unexpected deaths from malaria often occur in travellers to endemic areas returning to non-endemic areas, in whom the possibility of malaria has not been considered. These deaths are almost always due to *Plasmodium falciparum*.[92] Making an aetiological diagnosis is important, so that co-travellers can be warned. The diagnosis is made by demonstrating the parasites in a blood smear. The pathology is characterized by capillary obstruction in all organs, with the red blood cells harbouring developing stages of the parasite. The spleen is enlarged, and macrophages in this organ, as well as in other reticuloendothelial organs, contain malarial pigment and demonstrate erythrophagocytosis. The brain is a greyish colour, and both petechial haemorrhages and perivascular oedema may be present.

Other specific parasitic causes of death depend on geographic location, e.g. fulminant myocarditis due to Chaga's disease[93–95] in South America or cerebral infection due to trypanosomiasis (sleeping sickness) in Central and West Africa.

Intoxications from infectious agents

Although a few organisms may elaborate toxins in food, which, when eaten, causes nausea, vomiting and diarrhoea, e.g. *Staph. aureus*[96,97] and *Bacillus cereus*,[98,99] these diseases are rarely fatal. However, one such disease, namely botulism, is often fatal. Botulism, caused by *Clostridium botulinum*,[100,101] is characterized by widespread lower motor neurone paralysis six hours to eight days after eating contaminated food. Death is due to respiratory failure. The diagnosis is made by demonstration of the toxin in serum, or demonstrating the organism or the presence of toxin in remaining food, gastric contents or faeces. An infantile form of botulism, following ingestion of the organism which elaborates toxin *in-vivo*, has been considered a cause of some cases of the sudden infant death syndrome (SIDS). (See section on sudden infant death syndrome, p. 181.)

Other conditions due to the elaboration of bacterial toxins have been discussed above, e.g. diphtheria, whooping cough and tetanus.

Infection-related conditions

Reye's syndrome.[102] This is a disease of unknown aetiology affecting infants, children and teenagers, characterized by a toxic encephalopathy and fatty change in the viscera, in particular the liver. It usually follows a viral infection such as influenza or chickenpox, and there is an epidemiological association with the ingestion of salicylates preceding this infection. Clinically it manifests with vomiting, a decreasing level of consciousness and evidence of liver dysfunction. Pathologically there is cerebral oedema, and microvesicular fatty change in the liver.

Kawasaki disease (mucocutaneous lymph node syndrome).[103,104] This is an acute febrile illness of unknown aetiology, affecting infants and children, which has many clinical and epidemiological features of an infectious disease. It is characterized by high fever, red buccal mucosae, non-purulent conjunctivitis, cervical lymphadenopathy, erythematous rash, erythema and swelling of the hands and feet and subsequent cutaneous desquamation. The most serious complication is the formation of coronary artery aneurysms with consequent myocardial infarction. This accounts for the case-fatality rate of 1–2%.

Acquired immune deficiency syndrome (AIDS)

This syndrome is due to infection with Human T-cell lymphotropic virus type III (HTLV-III) otherwise known as LAV (lymphadenopathy-associated virus) or more recently named HIV (human immunodeficiency virus). The diagnosis is made by serology or more rarely isolation of the virus. The infected tissues are the brain as well as helper T-cells in the blood and the reticuloendothelial system. Destruction of these cells leads to immunodeficiency in the host and the patients die from overwhelming opportunistic infections such as *Pneumocystic carinii* pneumonia,[105] atypical mycobacterial infections,[106,107] disseminated conditions and other fungal, parasitic, viral and bacterial conditions. Other associated pathological features of AIDS include encephalopathy, CNS lymphoma and Kaposi's sarcoma.[108]

Cardiac lesions

The commonest cause of sudden and unexpected death in apparently healthy adults is cardiac disease, and the commonest cause of such disease is coronary arteriosclerosis. Deaths from coronary arteriosclerosis often take place during physical exertion. As a general rule the clinical features are those of a hyperacute congestive cardiac failure with symptoms such as dyspnoea and precordial or epigastric pain (p. 153). Death usually occurs within a few minutes. In an analysis of the autopsy findings in a large series of such cases Moritz and Zamcheck[109] found the following: the disease usually involved the main arterial trunks; complete occlusion of a coronary artery was found in about one half of the cases; thrombosis occurred in less than one third of the cases; the proportionate involvement of the left coronary artery as compared with the right coronary artery was at 2.5:1; and infarction of the myocardium was present in less than one fifth of the cases. Schlesinger and Zoll[110] have shown that occlusion of the coronary arteries may be overlooked by ordinary dissection methods. They found that zones of occlusion are usually less than 5 mm in length and the majority of occlusions occur within 3 cm of the orifices of the vessels. Moritz and Zamcheck and Schlesinger and Zoll emphasize that in the investigation of all rapid and unexpected deaths it is essential to examine the coronary arteries with special care and detail.

Hirvonen[111] has explained his experiences concerning the practical demonstration of recent myocardial lesions (infarctions) with various conventional and enzyme-histochemical methods. He found that besides the careful inspection of the heart, additional useful information can be obtained with ordinary H–E staining and β-hydroxybutyrate dehydrogenase reaction on frozen sections. Myocardial cells are darkly eosinophilic in the areas of infarction. Uneven staining in the dehydrogenase reactions was regarded as a sign of lesion in that section. β-hydroxybutyrate hydrogenase revealed the damage more clearly than succinate and malate dehydrogenase.

The enzyme reactions were usable as late as seven days after death if decomposition had not commenced.

Acute rheumatic carditis may be the cause of a sudden or rapid death in a young adult. There may be a clinical history of rheumatic fever and as a rule characteristic naked-eye lesions of the pericardium and endocardium are demonstrable. In certain cases, however, acute rheumatic carditis may be unaccompanied by naked-eye changes, but histological examination of the myocardium will reveal the typical Aschoff bodies of rheumatic fever. Rheumatic lesions may involve the aorta and the coronary arteries and such lesions may readily be overlooked. In one of our cases the only macroscopic change was a solitary rheumatic nodule which projected into the lumen of a coronary artery.

Another lesion which may result in rapid death is the acute toxic myocarditis of diphtheria. In such cases the primary lesion in the nose or throat may not be recognized clinically.

Apart from the known causes of myocarditis there is a group of conditions associated with sudden or rapid death, in which subacute inflammatory lesions are found in the myocardium. These conditions are of obscure aetiology and have been described as 'Fiedler's myocarditis', 'primary myocarditis', 'interstitial myocarditis', and 'idiopathic myocarditis'. Many such cases are now believed to be caused by Coxsackie viruses. Marcuse[112] found 36 of these cases in 3800 consecutive autopsies. According to Saphir[113,114] there are two distinctive types of this disease. The first type is characterized by the development of granulomatous lesions in the myocardium, and in the second type diffuse lesions are found in the myocardium. Some workers have claimed that the granulomatous lesions are of tuberculous or syphilitic origin but this has not been proved. The diffuse or interstitial type of myocarditis is seen most commonly in children and takes the form of a diffuse infiltration of the myocardium with lymphocytes, mononuclear cells, occasional neutrophils, and plasma cells.

The sudden onset of symptoms of acute cardiac failure with marked cyanosis, abdominal pain (from acute congestion of the liver), and vomiting and diarrhoea may suggest the possibility of acute poisoning, particularly when no naked-eye lesions are found in the heart. It is therefore essential, in all obscure cases of sudden death, to submit sections of the heart, suitably fixed in formol-saline, for histological examination.

Metabolic disorders

Uraemia. Gross lesions are usually demonstrable in the kidneys in a case of uraemia, but in acute diffuse glomerulonephritis the kidneys may appear to be normal on naked-eye examination. In such cases inquiries from the relatives or friends of the deceased will usually elicit some history of illness before death. A finding of generalized oedema may suggest the diagnosis which can be confirmed by a histological examination of sections of the kidneys. Specimens of cerebrospinal fluid collected at the time of the post-mortem examination may be submitted for chemical analysis for urea (p. 77).

Bilateral cortical necrosis of the kidneys may cause death after pregnancy or after certain infectious diseases such as scarlet fever. In these cases there is usually a clinical history of oliguria with symptoms suggestive of uraemia preceding death. Death may occur within a week of the onset of symptoms. No naked-eye changes may be observed in the kidneys at autopsy, but histological examination will show a coagulation necrosis of the cortex. Sheldon and Hertig[115] have described two cases of cortical necrosis following toxic separation of the placenta. In both of these cases the authors noted areas of vascular necrosis, similar to the changes seen in the kidneys, in the anterior lobe of the pituitary, the pituitary stalk, and the tuber cinereum.

Diabetes. There are no characteristic naked-eye changes in the pancreas in deaths from diabetes. Moreover, microscopic examination may fail to reveal lesions in the islets of Langerhans even if the organ is placed in special fixative solutions shortly after death. For these reasons a diagnosis of death from diabetes must depend upon the clinical history. Inquiries will often show that the deceased was comatose before he died, and suffered from symptoms suggestive of diabetes before the onset of the coma. It should be noted that diabetic coma is often precipitated by some acute infection, and local lesions such as carbuncles may be found at the autopsy. In middle-aged or older diabetics arteriosclerotic changes are commonly found in the vessels and death may be attributed to this cause unless a clear history of the deceased's last illness can be obtained.

Kimmelstiel and Wilson[116] have claimed that certain lesions of the kidneys are characteristic of diabetes. They state that these lesions are found in approximately one third of patients over the age of 40 who suffer from diabetes.

Chemical examinations of the blood and the urine after death are of limited value. Naumann[117] has shown, however, that examinations of cerebrospinal fluid collected by puncture of the cisterna magna within six hours of death may be of value in the post-mortem diagnosis of diabetes.

Disorders of the blood

Deaths which appear to be obscure and unexplained may be due to primary blood dyscrasias. As a general rule careful inquiry from relatives or friends will reveal that the deceased showed symptoms of illness, but in exceptional circumstances death may occur rapidly. Agranulocytosis or malignant neutropenia may develop rapidly and death may be precipitated by some acute fulminating infection, e.g. acute respiratory infection, and in such cases necrotic lesions may be observed in the pharynx and in the lungs. On histological examination, the striking feature of these lesions is the absence of neutrophil polymorph reaction to the foci of necrosis. Examinations of the bone marrow show that granulocytes are absent or scanty, but myeloblasts may be present; this condition of the bone marrow is known as 'maturation arrest'.[118]

In rapid deaths associated with agranulocytosis it may be advisable to submit the viscera for toxicological analysis as certain drugs may produce agranulocytosis.

Obscure causes of death from non-natural causes

Deaths due to allergy

Reactions to the injection of foreign proteins such as bacterial vaccines, drugs such as penicillin or insect venoms are liable to occur in persons who are known to be allergic subjects. In exceptional circumstances such reactions may lead to death. Most of these deaths are rapid and are preceded by symptoms and signs suggestive of hyperacute bronchial asthma. Other deaths may be delayed for several hours with predominant nervous symptoms such as coma or with symptoms of circulatory failure simulating traumatic shock.

Vance and Strassman[119] have recorded seven deaths from allergy. In all seven cases they found that the lungs were inflated and with the exception of one case, histological examination of the lungs showed infiltration of the bronchial walls with eosinophils.

Lund and Hunt[120] have reported a death from allergic shock which followed the injection of guinea pig protein. Small amounts of serum, taken from the heart of the deceased, were injected into the skin of three volunteers. The skin in the region of the intradermal injection was then scarified and the allergen (the guinea pig blood) was rubbed into this area. In two of the subjects intense local reactions developed promptly at the site of scarification. Lund and Hunt state that several facts must be established before a diagnosis of death from allergic shock can be justified:

1. The injected material must be non-toxic to 'normal' persons;
2. Before death the deceased must have shown characteristic allergic symptoms;
3. No other lesion which could have accounted for death must be found at autopsy;
4. A specific sensitizing substance corresponding to the allergen must be demonstrated in the serum of the deceased's blood by the passive transfer technique described.

Stefanini[121] has described biochemical and immunological observations which, correlated with the autopsy findings, may support a diagnosis of death from anaphylaxis.

Deaths due to drug idiosyncrasies

Death may follow upon the administration of drugs in amounts which are known to be innocuous to normal persons. Such deaths usually depend upon a drug idiosyncrasy, e.g. many persons are hypersensitive to cocaine and the use of relatively small doses of the drug may elicit characteristic symptoms of cocaine poisoning.

The diagnosis of death due to drug idiosyncrasy must be based mainly on clinical information. In those cases where pathological lesions are demonstrable at autopsy, other causes for such lesions must be excluded.

Deaths from chemical poisoning

Deaths from chemical poisoning where lesions are found at autopsy are discussed in Chapter 10. Many poisons, however, cause death without producing any characteristic pathological changes in the tissues. When no pathological changes which adequately account for a death are found at autopsy the possibility of poisoning must be considered.

The circumstances in which the death occurred or the symptoms presented by the deceased before he died may suggest the possibility of poisoning. The sudden onset of acute symptoms in an apparently healthy person, occurring within a short period of the ingestion of food or medicine, is suggestive of poisoning. This possibility is increased when several persons who have ingested the same food are affected in the same manner at approximately the same time.

A suspicion of poisoning may arise when there has been some alteration in the usual colour, taste, or smell of the food or medicine ingested by the deceased before he died.

Although the smptoms and signs caused by poisoning may be simulated by the clinical features of many natural disease processes, the following groups of symptoms are suggestive of poisoning:

1. The sudden onset of abdominal pain, nausea, vomiting, diarrhoea, and collapse;
2. The sudden onset of coma, particularly if accompanied by a reduced respiratory rate and constriction of the pupils;
3. The sudden onset of convulsions;
4. The occurrence of delirium, especially when it is accompanied by an increased respiratory rate and the dilatation of the pupils;
5. The occurrence of paralyses, especially paralyses of a lower motor neurone type;
6. The development of jaundice and hepatocellular failure;
7. The occurrence of oliguria with proteinuria and haematuria;
8. The development without obvious cause of a persistent cyanosis or some form of discoloration of the skin.

Procedure in cases of uncertainty

If the symptoms and signs shown by the deceased before his death are consistent with poisoning, and if all appropriate laboratory investigations have been undertaken with negative results, the question arises as to whether or not the medical practitioner should submit the retained viscera for toxicological analysis.* In many countries, in order to avoid unnecessary expense, it is laid down that viscera should not be sent for analysis merely because the medical practitioner can find no cause for death. There must be a reasonable suspicion that death was due to the administration of some poisonous substance with criminal intent or as the result of culpable carelessness. In cases of this nature the police should be informed of the difficulty in diagnosis and they should be requested to try to obtain further details concerning the death of the deceased. A report stating that the cause of death could not be determined should then be submitted to the responsible administrative officer (such as a magistrate, medical examiner or a coroner) and he should be informed that certain of the viscera have been retained for a possible toxicological analysis. If the administrative officer is satisfied from the police inquiries that there is no reason to suspect poisoning, he will usually instruct the medical practitioner to dispose of the viscera. The medical practitioner may then certify the cause of death as 'undetermined'.

Other obscure deaths from non-natural causes

Deaths from acute neurogenic cardiovascular failure are dealt with in Chapter 7. Deaths from diffuse neuronal injury are described at pages 273 and 274. Other obscure deaths form non-natural causes include air embolism (p. 372), fat embolism (p. 329), acute tubular necrosis (p. 333), and electrical injuries (p. 144).

SUDDEN INFANT DEATH SYNDROME AND NEAR SUDDEN INFANT DEATH SYNDROME

The term sudden infant death syndrome (SIDS) was defined at the Second International Conference in Seattle, Washington, in 1969 as 'the death of an infant in apparent good health who dies suddenly and unexpectedly and in whose case an autopsy does not reveal a commonly accepted cause of death'.[122] In many developed countries, SIDS is the commonest cause of death in children aged 1 month to 1 year.[123] In the USA the annual inci-

---

* The procedure which should be followed in the submission of viscera for toxicological analysis in cases of death suspected to be due to poisoning is dealt with at pages 214–216.

dence is 2 per 1000 live births,[124] manifesting first at 2–3 weeks of age with a peak incidence at 2–4 months of age. It is rare after the first year of life.[123,124]

Numerous epidemiological studies have attempted to identify risk factors.[122,125–128] Infants at increased risk for SIDS have parents who are poor[127,129] and young[130,131] (less than 20 years of age), unmarried mothers[124] or mothers who were ill during pregnancy,[132] who are smokers[128,131,133,134] or abusers of narcotics,[135] had poor prenatal care,[130] short inter-pregnancy intervals[136] and previous fetal loss.[125] Environmental factors, such as low temperature, are strongly associated with peak SIDS incidence[137] though deaths occur throughout the year.

Edidemiological studies have suggested that a genetic component might be important in the aetiology. The rate of SIDS varies between ethnic groups[124,138,139] and there is an increased incidence of blood group O[125] or group B[128,131] in mothers of SIDS victims. Subsequent siblings of SIDS victims have a tenfold increased risk compared to the general population,[140,141] similarly, surviving twins are at a 20-fold increased risk.[142] However, the concordance rate between twins is only 5%, independent of zygosity,[123] and SIDS is rarely familial.[123] Studies evaluating the genetic input, using physiological research techniques, failed to show a difference between parents of SIDS victims and parents of infants dying from known causes.[143–146]

In summary, any 'genetic component' remains unidentified and the risk in twins or siblings is not necessarily genetic.

Identified perinatal risk factors include maternal bleeding in the third trimester,[147] maternal sedation or anaesthesia during labour[147] and amnionitis.[148] Infants who later succumb to SIDS, more frequently are second or third in birth order,[129] have required oxygen and resuscitation at birth,[147] had a low birth weight and had signs of hypoxia at birth, especially seizures[149] and more often have required admission to a neonatal intensive care unit.[150]

SIDS victims are more often products of multiple births,[151] were premature, [152–154] and suffered intra-uterine growth retardation.[124]

All these features suggest that there is some form of prenatal insult or injury associated with certain cases of SIDS.

These sudden deaths are not entirely random, however. They occur mostly between midnight and 6 a.m. A low environmental temperature and a subsequent drop in body temperature has been put forward as a possibility for causing SIDS. Bernard Knight et al[155] related meteorological conditions in South Wales to the incidence of cot deaths over a considerable number of years and found that there was a definite statistical relationship between the rate of death and the temperature. It is true that, seasonally, most SIDS occur in the winter months, but most experts would consider that extreme periods of cold weather do not seem to be associated with an increase in the incidence of SIDS. Deaths, however, are often preceded by a mild upper respiratory tract infection[128,130,132,156] or mild gastrointestinal symptoms in the week preceding death.[127,129,153] There is a slight male preponderance[124,125,127,130,132,153] and the age of victims is similar to that of infants dying from respiratory tract infections, i.e. 1–4 months mainly.[157] The type of feeding (breast versus bottle) is not significant.[126,129,131] The infant might have been asleep in any position at the time of death.[127,131,141,158]

However, all these socio-economic and environmental 'risk factors' are not specific for SIDS, since they are also associated with known causes of death.[150,159]

Kelly and Shannon,[160] in a review of the literature, indicated several limitations to the published epidemiological data. The authors were able to review only two studies in which the data were collected prospectively[122,126,127,161] and in only two studies[125,128] were the data collected by a researcher who was unaware of the past history (control or SIDS victims) when the records were examined or when the parents were interviewed.

Kelly and Shannon,[160] in their summary of epidemiological investigations, suggested that in infant deaths from both known and unknown causes a number of perinatal and perimortal factors could be identified. However, when the highest risk factors are applied prospectively in only 1% of the high risk population does SIDS occur.[128,132]

Since 1972, however, autopsy evidence suggests that SIDS victims are probably subject to chronic alveolar hypoxia and arterial hypoxaemia for a significant period prior to death. Post-mortem findings are subtle and would not be detectable by routine methods.

In order to elucidate further the role of the apnoea theory of SIDS, researchers have paid particular attention to the brain stem and the carotid body, these being the anatomical sites of ventilatory control. Included in the studies was the pulmonary vasculature, liver, adrenal glands and brown fat deposits, all good target organs for the histological elucidation of changes related to chronic hypoxaemia.

The following pathological findings suggest chronic alveolar hypoxia:

1. Changes in the pulmonary arterioles. There is hyperplasia of smooth muscle in the media of pulmonary arterioles[157] but this finding is not specific for hypoxia, since it can occur with increased pulmonary blood flow or raised pulmonary arterial pressure. However, smooth muscle is found extending into small pulmonary arterioles, a site where these vessels are usually devoid of smooth muscle and this finding is apparently specific for alveolar hypoxia.[162] In 'near miss' SIDS* cases, who were subsequently SIDS victims, pulmonary arteriolar hyperplasia has been demonstrated by lung biopsy during the infant's life.[162]

---

* A 'near miss' SIDS infant[171,172] is an infant who ceases to breathe and although seems to have died suddenly and unexpectedly is however saved by timely intervention.

Right ventricular hypertrophy would be an expected finding if alveolar hypoxia was sufficiently severe to cause pulmonary arteriolar hypertension with smooth muscle hyperplasia. Naeye found right ventricular mass to be increased above control values[163] an observation not confirmed by other workers.[164]

2. Brain-stem studies[165,166] have shown abnormal astrocyte gliosis, especially in the 'watershed' zone of brain-stem circulation. The astroglial proliferation involved many cranial nerve nuclei, including medullary nuclei involved in autonomic nervous control and control of respiration.

Similar gliosis has been observed in pre-term infants with a history of prolonged periods of apnoea or who had congenital cyanotic heart disease.[162,166] The possibility that the gliosis may also result in abnormal regulation of breathing must, however, also be considered.

The degree of the brain-stem gliosis correlates with the degree of pulmonary arteriolar hyperplasia.

3. Changes in the carotid body of SIDS victims are controversial, with some authors reporting decreased glomic volume, while others record an increased glomic volume.[167,168]

4. Bone marrow hyperplasia and hepatic extramedullary haemopoiesis are well described autopsy findings.[169]

5. There is increased retention of peri-adrenal brown fat in SIDS victims.[163,170]

6. There is depletion of the adrenal medulla.[165]

7. Evidence of growth retardation in a pattern characteristic of chronic hypoxaemia has been demonstrated[123] and Sinclair-Smith et al[173] selected sections of costochondral junctions to detect features of growth retardation.

A variety of other subtle changes has been described at autopsy. The brain shows evidence of leukomalacia in 21.6% of SIDS victims[174] which can be attributed to chronic hypoxaemia. A reduction in the number of small myelinated fibres in the cervical vagus has been described[175] and it is suggested that this vagal defect could cause abnormalities of respiratory control, such as diminution of the Hering–Breuer reflex. Abnormal endocardial thickening has been reported in a small proportion of SIDS cases.[176] Fatty change in the liver is seen in 90% of SIDS victims[173,177] and splenic or thymic change (suggestive of a normal reaction to infection) is seen in 50% of SIDS cases.[173,178] This last change is not surprising, since over 50% of SIDS victims are known to have had an upper airway infection.

James[179] reported abnormalities in the intracardiac conducting system in SIDS victims, findings which have not been substantiated by other authors.[164,180]

Autopsy findings thus suggest that SIDS victims suffered chronic hypoxia with consequent pulmonary arteriolar hyperplasia and possible right ventricular hypertrophy. The resulting chronic hypoxaemia produces typical organ changes, including brainstem gliosis which could further exacerbate the hypoxaemia by interfering with the normal regulation of pulmonary ventilation. The tissue pathology suggests that the hypoxia precedes the sudden death of an infant by, at least, several weeks. However, the above changes are detected in only 60% of SIDS victims. The rest leave even fewer clues as to the cause of death.[155]

Clues are, however, constantly presenting themselves; one of these is the relationship between carbon monoxide and SIDS[181]—a relationship not as bizarre as it may initially seem to be. Any non-electric heating appliance may produce carbon monoxide when the domestic environment is at its lowest, as may occur during the winter months. The carbon monoxide concentration produced may be sufficient to significantly raise an infant's carbon monoxide level. Concentrations as low as 10 p.p.m. can more than treble the endogenous level of an infant's carboxyhaemoglobin. This may account for the high incidence of SIDS in low socio-economic classes', as well as the seasonal variation. Further, the carbon monoxide excretion rate is considerably slower in males than females and this in turn could account for the male to female ratio.

A further example of SIDS and carbon monoxide poisoning is that the mild illnesses seen before death, the autopsy evidence of hypoxaemia and other abnormalities, are consistent with carbon monoxide poisoning.

Atypical examples of SIDS may, in turn, offer clues to a possible aetiology. Mason and Bain[177] documented a case of fatal Reye's syndrome, presenting as the second sudden infant death in a family and concluded that the differentiation of Reye's syndrome from SIDS did very little to solve the aetiological problems of either. Documentation of such clues may aid in unravelling the SIDS enigma.

Many aetiological hypotheses have been postulated to explain the syndrome of sudden infant death. Steinschneider[182] formulated the apnoea hypothesis in an attempt to account for the autopsy findings described above. Irregular breathing patterns with periods of apnoea and bradycardia occur frequently in preterm infants during sleep and this may persist beyond the neonatal period.[183] It has been suggested that some SIDS victims may well have had several of such abortive apnoeic spells before the terminal apnoea.[184]

Further support for Steinschneider's apnoea hypothesis are various patterns of hypoventilation suggesting an abnormal control of respiration which has been observed in 'near miss' SIDS victims, who subsequently succumbed to SIDS.[182,185]

Thus, 40% of SIDS victims do not have even subtle signs of chronic hypoxaemia at autopsy. Some workers have found a strong association between influenza type A epidemics and SIDS[137] but no studies have demonstrated evidence of systemic viral infection (either by viraemia or raised interferon levels) at autopsy.[186] Arnon found *Clostridium botulinum* organisms and/or toxin in 4.3% of SIDS victims[123] but *C. botulinum* also occurs in stools of infants dying from known causes.[173,187]

Although studies of the immune system in SIDS have failed to demonstrate any abnormalities,[188,189] recently an autoaggressive aetiology has been postulated,[190] where a precipitating factor such as an allergen or micro-organism within the host may result in the production of an aberrant clone of cells, producing antibodies against the hosts' cells. This could apparently account for the fairly rapid death, within only a few days, and warning signs are likely to be either absent or of short duration.

The above postulated mechanism could be the final common pathway of different aetiologies, a challenge for future investigation.

Occasional cases of SIDS are attributed to cardiac arrhythmias such as the Wolf–Parkinson–White syndrome,[191] or the prolonged QT interval syndrome.[192]

Similarly, sporadic cases of infanticide are initially mis-diagnosed as SIDS.[155] Sophisticated radiological techniques have been used to demonstrate that extreme neck extension might cause bilateral vertebral artery compression in infants with atlanto-occipital instability; when the posterior arch of the atlas inverts through the foramen magnum upon neck extension, compression of the vertebral arteries can occur.[193]

Studies of electrolytes and metabolites in blood[194,195] and vitreous humour[161]; have not demonstrated any abnormalities in SIDs victims, and detailed toxicological analyses have not revealed toxic levels of any known substances or drugs detectable by sophisticated methods.[196]

Thus it appears that SIDS babies are subtly physiologically handicapped from before birth.[128] This handicap, involving brain-stem function, manifests as subtle abnormalities of feeding or temperature regulation[123] and defective central control of ventilation in many victims. Prenatal factors, such as amnionitis,[148] maternal cigarette smoking[128,131,133,134] or methadone dependence can affect the fetal brain-stem and only months later, after birth, does the infant suffer the effects of chronic hypoxaemia and subtle brain dysfunction.

In most sleep stages, metabolic heat generation and thermoregulation are normal. However, during rapid eye movement (REM) sleep, thermoregulation and other hypothalamic functions may be less precisely regulated or may even cease and, further, sweating may decline markedly during the REM stage of sleep in a warm environment. Stanton[197] reported 34 cases of overheating in relation to SIDS and concludes that the stress of an infection may cause a rapid rise in body temperature, which, in a warm environment, may convert a potential danger into a lethal disadvantage.

REFERENCES

1 Bass J W, Steele R W, Wiebe R A. Acute epiglottitis: A surgical emergency. J Am Med Assoc 1974; 229:671.
2 Branefors-Helander P, Jeppsson P–H. Acute epiglottitis: A clinical, bacteriological and serological study. Scand J Infect Dis 1975; 7:103.
3 Cramblett H G. Croup (epiglottitis, laryngitis, laryngotracheobronchitis). In: Kendig E L Jr, Chernick V. eds. Disorders of the respiratory tract in children. 3rd ed. Philadelphia: W B Saunders 1977: p 353.

4 Buchan K A, Marten K W, Kennedy D H. Aetiology and epidemiology of viral croup in Glasgow 1966–1972. J Hyg (Camb) 1974; 73:143.

5 Urquhart G E D, Kennedy D H, Ariyawansa J P. Croup associated with parainfluenza type 1 virus: Two subpopulations. Br Med J 1979; 1:1604.

6 Zach M, Erban A, Olinsky A. Croup, recurrent croup, allergy and airways hyperreactivity. Arch Dis Child 1981; 56: 336–341.

7 McCloskey R V, Eller J J, Green M, et al. The 1970 epidemic of diphtheria in San Antonio. Ann Intern Med 1971; 75:495.

8 Fisher A M, Cobb S. The clinical manifestations of the severe form of diphtheria. Bull Johns Hopkins Hosp 1948; 83:297.

9 Ward J, Gorman G, Phillips C, et al. Haemophilus influenzae type b disease in a day-care center. J Pediatr 1978; 92:713.

10 Robbins J B, Schneerson R, Argaman M, et al. Haemophilus influenzae type b: disease and immunity in humans. Ann Intern Med 1973; 78:259.

11 Beyer N H, Weinstein L. Diptheritic myocarditis. N Engl J Med 1948; 239:913.

12 Isaac-Renton J L, Boyke W J, Chan R, et al. Corynebacterium diphtheriae septicaemia. Am J Clin Pathol 1981; 75:631.

13 Hoeprich P D. Etiologic diagnosis of lower respiratory tract infections. Calif Med 1970; 112:1.

14 Wohl M E B, Chernick V. Bronchiolitis. Am Rev Resp Dis 1978; 118:759.

15 Henderson F W, Clyde W A Jr, Collier A M, Denny F W. The etiologic and epedemiologic spectrum of bronchiolitis in paediatric practice. J Paediatr 1979; 95:183.

16 McConnochie K. Bronchiolitis: What's in the name? Am J Dis Child 1983; 137:11.

17 Anas N, Boettrich C, Hall C B, Brooks J G. The association of apnea and respiratory syncytial virus infection in infants. J Pediatr 1982; 101:65.

18 Mogabgab W J. Mycoplasma pneumoniae and adenovirus respiratory illnesses in military and university personnel 1959–1966. Am Rev Res Dis 1968; 97:345.

19 Grayston J T, Alexander E R, Kenny G E, et al. Mycoplasma pneumoniae infections: clinical and epidemiological studies. J Am Med Assoc 1965; 191:97.

20 Fekety F R, Caldwell J, Gump D, et al. Bacteria, viruses and mycoplasmas in acute pneumonia in adults. Am Rev Resp Dis 1971; 104:499.

21 Helms C M, Viner J P, Sturm R H. Comparative features of pneumococcal, mycoplasmal and legionnaire's disease pneumonias. Ann Intern Med 1979; 90:543.

22 Ebright J R, Rytel M W. Bacterial pneumonia in the elderly. J Am Geriatr Soc 1980; 28:220.

23 Verghese A, Berk S L. Bacterial pneumonia in the elderly. Medicine 1983; 62:271.

24 Lerner A M, Jankauskas K. The classic bacterial pneumonias. Disease-A-Month Feb 1975.

25 Respiratory syncytial virus—Missouri. Morbid Mortal Wkly Rep 1977; 26:351.

26 Breitfeld V, Hashida Y, Sherman F E, et al. Fatal measles infections in children with leukaemia. Lab Invest 1973; 28:279.

27 Tillotson J R, Lerner A M. Pneumonias caused by gram negative bacilli. Medicine 1966; 45:65.

28 Valdivieso M, Gil-Extremera G, Zornoza J, et al. Gram-negative bacillary pneumonia in the compromised host. Medicine 1977; 56:241.

29 Hausmann W, Karlish A J. Staphylococcal pneumonia in adults. Br Med J 1956; 2:845.

30 The Center for Diseases Control, Atlanta, Georgia. Legionnaire's disease. Diagnosis and management. Ann Intern Med 1978; 88:363.

31 Yu V L, Kroboth F J, Schonnard J, et al. Legionnaire's disease. New clinical perspective from a prospective pneumonia study. Am J Med 1982; 73:357.

32 Fraser D W, Tasi T F, Orenstein W, et al. Legionnaire's disease. Description of an epidemic of pneumonia. N Engl J Med 1977; 297:1189.

33 Kirby B D, Snyder K M, Meyer R D et al. Legionnaire's disease. A cluster of cases, abstract. Clin Res 1978; 26:399A.

34 Follansbee S E, Busch D F, Wofsy C B et al. An outbreak of Pneumocystis carinii pneumonia in homosexual men. Ann Intern Med 1982; 96 (1):705.

35 Gottlieb M S, Schroff R, Schanker H M, et al. Pneumocystis carinii pneumonia and mucosal candidiasis in previously healthy homosexual men: Evidence of a new acquired cellular immunodeficiency. N Engl J Med 1981; 305:1425.

36 Brooksaler F, Nelson J D. Pertussis: A reappraisal and report of 190 confirmed cases. Am J Dis Child 1967; 114:389.

37 Brooks G F, Buchanan T M. Pertussis in the United States. J Infect Dis 1970; 122:123.

38 Morse S I. Pertussis in adults, Editorial. Ann Intern Med 1968; 68:953.

39 Kaplan J E, Gary G W, Baron R C, et al. Epidemiology of Norwalk gastroenteritis and the role of Norwalk virus in outbreaks of acute nonbacterial gastroenteritis. Ann Intern Med 1982; 96:756.

40 Murphy A M, Grohmann G S, Christopher P J, et al. An Australia-wide outbreak of gastroenteritis from oysters caused by Norwalk virus. Med J Austr 1979; 2:329.

41 Middleton P J, Szymanski M T, Abbott G D, et al. Orbivirus acute gastroenteritis of infancy. Lancet 1974; 1:1241.

42 Davidson G P, Bishop R F, Townley R R, et al. Importance of a new virus in acute sporadic enteritis in children. Lancet 1975; 1:242.

43 Paniker L K J, Mathew S, Mathan M. Rotavirus and acute diarrheal disease in a Southern Indian coastal town. Bull WHO 1982; 60:123.

44 Middleton P J, Pathogenesis of rotaviral infection. J Am Vet Assoc 1978; 173:544.

45 Carlson J A K, Middleton P J, Szymanski M, et al. Fatal rotavirus gastroenteritis. An analysis of 21 cases. Am J Dis Child 1978; 132:477.

46 Edelman R, Levine M M. Summary of a workshop on enteropathogenic Escherichia coli. J Infect Dis 1983; 147:1108.

47 Tulloch E F, Ryan K J, Formal S B, et al. Invasive enteropathic Escherichia coli dysentery: An outbreak in 28 adults. Ann Intern Med 1973; 79:13.

48 Sack R B. Human diarrheal disease caused by enterotoxigenic Escherichia coli. Ann Rev Microbiol 1975; 29:333.

49 Taylor W R, Schell W L, Wells J G, et al. A foodborne outbreak of enterotoxigenic Escherichia coli diarrhea. N Engl J Med 1982; 306:1093.

50 Nolan C, Harris N, Ballard J, et al. Outbreak of Yersinia enterocolitica—Washington State. Morbid Mortal Weekly Rep 1982: 31:562.

51 Marks M I, Pai C H, LaFleur L, et al. Yersinia enterocolitica gastroenteritis: A prospective study of clinical, bacteriologic, and epidemiologic features. J Pediatr 1980; 96:26.

52 Blaser M J, Reller L B Campylobacter enteritis. N Engl J Med 1981; 305:1444.

53 Skirrow M B. Campylobacter enteritis: The first five years. J Hygiene 1982; 89 (2):175.

54 Ahnen D J, Brown W R. Campylobacter enteritis in immune-deficient patients. Ann Intern Med 1982; 96:187.

55 Drake A A, Gilchrist M J R, Washington J A, et al. Diarrhea due to Campylobacter fetus subspecies jejuni. A clinical review of 73 cases. Mayo Clin Proc 1981; 56:414.

56 Blaser M J, Wells J G, Feldman R A. Campylobacter enteritis in the United States: A multicenter study. Ann Intern Med 1983; 98:360.

57 Benenson A S, Islam M R, Greenough 111 W B. Rapid identification of Vibrio cholerae by darkfield microscopy. Bull WHO 1964; 30:827.

58 Larson H E, Price A B, Honour P, et al. Clostridium difficile and the aetiology of pseudomembranous colitis. Lancet 1978; 1:1063.

59 Wilson K H, Kennedy M J, Fekety F R. Use of sodium taurocholate to enhance spore recovery on a medium selective for Clostridium difficile. J Clin Microbiol 1982; 15:443.

60 Peikin S R, Galdibini J, Bartlett J G. Role of Clostridium difficile in a case of nonantibiotic-associated pseudomembraneous colitis. Gastroenterology 1980; 79:948.

61 Welch D F, Marks M I. Is Clostridium difficile pathogenic in infants? J Paediatr 1982; 100:393.

62 Cudmore M A, Silva J, Fekety R, et al. Clostridium difficile colitis associated with cancer chemotherapy. Arch Intern med 1982; 142:333.

63 Osterholm M T, Forfang J C, Ristinen T L, et al. An outbreak of foodborne giardiasis. N Engl J Med 1981; 304:24.

64 Balikian J P, Bitar J G, Rishani K K, Kabakian H A. Fulminant necrotising amebic colitis in children. Am J Proctol 1977; 28(1): 69–73

65 Aikat B K, Bhusnurmath S R, Pal A K, et al. The pathology and pathogenesis of fatal

hepatic amoebiasis; A study based on 79 autopsy cases. Trans R Soc Trop Med Hyg 1979; 73:188.

66 Meisel J L, Perem D R, Meligro C, et al. Overwhelming watery diarrhea associated with a Cryptosporidium in an immuno-suppressed patient. Gastroenterology 1976; 70:1156.

67 Kaye D. Infecting microrganisms. In: Kaye D. ed. Infective endocarditis, Baltimore: University Park Press. 1976: p 43.

68 Tiula E, Leinikki P. Fatal cytomegalovirus infection in a previously healthy boy with myocarditis and consumption coagulopathy as presenting signs. Scand J Infect Dis 1972; 4:57.

69 Swartz M N, Dodge P R. Bacterial meningitis: A review of selected aspects. N Engl J Med 1965; 272:725.

70 Dillon H C, Gray B M. Bacterial meningitis in children. Guidelines to Antibiotic Therapy 1977; 2:3.

71 Iwarson S, Lindin-Janson G, Svensson R. Listeric meningitis in the non-compromised host. Infection 1977; 5;204.

72 Davis L E, Johnson R T. A possible explanation for the localization of herpes simplex encephalitis? Ann Neurol 1979; 5: 2.

73 Dupont J R, Earle K M. Human rabies encephalitis: A study of forty-nine fatal cases with a review of the literature. Neurology 1965; 15:1023.

74 Weinstein L, Shelokov A, Seltser R, et al. A comparison of the clinical features of poliomyelitis in adults and in children. N Engl J Med 1952; 246:296.

75 Debré R, Thieffry D R. Symptomatology and diagnosis of poliomyelitis. In: Poliomyelitis. WHO Monograph Series No. 26, Geneva, 1955: p 109.

76 Schonberger L B, Bregman D J, Sullivan-Bolyai J Z, et al. Guillain-Barré syndrome following vaccination in the national influenza immunization program, United States 1976–1977. Am J Epidemiol 1979; 110:105.

77 Server A C, Johnson R T. Guillain-Barré syndrome. In: Remington J S, Schwartz M N eds. Current Clinical Topics in Infectious Diseases Vol 3. New York: McGraw-Hill, 1982: p 74.

78 Weinstein L. Tetanus. N Engl J Med 1973; 289:1293.

79 Kirschbaum W R. Jakob-Creutzfeldt disease. New York: Elsevier. 1968.

80 Brody J A, Gibbs C J. Chronic neurological diseases: Subacute sclerosing panenchephalitis, progressive multifocal leukoencephalopathy, kuru, Creutzfeldt-Jakob disease. In: Evans A S ed. Viral infections of humans. New York: Plenum, 1976: p 519.

81 Becker W B, Kipps A, McKenzie D. Disseminated herpes simplex virus infection: Its pathogenesis based on virological and pathological studies in 33 cases. Am J Dis Child 1968; 115:1.

82 Dennis L H, Reisberg B E, Crosbie J. The original haemorrhagic fever: Yellow Fever. Br J Haematol 1969; 17:455.

83 McCormick J B, Johnson K M. Lassa fever: Historical review and contemporary investigation. In: Pattyn S R. ed. Ebola virus haemorrhagic fever. New York: Elsevier/North-Holland, 1978: p 278.

84 Martini G A. Marburg virus disease: The clinical syndrome. In: Martini G A, Siegert R. eds. Marburg virus disease. Berlin: Springer-Verlag, 1971: p. 1.

85 Gear J H S, Ryan J, Rossouw E. A consideration of the diagnosis of dangerous infectious fevers in South Africa. S Afr Med J 1978; 53:235.

86 Maiztegui J I. Clinical and epidemiological patterns of Argentine haemorrhagic fever. Bull WHO 1975; 52:567.

87 Stinebaugh B J, Schloeder F X, Johnson K M, et al. Bolivian haemorrhagic fever: A report of four cases. Am J Med 1966; 40:217.

88 Mosley J W. Hepatitis type B and non-B. Epidemiologic background. J Am Med Assoc 1975; 233:967.

89 Krugman S, Overby L R, Mushahwar I K, et al. Viral hepatitis, type B. Studies on the natural history and prevention re-examined. N Engl J Med 1979; 300:101.

90 Alter H J, Purcell R H, Feinstone S M, et al. Non-A, non-B hepatitis. Its relationship to cytomegalovirus, to chronic hepatitis, and to direct and indirect test methods. In: Szmuness W, Alter H J, Maynard J E. eds. Viral Hepatitis 1981 International Symposium. Philadelphia: Franklin Institute Press, 1982: p 279.

91 Saah A J, Hornick R B. Rickettsiosis. In: Mandell G L, Douglas R G, Bennett J E.
    eds: Principles and practice of infectious diseases. 2nd ed. New York: Wiley
    Medical 1985: p 1081.
92 Wyler D J. Malaria—resurgence resistance and research. N Engl J Med 1983; 308:875.
93 Cossio P M, Diez C, Szarfman A, et al. Chagasic cardiopathy—demonstration of a
    serum gamma globulin factor which reacts with endocardium and vascular structures.
    Circulation 1974; 49:13.
94 Brener Z. Recent developments in the field of Chaga's disease. Bull WHO 1982;
    60:463.
95 Andrade Z A, Andrade S G, Oliveira G R, et al. Histopathology of the conducting
    tissue of the heart in Chaga's myocarditis. Am Heart J 1978; 93:316.
96 Feig M. Staphylococcal food poisoning: A report of two related outbreaks, and a
    discussion of the data presented. Am J Public Hlth 1950; 40:279.
97 Holmberg S D, Blake P A. Staphylococcal food poisoning in the United States: New
    facts and old misconceptions. J Am Med Assoc 1984; 251:487.
98 Terranova W, Blake P A. Bacillus cereus food poisoning. N Engl J Med 1978; 298:143.
99 Holmes J R, Plunkett T, Pate P, et al. Emetic food poisoning caused by Bacillus
    cereus. Arch Intern Med 1981; 141:766.
100 Midura T F, Arnon S S. Infant botulism: Identification of Clostridium botulinum and
    its toxin in feces. Lancet 1976; 2:934.
101 Arnon S S, Midura T F, Clay S A, et al. Infant botulism: Epidemiological, clinical and
    laboratory aspects. J Am Med Assoc 1977; 237:1946.
102 Morens D M, Sullivan-Bolyai J Z, Slater J E, et al. Surveillance of Reye Syndrome in
    the United States, 1977. Am J Epidemiol 1981; 114:406.
103 Melish M E. Kawasaki syndrome (mucocutaneous lymphnode syndrome). Peds Rev
    1980; 2:107.
104 Bell D M, Morens D M, Holman R C, et al. Kawasaki syndrome in the United States.
    Am J Dis Child 1983; 137:211.
105 Gottlieb M S, Schroff R, Schauber H M, et al. Pneumocystis carinii pneumonia and
    mucosal candidiasis in previously healthy homosexual men. N Engl J Med 1981;
    305:1425.
106 Zakowski P, Fligiel S, Berlin G W, Johnson B L. Disseminated Mycobacterium avium-
    intracellulare infection in homosexual men dying of acquired immunodeficiency. J
    Am Med Assoc 1982; 248:2980.
107 Macher A M, Kovacs J A, Gill V, et al. Bacteremia due to Mycobacterium avium-
    intracellulare in the acquired immunodeficiency syndrome. Ann Intern Med 1983;
    99:782.
108 Friedman-Kien A E, Laubenstein L J, Rubinstein P, et al. Disseminated Kaposi's
    sarcoma in homosexual men. Ann Intern Med 1982; 96:693.
109 Moritz A R, Zamcheck N. Sudden and unexpected deaths of young soldiers. Diseases
    responsible for such deaths during World War II. Arch Pathol 1946; 42: 459–494.
110 Schlesinger M J, Zoll P M. Incidence and localisation of coronary artery occlusion.
    Arch Pathol 1941; 32: 178–188.
111 Hirvonen J. Practical approach to the diagnosis of sudden unexpected death of cardiac
    origin. Forens Sci 1976; 8: 49–52.
112 Marcuse P M. Non-specific myocarditis. Arch Pathol 1947; 43: 602–610.
113 Saphir O. Myocarditis: a general review with an analysis of 240 cases. Arch Pathol
    1941; 32: 1000–1051.
114 Saphir O. Myocarditis: a general review with an analysis of 240 cases. Arch Pathol
    1942; 33: 88–137.
115 Sheldon W H, Hertig A T. Bilateral cortical necrosis of the kidney: a report of two
    cases. Arch Pathol 1942; 34: 866–874.
116 Kimmelstiel P, Wilson C. Benign and malignant hypertension and nephrosclerosis: a
    clinical and pathological study. Am J Path 1936; 12: 45–82.
117 Naumann H N. Diabetes and uraemia diagnosed at autopsy by testing cerebro-spinal
    fluid and urine. Arch Pathol 1949; 47: 70–77.
118 Wintrobe M M. Clinical Haematology. 2nd ed. Philadelphia: Lea & Febiger. 1947:
    p 795.
119 Vance B M, Strassman G. Sudden death following injection of foreign protein. Arch
    Pathol 1942; 34: 847–865.

120 Lund H, Hunt E L. Post-mortem diagnosis of allergic shock: the value of the Prausnitz-Kustner reaction. Arch Pathol 1941; 32: 664–669.

121 Stefanini M. Death due to anaphylactic reaction, with presentation of pertinent biochemical parameters: A case report. Forens Sci Int 1979; 13: 137–144.

122 Beckwith J B. Observations of the pathological anatomy of SIDS. In: Bergman A B, Beckwith J B, Ray C G. eds. Proceedings of the Second International Conference on Causes of SIDS. Seattle: University of Washington Press. 1970.

123 Naeye R L. Sudden infant death. Sci Am 1980; 242: 52–58.

124 Kraus J F, Borhani N O. Post-neonatal sudden unexplained death in California—A cohort study. Am J Hyg 1972; 95:497.

125 Arsenault P S. Maternal and antenatal factors in the risk of SID syndrome. Am J Epidemiol 1980; 11:278.

126 Biering-Sørensen F, Jørgensen T, Hilden J. SID in Copenhagen 1956–1971; I. Infant feeding. Acta Paediatr Scand 1978; 67:129.

127 Biering-Sørensen F, Jørgensen T, Hilden J. SID in Copenhagen 1956–1971; II. Social factors and morbidity. Acta Paediatr Scand 1979; 68:1.

128 Naeye R L, Ladis B, Drage J S. Sudden infant death syndrome. Am J Dis Child 1976; 130:1207.

129 Froggatt P, Lynas M A, Marshall T K. Epidemiology of sudden unexpected death in infants (cot death). Report of a collaborative study in Northern Ireland. Ulster Med J 1971; 40:116.

130 Peterson D R, van Belle G, Chinn N M. Epidemiologic comparisons of the SID syndrome with other major components of infant mortality. Am J Epidemiol 1979; 110:699.

131 Steele R, Langworth J T. The relationship of antenatal and postnatal factors to SID in infancy. Can Med Assoc J 1966; 94:1165.

132 Froggat P, Lynas M A, Marshall T K. Sudden death in babies: Epidemiology. Am J Cardiol 1968; 22:457.

133 Bergman A B, Wiesnes L A. Relationship of passive cigarette-smoking on SID syndrome. Pediatrics 1976; 58:665.

134 Oakley J R, Tavare C J, Stanton A N. Evaluation of the Sheffield system for identifying children at risk from unexpected death in infancy. Arch Dis Child 1978; 53:649.

135 Butler N R, Goldstein H, Ross E M. Cigarette smoking in pregnancy. Its influence on birth weight and maternal mortality. Br Med J 1972; 2:127.

136 Spiers P S, Wang L. Short pregnancy interval, low birth weight and the SID syndrome. Am J Epidemiol 1976; 104:15.

137 Bonser R S A, Knight B H, West R R. SIDS in Cardiff, association with epidemic influenza and with temperature—1955–1974. Int J Epidemiol 1978; 7 (4): 335–340.

138 Fleshman J K, Peterson D R. The SID syndrome among Alaskan natives. Am J Epidemiol 1977; 105:555.

139 Valdes-Dapena M, Birle J, McGovern J A, et al. Sudden unexpected death in infancy: A statistical analysis of certain socioeconomic factors. J Pediatr 1968; 73:387.

140 Cooke R T, Welch R G. A study in cot death. Br Med J 1964; 2:1549.

141 Peterson D R, Chinn N M, Fisher L D. The sudden infant death syndrome: Repetitions in families. J Pediatr 1980; 97:265.

142 Speer L. Aborted crib death? J Am Med Assoc 1973; 223:1512.

143 Kanarek D J, Kelly D H, Shannon D C. Ventilatory chemoreceptor response in parents of children at risk for SID syndrome. Pediatr Res 1981; 15:1402.

144 Schiffman P L, Westlake R E, Santiago T V, Edelman N H. Ventilatory control in parents of victims of SID syndrome. N Engl J Med 1980; 302:486.

145 Shannon D C, Kelly D H, O'Connell K. Abnormal regulation of ventilation in infants at risk for SID syndrome. N Engl J Med 1977; 297:747.

146 Zwillich C, McCullough R, Guilleminault C, et al. Respiratory control in the parents of SID syndrome victims. Ventilatory control in SIDS parents. Pediatr Res 1980; 14:762.

147 Protestos C D, Carpenter R D, McWeeny P M, Emery J L. Obstetric and perinatal histories of children who died unexpectedly (cot death). Arch Dis Child 1973; 48:835.

148 Naeye R L. Placental abnormalities in victims of SID syndrome. Biol Neonate 1977; 32:189.

149 Anderson-Huntington R B, Rosenblith J F. Central nervous system damage as a possible component of unexpected deaths in infancy. Dev Med Child Neurol 1976; 18: 480–492.

150 Kulkarni P, Hall R T, Rhodes P G, Sheehan M B. Postneonatal infant mortality in infants admitted to a neonatal intensive care unit. Pediatrics 1978; 62:178.

151 Kelly D H, Walker A M, Cahen L, Shannon D C. Periodic breathing in siblings of SID syndrome victims. Pediatrics 1980; 66:515.

152 Naeye R L, Messmer J, Spech T T, Merritt T A. SID syndrome temperament before death. J Pediatr 1976; 88:511.

153 Richards I D G, McIntosh H T. Confidential inquiry into 226 consecutive infant deaths. Arch Dis Child 1972; 47:697.

154 Spiers P S. Previous fetal loss and risk of SID syndrome in subsequent offspring. Am J Epidemiol 1976; 103:355.

155 Knight B. Sudden death in infancy: The 'cot death' syndrome. London: Faber and Faber. 1983; pp 66–103.

156 Jørgensen T, Biering-Sørensen F, Hilden J. SID in Copenhagen 1956–1971; III. Perinatal and perimortal factors. Acta Paediatr Scand 1979; 68: 11–22.

157 Naeye R L, Pulmonary arterial abnormalities in the SID syndrome. N Engl J Med 1973; 289:1167.

158 Carpenter R G, Gardner A, McWeeny P M, Emery J L. Multistage scoring system for identifying infants at risk of unexpected death. Arch Dis Child 1977; 52:606.

159 McWeeny P M, Emery J L. Unexpected postneonatal deaths (cot deaths) due to recognizable disease. Arch Dis Child 1975; 50: 191–196.

160 Kelly D H, Shannon D C. Sudden infant death syndrome and near sudden infant death syndrome: A review of the literature, 1964 to 1982. Paediatr Clin N Am 1982; 29: 1241–1261.

161 Blumenfeld T A, Mantell C H, Catherman R L, Blanc W A. Postmortem vitreous humor chemistry in SID syndrome and in other causes of death in childhood. Am J Clin Pathol 1979; 71:219.

162 Williams A J, Shannon D C, Rabinovitch M, et al. Pulmonary vascular muscle hyperplasia associated with impaired ventilatory control in SID syndrome. Am Rev Resp Dis 1980; 121:419.

163 Naeye R L, Whalen P, Ryser M, Fisher R. Cardiac and other abnormalities in the SID syndrome. Am J Pathol 1976; 82:1.

164 Valdes-Dapena M A, Greene M, Basvanard N, et al. The myocardial conduction system in sudden death in infancy. N Engl J Med 1973; 289:1179.

165 Naeye R L. Brain-stem and adrenal abnormalities in the SID syndrome. Am J Clin Pathol 1976; 66: 526.

166 Takashima S, Armstrong D, Becker L, Bryan A C. Cerebral hypoperfusion in the SID syndrome? Brainstem gliosis and vasculature. Ann Neurol 1978; 4:257.

167 Cole S, Lindenberg L B, Galioto F M, et al. Ultrastructural abnormalities of the carotid body in SID syndrome. Pediatrics 1979; 63:13.

168 Naeye R L, Fisher R, Ryser M, Whalen P. Carotid body in SID syndrome. Science 1976; 91:567.

169 Naeye R L. Hypoxemia and the SID syndrome. Science 1974; 186:837.

170 Valdes-Dapena M A, Gillane M M, Catherman R. Brown fat retention in SID syndrome. Arch Pathol Lab Med 1976; 100:547.

171 Kelly D H, Shannon D C, O'Connell K. Care of infants with near-miss SID syndrome. Pediatrics 1978; 61:511.

172 Kelly D H, Shannon D C. Periodic breathing in infants with near-miss SID syndrome. Pediatrics 1979; 63:355.

173 Sinclair-Smith C, Dinsdale F, Emery J. Evidence of duration and type of illness in children found unexpectedly dead. Arch Dis Child 1976; 51:424.

174 Takashima S, Armstrong D, Becker L E, Huber J. Cerebral white matter lesions in SID syndrome. Pediatrics 1978; 62:155.

175 Sachis P N, Armstrong D L, Becker L E, Bryan A C. The vagus nerve and SID syndrome. A morphometric study. J Pediatr 1981; 98:278.

176 Williams R B, Emery J L. Endocardial fibrosis in apparently normal infant hearts. Histopathology 1978; 2: 283–290.

177 Mason J K, Bain A D. Reye's syndrome presenting as atypical SID syndrome? Forens Sci Int 1982; 20: 39–44.

178 Borzanji A A, Emery J L. Quantitative study of the lymphatic tissue and germinal centers in the spleen in infants dying from unexpected causes (cot deaths). Histopathology 1977; 1:445.

179 James T N. Sudden death in babies: New observations in the heart. Am J Cardiol 1968; 22:479.

180 Lie J T, Rosenberg H S, Erickson E E. Histopathology of the conduction system in the sudden infant death syndrome. Circulation 1976; 53:3.

181 Cleary J. Carbon monoxide and cot death. Lancet 1984; 2:1403.

182 Steinschneider A. Prolonged apnea and the SID syndrome: Clinical and laboratory observations. Pediatrics 1972; 50:646.

183 Moore A. Sudden infant death syndrome. Br J Hosp Med 1981; 26: 37–45.

184 Allen E M. SID syndrome. N Z Med J 1982; 95: 183–184.

185 Guilleminault C, Ariagno R, Korobkin R, et al. Mixed and obstructive sleep apnea and near-miss for SID syndrome: 2 Comparison of near-miss and normal control infants by age. Pediatrics 1979; 64:882.

186 Seto D S Y, Carver D H. Circulating interferon in SID syndrome. Proc Soc Exp Biol Med 1978; 157:378.

187 Arnon S S, Midura T F, Damus K. Intestinal infection and toxin production by Clostridium botulinum as one cause of SID syndrome, Lancet 1978; 1:1273.

188 Ogra P L, Ogra S S, Coppola P R. Secretory component and SID syndrome. Lancet 1975; 2:387.

189 Turner J K, Baldo B A, Carter R F, Kerr H R. SID syndrome in South Australia: Measurement of serum IgE antibodies to three common allergens. Med J Aust 1975; 2:855.

190 Burch P R J, Chesters M S. Age-specific cot-death rates. Lancet 1984; 2:1404.

191 Keeton B R, Southall E, Rutter N, et al. Cardiac conduction disorders in six infants with 'near-miss' SID. Br Med J 1977; 2:600.

192 Maron B J, Clark E E, Goldstin R E, Epstein S E. Potential role of QT interval prolongation in SID syndrome. Circulation 1976; 54:423.

193 Gilles F H, Bina M, Sotrel A. Infantile atlantoccipital instability. Am J Dis Child 1979; 133: 30–37.

194 Naeye R L, Fisher R, Rubin R, Nemers I M. Selected hormone levels in victims of the SID syndrome. Pediatrics 1980; 65:1134.

195 Hillman L S, Erickson M, Haddad J G. Serum 25-hydroxyvitamin D concentrations in sudden death syndrome. Pediatrics 1980; 65:1137.

196 Smialek J E, Monforte J R. Toxicology and SID. J Forens Sci 1977; 22:757.

197 Stanton A N. Overheating and cot death. Lancet 1984; 2:1199.

9

Deaths associated with anaesthetic procedures

The performance of a surgical operation and the administration of an anaesthetic are never without risk to the life of a patient. In 1982, Lunn and Mushin[1] reviewed the mortality associated with anaesthesia. The review included all deaths occurring within six days of surgery. Lunn and Mushin[1] estimated the mortality directly related to anaesthesia to be 1 in 166 (0.6%). Following a ten year study from 1967 to 1976, Harrison[2] found that anaesthesia contributed in some degree to mortality in 2.2 per 10 000 anaesthetics, and that this represented 2.2% of the total mortality from surgery, which was 10.15 per 1000. Comparing the findings of Lunn and Mushin and Harrington, it might appear that there has been an increase in mortality. It has been suggested that such an increase may be attributed to the greater complexity of surgery now attempted and the larger numbers of moribund patients now accepted for anaesthesia.

The main factors which determine this risk are the type of anaesthesia, the nature of the operation and the physical condition of the patient. When a suitable form of anaesthetic is competently administered; when the operation is performed by a skilful surgeon; and when the preoperative physical condition of the patient is good, the risk to life is minimal. There may be serious risk to the life of a patient, however, when an unsuitable form of anaesthetic is administered; when an operation is unskilfully performed; or when the general condition of the patient is poor before the operation.

PROCEDURES RELATING TO 'ANAESTHETIC' DEATHS

In many countries, deaths which occur under the influence of anaesthesia, or of which the administration of an anaesthetic has been a contributory cause, are not regarded as deaths from natural causes. Accordingly, enquiries or inquests are held into such 'anaesthetic' deaths.

Although other factors are often responsible for a death under anaesthesia, the terms of legislative provisions are such that there is a tendency at inquest proceedings to place the entire responsibility for such a death upon the anaesthetist. The fact that deaths occurring in association with surgical procedures are often not due to the administration of the anaes-

194

thetic, tends to operate unfairly towards anaesthetists in those jurisdictions where formal public enquiries or inquests are held.

In most countries, the following types of death have to be notified to the relevant administrative or judicial authorities: deaths that occur during the administration of an anaesthetic, or deaths which occur after the administration of an anaesthetic has been completed when the anaesthetic may be regarded as a contributory cause of death.

It is generally accepted that once the patient has recovered consciousness, or been restored to his condition prior to the administration of the anaesthetic, that anaesthesia is not responsible for the subsequent demise of the patient. Under certain circumstances, anaesthesia may contribute to delayed deaths as in the case of aspiration of material into the lungs with late complications, or liver failure induced by the administration of anaesthetic drugs such as halothane[3].

When a death occurs in any of these circumstances one of the medical practitioners is required to report the death to the administrative or judicial authorities. On receiving this information the responsible officer may instruct a pathologist to ascertain the cause of death. At the same time detailed clinical information should be obtained from all the medical practitioners who attended to the deceased.

In all cases a careful and complete autopsy should be undertaken by a pathologist. In certain cases it may be possible to ascertain the cause of death from the autopsy findings alone, but in most cases the cause of death has to be determined from a consideration of the clinical features as well as the autopsy findings.

CLASSIFICATION OF THE CAUSES OF 'ANAESTHETIC' DEATHS

'Anaesthetic' deaths may be divided into two broad groups, namely:

(1) deaths which occur during the administration of an anaesthetic but which are not due to the anaesthetic; and

(2) deaths which are the direct result of the administration of an anaesthetic.

Deaths which occur during the administration of an anaesthetic but which are not due to the anaesthetic

Deaths due to the injury or disease which necessitated the operation and administration of an anaesthetic

When the injury (or disease) which necessitated the operation is, by itself, of a sufficiently serious nature to account for death, the injury (or disease) may be regarded as the principal factor which caused the death, even though the operation and the anaesthetic may have precipitated the death. Many anaesthesia-related deaths are classifiable in this subgroup.

Deaths due to diseases other than those for which the operation was undertaken, but which were diagnosed before the operation was commenced

A patient who is known to have a disease of a serious nature which by itself could cause death (e.g. valvular disease of the heart) may have to undergo an operation for another disease or injury. In these circumstances the risk to life may be greatly increased, but it may be desirable for the patient to undergo the operation and the administration of the anaesthetic. Should death then occur it may be considered to be due essentially to natural causes even though the operation and the anaesthetic may have precipitated the death. However, a competent anaesthetist would be expected to make due allowance for such pre-existing disease.

Deaths due to disease other than that for which the operation was undertaken, but which was not diagnosed before the operation was commenced

A post-mortem examination on a person who died in the perioperative period may reveal a lesion of a serious nature which could have been an important contributory factor in causing the death of the patient, but which was not diagnosed before the operation was undertaken. In a case of this nature it has to be determined whether the condition could reasonably have been diagnosed by a proper preoperative clinical examination. There are several diseases of a potentially serious nature, e.g. coronary artery arteriosclerosis, which may be clinically latent and which may not be detectable even after the most careful routine clinical examination. The failure to make a preoperative diagnosis of such a condition does not necessarily imply that the practitioner in attendance was negligent.

Surgical deaths

A surgical mishap during the administration of an anaesthetic may be responsible for the death of a patient. Such an incident, e.g. the accidental incision of a large blood vessel or aneurysm, is the direct responsibility of the surgeon.

Deaths which are the direct result of the administration of an anaesthetic

General

The state of general anaesthesia of necessity deprives the patient of the majority of his protective reflexes. Consequently, homeostatic mechanisms are disturbed, particularly those pertaining to the respiratory and cardiovascular systems. In addition, the anaesthetic agents and equipment themselves may pose hazards to the patient and a high degree of vigilance is demanded of the anaesthetist. A comprehensive review of the hazards of anaesthetics has been published in a special postgraduate educational issue of the *British Journal of Anaesthesia*.[4]

Deaths due to respiratory failure

General. In all recent studies of anaesthesia-related mortality, problems pertaining to the respiratory system were the single largest cause of death.[2,5–8] Respiratory failure in the anaesthesized patient may develop insidiously, as respiratory distress may not be obvious and cyanosis is a late sign. A serious degree of hypoxia may develop unless the anaesthetist maintains a high level of vigilance.

Airway obstruction. Loss of protective reflexes as a result of anaesthesia frequently leads to obstruction of the upper airway by the soft tissues of the mouth and pharynx. Irritation of the larynx in a lightly anaesthetized patient may provoke laryngeal spasm and consequent hypoxia; this is, however, seldom fatal as the spasm usually abates before the hypoxia becomes lethal. The larynx and trachea may become obstructed as a result of the impaction of foreign bodies such as swabs or dentures.

It must be remembered that foreign bodies may be dislodged from their site of impaction during the removal of thoracic organs from the chest cavity.[9] Endotracheal intubation is no guarantee of safety as the tubes may become obstructed in various ways, resulting in occlusion of the airway. Inadvertent misplacement of the endotracheal tube may result in airway obstruction going undetected until catastrophe occurs. Complications related to endotracheal intubation have recently been reviewed,[10] and problems related to endotracheal intubation were found to be among the commonest causes of anaesthesia-related mishaps.[8,11] Bronchiolar spasm may contribute to airway obstruction and may be due to many factors including pre-existing asthma, hypersensitivity to drugs, aspiration of gastric contents and fluid overload. On its own, however, this should seldom produce fatal hypoxia if properly managed.

Pneumothorax. Rupture of the lungs may result from the application of excessive pressure to the airway, but may also occur at normal ventilatory pressure if there is a pre-existing weakness in the lung. Positive pressure ventilation will rapidly convert a simple pneumothorax into a tension pneumothorax one with life-threatening consequences. The use of nitrous oxide will cause a pneumothorax to expand rapidly and may contribute to a fatal outcome.[12]

Aspiration of gastric contents. Active vomiting may be provoked by oropharyngeal manipulations in a lightly anaesthetized patient, but this seldom leads to serious aspiration as laryngeal protective mechanisms are still intact. Passive regurgitation during deep anaesthesia or following neuromuscular paralysis is a more serious event, and may lead to lethal pulmonary contamination.[13] Although massive regurgitation may lead to airway obstruction, this is an uncommon cause of death. More often, aspiration leads to a fatal outcome as a result of the subsequent broncho-pneumonia, or as a result of the development of non-cardiogenic pulmonary oedema now described as the adult respiratory distress syndrome. This complication, first described by Mendelson in 1946,[14]is particularly likely when the pH of the gastric contents is below 3.5, and is the commonest cause of anaesthesia-related mortality in obstetrics.[15]

The diagnosis of death as a result of aspiration has to be based on clinical features alone, as the amount of material found in the respiratory tract may be very small or absent if death is delayed by several days. Even when a large amount of material is found in the trachea it may be difficult to exclude the possibility of the material having 'welled up' and entered the trachea during the 'agonal' phase of death from some other cause. A similar process of regurgitation may occur after death, particularly in cases of putrefaction[16,17]

Respiratory depression. Ventilatory effort may be impaired during anaes-thesia either as a result of depression of the respiratory centre, or through muscular weakness. Almost all anaesthetic agents are respiratory depres-sants, and overdosage will result in inadequate ventilation, particularly in debilitated patients and those at the extremes of age. Inadequate ventilatory support following the use of neuromuscular blocking drugs has been cited as a frequent cause of death due to anaesthesia, and the effect of these drugs is potentiated by volatile anaesthetic agents. Postoperative ventilatory failure is often the result of inadequate reversal of these drugs,[2] whose actions may be prolonged by acidosis, some antibiotics and pre-existing neuromuscular disease.[18] Ventilatory failure may also follow epidural or spinal anaesthesia when the block extends into the high thoracic or cervical segments.

Equipment failure. Death may result from failure of the oxygen supply to the patient through misconnection of the pipelines, empty oxygen cylin-ders, leaks from the machine or disconnection of the anaesthetic circuit. The latter is particularly hazardous when the patient is paralysed with muscle relaxants, and artificial ventilation is being employed. Hypoxic mixtures may also be administered as a result of inaccuracies in the flow-meters, or through operator error.

Deaths due to cardiovascular failure during anaesthesia

General. All forms of anaesthesia alter cardiovascular homeostatic mech-anisms to a greater or lesser extent. Disorders of circulatory homeostasis form the second largest group of anaesthesia-related deaths.[2,5] General anaesthetic agents lower peripheral vascular resistance by depressing sympathetic outflow from medullary centres. In addition, they all display some calcium antagonism, and thus have direct vasodilator properties, as well as exerting a depressant action on the myocardium. These principal actions may be masked with some agents by a concomitant release of catecholamines.

Hypovolaemia. Unrecognized or inadequately managed hypovolaemia is the commonest cause of anaesthesia-related death attributable to the cardiovascular system. Deaths due to hypovolaemia may arise in a number of ways. Failure to recognize or to make adequate provision for preoperative hypovolaemia accounts for a significant proportion of these mishaps. The dosage of an anaesthetic drug or spinal or epidural anaesthetic which is safe in a normal patient may—through vasodilatation—convert a compensated hypovolaemia into an uncompensated lethal form. Inadequate volume replacement for intraoperative losses may contribute to death from surgically induced haemorrhage, although in some cases, operative bleeding may be such as to render adequate replacement impossible. Replacement of large quantities of blood lost leads to deficiencies in clotting factors of the blood and shock leads to the liberation of fibrinolysins which may cause death from uncontrollable haemorrhage unless adequate precautions are taken.

Where death has occurred from such hypovolaemia, autopsy is frequently unhelpful in establishing the cause. Over-enthusiastic fluid therapy may also contribute to anaesthesia-related mortality from pulmonary oedema or cardiac failure.

Cardiac arrhythmias. Fatal cardiac arrhythmias during anaesthesia may result from a number of factors, such as pre-existing disease, abnormal reactions to drugs, unskilful anaesthesia, surgical stimulation, or a combination of these. Elevated catecholamine levels from either endogenous or exogenous sources may precipitate arrhythmias particularly in combination with hypoxia, hypercarbia and halothane and from the injection of adrenaline. Forceful dilatation of the cervix, stimulation of the pharynx, larynx, abdominal and thoracic organs and the muscles of the eye may all result in vagal inhibition of the heart or in the release of catecholamines leading to arrhythmias.[19,20] Electrolyte disturbances, particularly of extracellular potassium and magnesium predispose to the development of dysrhythmias. The administration of suxamethonium may provoke arrhythmias by releasing large amounts of potassium especially in patients with burns or muscular denervation.

Diminished myocardial contractility. Myocardial performance may be impaired by a number of factors, including metabolic disorders, electrolyte imbalances, hypoxia, hypothermia, drugs and acute myocardial ischaemia. Although most anaesthetic drugs exert their principal depressant actions on vascular tone, almost all interfere with myocardial contractility to some degree, and overdosage will produce negative inotropic effects. Disruption of myocardial integrity by ischaemia will have profound effects on contractility, and anaesthesia and surgery may precipitate ischaemia in susceptible subjects. Pre-existing disease of the myocardium will predispose to reductions in contractility, and imbalance of oxygen demand to supply will lead to ischaemia and possible infarction. The myocardial risk factors for non-cardiac surgery have been evaluated by Goldman et al.[21]

Miscellaneous causes. Mishaps related to the cardiovascular and respiratory systems account for the vast majority of anaesthesia-related deaths. There are, however, a number of other conditions which contribute to anaesthesia-related mortality to a significant degree.

Complications of regional anaesthesia

Regional anaesthesia may contribute to a fatal outcome through systemic toxicity of the agents used, or as a result of complications of the technique. Systemic toxicity is most commonly manifested in the central nervous system, producing convulsions. Subconvulsant doses rarely produce significant cardiac depression, although intractable cardiac arrest has been reported with bupivicaine administered for intravenous regional anaesthesia. Systemic toxicity of these drugs may be related to overdosage, although it is more commonly associated with inadvertent intravascular injection. Regional procedures around the spinal column such as epidural, spinal and paravertebral blocks may cause death through cardiovascular collapse from autonomic blockade, or by respiratory paralysis or both. Procedures involving the chest wall such as supraclavicular brachial plexus block or intercostal block may produce a potentially fatal pneumothorax, and procedures in the neck may block the phrenic nerve, which may lead to respiratory failure in a patient with pulmonary disease.

Adverse drug reactions. The role of adverse reactions to drugs in anaesthesia-related mortality has been debated.[22,23] Adverse reactions to anaesthetic drugs are not uncommon, but infrequently lead to death as full resuscitative facilities and expertise should be immediately available in the theatre environment. The frequency of these reactions has recently been estimated at about 0.2% of all anaesthetics and although some are of the minor histaminoid type, most presented with life-threatening bronchospasm and acute hypotension. The majority of reactions involved intravenous induction agents and/or muscle relaxants but there was little evidence to suggest that they were immune mediated or drug specific.[24] Death due to massive hepatitis following the use of halothane is a much-debated and complex topic. On balance it would appear that halothane is capable of producing hepatic injury in susceptible patients under certain conditions, but that the condition is extremely rare with an incidence of less than 1:10000.[25]

Malignant hyperthermia[2] (see p. 28). This very rare inherited condition is important in anaesthetic practice as the syndrome is triggered by various anaesthetic agents and carries a high mortality. The diagnosis requires a careful family history of anaesthesia-related disaster and is confirmed on muscle biopsy. Once the diagnosis is made, the use of dantroline sodium and avoidance of trigger agents will prevent occurrence of the syndrome. Where the condition occurs unexpectedly, it is characterized by a rapid rise in body temperature with muscle rigidity, followed by severe metabolic disturbance and death. Prompt administration of dantroline will usually abort the attack.

Others. Other factors may contribute to anaesthesia-related mortality, but they are all rare. The most important of these is air embolism which most commonly occurs during neurosurgical procedures undertaken in the sitting position, with the air entering the venous system through vessels in the skull bones.

Electrocution due to defective equipment has caused deaths in the operating theatre. Even very small currents may lead to ventricular fibrillation, e.g. in the presence of intracardiac leads and catheters. The hazards of electrocution in the operating theatre have been recently reviewed by Hull.[26]

Fires and explosions related to the use of inflammable anaesthetic agents have caused fatalities. These agents have virtually disappeared from modern anaesthetic practice, but surgical spirit, drapes and nebulizers have all been responsible for fires.[27]

AUTOPSY FINDINGS IN 'ANAESTHETIC' DEATHS

The causes of 'anaesthetic' deaths have been classified in the preceding section of this chapter. The findings at autopsy will vary according to the cause of death. Unfortunately, however, there are no diagnostic findings at autopsy in most instances because there are no pathognomic pathological changes found in deaths caused by anoxia nor in acute cardiovascular collapse unless there is some underlying cause, such as a myocardial infarction.

Engorgement of the dependent portions of the viscera is commonly seen when death follows prolonged anaesthesia. The distribution of this engorgement in the viscera depends upon the posture of the patient during the operation. Dependent engorgement should not be confused with the congestive changes of pathological processes.

INQUESTS OR ENQUIRIES AND 'ANAESTHETIC' DEATHS

A study of the classification of the causes of 'anaesthetic' deaths set out in this chapter shows that factors other than the administration of the anaesthetic are often responsible for the death of a patient. Moreover, some of the deaths which are the direct result of the administration of an anaesthetic cannot be anticipated or prevented.

One of the purposes of an inquest is to determine whether there is any *prima facie* evidence of criminal liability on the part of the anaesthetist or any other person who attended to the patient. The onus of proof of the negligent killing of persons differs in criminal and delictual (or civil) law. Whereas in criminal law the negligence must be established beyond reasonable doubt, in civil law the negligence must be established upon a preponderance of probability. In applying these criteria, a magistrate or presiding judicial officer is likely to consider the following questions:

1. Was *informed* consent obtained for the operation and the administration of the anaesthetic?
2. Was an operation and/or the administration of an anaesthetic necessary in the circumstances?
3. Was the patient properly examined before the operation and was his fitness to undergo the operation assessed with reasonable skill and care?
4. Was the patient suitably prepared for the operation and the administration of the anaesthetic?
5. Was a suitable form of anaesthetic administered?
6. Was the anaesthetic administered and the operation performed with reasonable skill and care?
7. Were suitable and adequate arrangements made before the operation to deal with any emergency which might arise during the administration of the anaesthetic?
8. When the emergency arose, were suitable steps taken immediately to resuscitate the patient?
9. Were suitable and adequate arrangements made to ensure the safe recovery of the patient?

REFERENCES

1 Lunn J N, Mushin W W. Mortality associated with anaesthesia (monograph). London: Nuffield Provincial Hospitals Trust. 1982.
2 Harrison G G. Deaths attributable to anaesthesia. A 10-year survey (1967–1976). Br J Anaesth 1978; 50: 1041–1046.
3 Sherlock S. Halothane hepatitis. Lancet 1978; 2: 364–365.
4 Hull C J, Norman J. eds. Hazards of Anaesthesia. Br J Anaesth 1978; 50:639.
5 Cooper J B, Newbower R S, Long C D, McPeek B. Preventable anesthesia mishaps: a study of human factors. Anesthesiology 1978; 49: 309–406.
6 Craig J, Wilson M E. A survey of anaesthetic misadventures. Anaesthesia 1981; 36: 933–936.
7 Solazzi R W, Ward R J. The spectrum of medical liability cases. Int Anesthes Clin 1984; 22: 43–51.
8 Holland R. Anesthetic mishaps in Australia. Int Anesthes Clin 1984; 22: 61–71.
9 Robertson I. A swab in the bronchus—a medico-legal problem. J Forens Med 1961; 8: 157–160.
10 Harmer M. Complications of tracheal intubation. In: Latto I P, Rosen M. eds. Difficulties in tracheal intubation. London: Balliere Tindall. 1985: pp 36–47.
11 Green R A, Taylor T H. An analysis of anesthesia medical liability claims in the United Kingdom, 1977–1982. Int. Anesthes Clin 1984; 22: 73–89.
12 Coleman A J. Uptake and distribution of anaesthetic agents. In: Churchill-Davidson H C. ed. A practice of anaesthesia. London: Lloyd-Luke (Medical Books). 1984: pp 223–238.
13 Morton H J V, Wylie W D. Anaesthetic deaths due to regurgitation or vomiting. Anaesthesia 1951; 6: 190–201.

14 Mendelson C L. The aspiration of stomach contents into the lungs during obstetric anaesthesia. Am J Obstet Gynecol 1946; 52: 191–205.

15 Hunter A R, Moir D D. Confidential enquiry into maternal deaths. Br J Anaesth 1983; 55: 367–369.

16 Gardner A M N. Aspiration of food and vomit. Quart J Med 1958; 27: 227–242.

17 Shapiro H. The significance of foreign matter seen in the respiratory tract after death. J Forens Med 1958; 5: 161–162.

18 Vickers M D, Wood-Smith F G, Stewart H C. Drugs in anaesthetic practice, 5th ed. London: Butterworths. 1978: pp 273–305.

19 Reid L C, Brace D E. Irritation of the respiratory tract and its reflex effect upon the heart. Surg Gynec Obstet 1940; 70: 157–162.

20 Simpson K. Deaths from vagal inhibition. Lancet 1949; 256: 558–560.

21 Goldman L, Caldera D L, Nussbaum S R. et al. Multifactorial index of cardiac risk in non-cardiac surgical procedures. N Engl J Med 1977; 297: 845–896.

22 Hamilton W K. Unexpected deaths during anesthesia: wherein lies the cause? Anesthesiology 1979; 50: 381–383.

23 Keats A S. What do we know about anesthetic mortality? Anesthesiology 1979; 50: 387–392.

24 Watkins J. Adverse anaesthetic reactions. An update from a proposed national reporting and advisory service. Anaesthesia 1985; 40: 797–800.

25 Strunin L, Davies J M. The liver and anaesthesia. Can Anaesth Soc J 1983; 30: 208–217.

26 Hull C J. Electrocution hazards in the operating theatre. Br J Anaesth 1978; 50: 647–657.

27 Vickers M D. Fire and explosion hazards in operating theatres. Br J Anaesth 1978; 50: 659–684.

10

Poisoning and forensic medicine

This chapter deals with poisoning in relation to forensic medicine, as follows:

1. The clinical aspects of poisoning—clinical toxicology;
2. Suspected poisoning;
3. The post-mortem detection of poisons;
4. The submission of specimens for chemical analysis;
5. The interpretation of toxicological findings;
6. The concept of the fatal dose.

THE CLINICAL ASPECTS OF POISONING—CLINICAL TOXICOLOGY

In his work on *poisoning by chemicals in agriculture and public health*, Fourie[1] writes as follows:

> There are more than five million chemical compounds in the world, of which approximately 80 000 or any permutation thereof, are used daily in the industrial, domestic, pharmaceutical and agricultural sectors of society. It is estimated that these numbers grow by as much as 1000 compounds per annum, either by synthetic preparations or by isolation from naturally occurring plant or animal life.

The complexities involved in the presentation of information about available potentially poisonous commercial and household products in various countries led to a coincident presentation of the problem by Gleason *et al*[2] in 1967 and the establishment of Poison Centres of Information in many large cities in the world.

There is widespread accidental poisoning of children following ingestion of commercial and household products. Accidental poisoning of adolescents and adults occurs, not only following the ingestion of commercial and household products, but also from the widespread use of poisonous chemicals and pesticides in the field of agriculture and public health.

Clinical toxicology and toxicology are major subjects with a broad base in human medicine and veterinary medicine. In books on forensic medicine, regardless of tradition, it is impractical to set out a catalogue of the names, modes of action and effects of all or even a selection of poisons. Accordingly we have advised students of medicine and medical practitioners to rely upon reference to regional poison centres or to have access to a major and comprehensive treatment manual.

In order to appreciate the magnitude of the problem of accidental and suicidal poisoning in relation to the availability of innumerable chemical compounds, the following extract is taken from Gosselin, Smith, Hodge and Braddock.[3]

> The original purpose of this book was to assist the physician in dealing quickly and effectively with acute chemical poisonings arising through misuse of consumer products. The book provides (a) a list of trade name products together with their ingredients, (b) addresses and telephone numbers of companies for use when descriptions of products are not available, (c) sample formulas of many types of products with an estimate of the toxicity of each formula, (d) toxicological information including an appraisal of toxicity of individual ingredients, and (e) recommendations for treatment and supportive care.
>
> We suggest that the physician take time to understand the organization of the material in the seven sections of the book before an emergency arises. An illustrative chart, *How to Use This Manual*, appears inside the front cover. A study of this guide, with hypothetical cases in mind, is recommended. The contents of each section are briefly described below.
>
> Over the years a second purpose of this reference manual has received increasing emphasis, namely to acquaint therapists and others with the pathophysiological mechanisms induced by various poisons, insofar as they are understood. The book now contains detailed documentation not only of published case reports but of clinical and experimental research papers as well, which should make this compilation more useful to the professional toxicologist. Such citations are now extensive in both *Sections II and III* and to some extent in *Section IV* (see below), but with few exceptions the literature coverage in this edition does not extend beyond 1982. We have taken pains to point out areas of uncertainty or disagreement where they exist because these areas represent important gaps in knowledge and therefore opportunities for future research. Although the primary emphasis is on acute toxicity, issues of chronic toxicity and teratogenic, carcinogenic and mutagenic effects have not been totally neglected.
>
> *Section I. First Aid and General Emergency Treatment*
> As a synopsis of the physician's role in chemical poisonings from the first phone call to the final disposition, this section outlines in sequence the general emergency procedures and precautions required in all cases of acute poisoning. Included are references to relevant material in other sections.
>
> *Section II. Ingredients Index*
> This section contains an alphabetical list of chemical substances (ingredients) commonly found in commercial products used by the consumer in and around the home and farm. Ingredients are also indexed by CAS (Chemical Abstract Service) registry numbers. The acute toxicity of each ingredient has been estimated ('toxicity rating'). Included for almost every ingredient is a brief description of toxic effects and/or cross references to more detailed information in *Sections III and IV*. Consult the Introduction to *Section II* for more information.

Section III. Therapeutics Index
Section III summarizes clinical and experimental data on 85 compounds (or classes of compounds) which are named '*reference congeners*' in *Section II* because each typifies a group of related substances. This section stresses toxic signs and symptoms and recommended programs of therapy.

Section IV. Supportive Treatment
In this section techniques of supportive treatment are discussed, with particular emphasis on those problems encountered frequently in clinical toxicology.

Section V. Trade Name Index
Here are listed alphabetically over 15 000 trade names of products which might be ingested accidentally or suicidally. For almost all items the category of use is indicated, e.g., rodenticide, silver polish, hair dye. In most cases the ingredients are stated, with asterisks marking those components expected to be responsible for harmful effects. With each product the manufacturer's name is given.

Section VI. General Formulations
This section presents formulas for the diverse types of products listed in the *Trade Name Index*. These formulas are believed to be 'basic,' 'typical,' or 'representative' and give some guidance to physicians when the trade name of an ingested substance is not known or when information about its ingredients cannot be obtained easily. A method of estimating a toxicity rating for each product is described in the introduction to this section.

Section VII. Manufacturers' Index
The names, addresses and, when available, telephone numbers of all manufacturers of products appearing in the *Trade Name Index* are listed for the convenience of physicians who wish to phone or write for further information.

The products listed in this book represent a wide sampling of the many thousands of items available on the market and used in homes, on farms, in small businesses, in institutions and industries—wherever toxic materials might be accessible to the public. Many of the products are relatively harmless, but are included because an attending physician needs assurance that an ingested substance is innocuous, if it is, as well as information concerning the ingredients of a product that is potentially poisonous.

Where to limit the list of trade name descriptions has been a problem. Our initial objective—to describe only products used in homes and on farms, which automatically excluded materials marketed solely for industrial use—has been modified somewhat. Many 'industrial' products can now be purchased by do-it-yourself workers, hobbyists, and owners of small businesses, and so, in the absence of industrial health safeguards, become accessible to small children. On the other hand, the wide use of commercial products in institutional and industrial environments has greatly expanded the need of physicians for toxicological information about these products.

Many commercial commodities were deliberately excluded, e.g., structural materials and objects which are hazardous only because of possible physical injury, e.g. broken glass. Most poisonous plants and animal venoms have been omitted. Foods, food products, and dietary supplements are not listed unless the contents of vitamin A, vitamin D, or iron are high.

In preparing this material it was recognized that changes in formulas are frequent, that new products are marketed daily and old ones discontinued. To achieve some degree of accuracy in describing the merchandise presented in this index, contributing manufacturers are given repeated opportunities to edit descriptions of their products throughout the years between the publication of the last edition in 1976 and the appearance of the present volume. A similar procedure is planned to keep this index up to date.

The present volume represents the culmination of studies and work that have continued without interruption since the first edition was published. The authors recognize the limitations of a reference volume appearing once in five to eight years to deal with a subject that changes so rapidly. In years past we have attempted to cope with this problem by preparing monthly a bulletin with the same format as the parent volume *Clinical Toxicology of Commercial Products* (*CTCP*). Such a mechanism we now believe is an anachronism in this electronic and computerized age. Beginning with the 4th edition we prepared various parts of this manual in machine-readable form. These parts now include *Section II, Section V* and the bibliographies to each congener in *Section III*. This material we refer to as the *CTCP Data Base*. An earlier version of this data base constituted one of the modules of the NIH-EPA Chemical Information System (CIS) which was available online nationwide and worldwide to subscribers who had access to the communications network Telenet. Other computerized versions of this data base are expected to be developed and marketed in the future.

The authors have often been told that their task is an impossible one. If the book were as all-inclusive as its title purports, i.e., if the purpose were to describe all commercial products with toxic potentialities, we would heartily agree with our critics. The coverage is admittedly incomplete. The goal has been to list the hardy perrennials and the current annuals and to omit the obsolescent and evanescent thousands. For instance, hundreds of cosmetic products come on and go off the market annually. Although most of these are not included by name, the book by no means neglects them; thus the ingredients in sample or prototype formulations are listed in *Section VI*, together with estimates of the toxicities of the products. Because there are many similarities in the formulas of such products as perfumes and cold wave lotions, whoever the manufacturer, the *General Formulations Section* seems to offer the best solution to the problem of saving space while providing physicians with needed information.

Material in all sections has been extensively revised and in many places completely rewritten. Toxicity data are more extensive and more intensive than in earlier editions.

As already noted, all product information has been brought up to date; final changes were introduced during 1983. The pages of each section are numbered in sequence separately from all other sections; the appropriate section number and title appearing at the top of each page to serve to designate the section. This convention was adopted to simplify the printing process and so to reduce its cost. Citations to the medical and toxicological literature are located throughout *Section II* with references at the end of the section. References are given throughout *Section III* and occasionally in *Sections IV and VI*. In addition, general references useful in clinical toxicology are listed in *Section I* (pp 17 and 18).

SUSPECTED POISONING

Poisoning may be (1) accidental, (2) suicidal, or (3) criminal.

1. Accidental poisoning

When a patient has been accidentally poisoned the medical practitioner is not required to take any action unless the poisoning has arisen in the course of the patient's employment. In most countries there are provisions in Public Health and Workmen's Compensation enactments whereby a medical practitioner is required to notify the authorities in the event of poisoning arising in the course of a patient's employment. In certain circumstances legal action may be instituted when poisoning is due to negligence, or when there has been a breach of the law in regard to the keeping and disposal of poisons. In such cases, if the medical practitioner is approached by an investigating officer, it is his duty to give the officer any information which he may have obtained relating to the poisoning.

If the patient dies, the practitioner must refuse to sign a death certificate.

2. Suicidal poisoning

In certain countries attempted suicide is a criminal offence. In other countries attempted suicide is not a crime. In countries where attempted suicide is not a crime, in dealing with a patient who has attempted to commit suicide, the medical practitioner must exercise professional secrecy and confine himself to the treatment of his patient. In certain circumstances it may be necessary for the patient's own protection to take action to prevent further attempts at suicide. If the patient appears to be suffering from a mental illness, further action may be necessary in order to ensure that the patient receives proper care and treatment. If a question arises in regard to the circumstances in which the poison was obtained it may be the duty of the medical practitioner to give information as in cases of accidental poisoning.

If the patient dies the medical practitioner must refuse to sign a death certificate.

3. Suspected criminal poisoning

General considerations

When a medical practitioner suspects that a patient is being criminally poisoned he is placed in a difficult position. On the one hand there is the unhappy prospect of unwelcome publicity, actions for damages, and perhaps the ruin of a practice if a mistaken accusation of poisoning is made. On the other hand there is the undoubted duty placed on the medical practitioner to protect and save the life of his patient. In the well-known Scottish poisoning case of Reg. *v.* Pritchard[4] the victim's physician was severely criticized by the Judge for his behaviour, in that he took no action when he had become convinced that his patient was being poisoned. The Judge said that no considerations of professional etiquette could stand in the way of the far higher duty 'owed by every right-minded man to his neighbour' to prevent the destruction of human life, in which duty the medical practitioner had failed.

The clinical difficulties of diagnosis are well known. The symptoms of poisoning may simulate a disease process, e.g. arsenical poisoning may be mistaken for gastro-enteritis, and strychnine poisoning may be mistaken for tetanus. Conversely the symptoms of a disease process may simulate acute poisoning, e.g. the sudden onset of an acute intestinal affection such as intestinal obstruction may be mistaken for irritant metal poisoning.

The medical practitioner should also be on his guard against simulated poisoning which is often the result of hysterical delusions. In certain circumstances patients may poison themselves in an attempt to throw suspicion on other persons.

Suggested procedure when criminal poisoning is suspected

1. When criminal poisoning is suspected every effort must be made to move the patient to a hospital or nursing home, where the necessary treatment and investigation can be undertaken with safety and discretion.

2. If the patient refuses to be moved, the medical practitioner should try to get him to agree to employ a nurse. This nurse should then be made solely responsible for the preparation and serving of all the patient's meals and the custody and administration of all his medicines. If a nurse who is not known to the medical practitioner is already employed by the patient, it may be advisable to dispense with her services and to employ a nurse in whom the medical practitioner has confidence.

3. If a particular person is suspected, attempts should be made to circumvent him (or her) by changes of diet and the alteration of meal times. It is also advisable to allow such a person to visit the patient only in the presence of a nurse or physician.

The medical practitioner should observe whether any person appears unduly attentive to the patient, e.g. a suspicion may arise when a person insists on preparing all the food and giving it to the patient personally. Suspicion may also be aroused if the person on various pretexts insists on throwing away all the food which the patient leaves.

4. If it is suspected that medicine is being poisoned it may be possible to devise some simple test whereby the presence of poison is demonstrated by a change in the colour or taste of the medicine.

5. Detailed notes should be kept of the case history as the medical practitioner may be called upon to give evidence in legal proceedings many months after the poisoning or death of the patient.

6. Specimens of faeces, vomited material, and hair should be taken whenever possible for toxicological examination. It is advisable to retain samples of the food for toxicological analysis.

Considerable ingenuity may be required in order to avoid causing anxiety to the patient or putting the poisoner on his guard.

The specimen which is most easily obtained is a specimen of urine. The medical practitioner should collect such a specimen himself. He should satisfy himself that the container which he intends using is chemically clean, and after he has collected the specimen he should personally seal the container and see that it is properly labelled for purposes of identification. No preservative should be added to the urine. Instructions for the forwarding of specimens for toxicological analysis are given at page 214.

7. If the patient's condition becomes grave the medical practitioner should insist on his removal to hospital, in spite of all protests.

8. It is advisable for the medical practitioner to take a colleague into his confidence. In certain circumstances the patient and/or his relatives should be told of the medical practitioner's suspicions, but this should be done with extreme care. The medical practitioner should only inform the relatives if he is completely satisfied that they can be trusted to act discreetly.

9. When the medical practitioner is convinced that his patient is being poisoned he should inform the police. The medical practitioner should place himself at the disposal of the police authorities.

If the patient dies the medical practitioner must refuse to give a death certificate.

Difficulties arising in practice

The difficulties with which a medical practitioner may be faced are well illustrated in the case of Rex v. Lee:[5]

> A medical practitioner was asked to attend to a patient whom he had known in the army and whom he had previously treated for a gastric ailment. The patient showed signs of some acute gastric disturbance. The medical practitioner was introduced to the patient's reputed wife, who appeared to be genuinely disturbed about her 'husband's' condition, and who was anxious that everything possible should be done for him. The medical practitioner began to suspect chronic arsenical poisoning when the symptoms failed to respond to treatment. His position became one of extreme difficulty. The patient's 'wife' was solely responsible for the nursing and for the preparation of the patient's food. The patient consistently and obstinately refused the services of a trained nurse and refused to go to hospital. At that stage any suggestion to the patient of the medical practitioner's suspicions would undoubtedly have led to the immediate dismissal of the medical practitioner and a possible action for defamation. The symptoms (as is so often the case in arsenical poisoning) were protean.
>
> The medical practitioner decided to take no action until he could obtain a clearer diagnosis. A sample of vomited material was obtained, but for various reasons the toxicologist to whom it was submitted felt that an analysis would not be satisfactory. Before a urine sample could be obtained, the patient developed what appeared to be a scarlatina rash and he was removed by the Public Health authorities to an isolation hospital.
>
> Tests for scarlatina proved negative, the patient rapidly recovered, and was discharged. Several months later the medical practitioner was again called to see the patient, but when he arrived the patient was moribund and died within a few hours. The medical practitioner correctly refused to sign a death

certificate and reported the matter to the magistrate. After police investigations the 'wife' of the deceased man was charged and convicted of the murder of her reputed husband by arsenical poisoning.

THE POST-MORTEM DETECTION OF POISONS

The procedure that should be followed at exhumation in a case of suspected poisoning is described at page 78.

In cases of accidental and suicidal poisoning, a medical practitioner is usually informed by the police of a suspicion of poisoning before he commences the autopsy. In homicidal poisoning, however, there is commonly no suspicion of poisoning before the autopsy is performed. In a proportion of these cases some pathological change suggestive of poisoning may be detected at the autopsy, but many poisons, such as the alkaloids, produce no characteristic tissue changes (below). For this reason cases of poisoning may be overlooked in spite of a careful post-mortem examination; and this is more likely to occur if some pre-existing lesion which could have caused death is found on dissection.

Although it is often difficult to determine whether a person has been poisoned or not, attention may be directed to some of the post-mortem signs which occur in cases of poisoning.

General

The pathological manifestations of chemical poisons have been divided into four groups by Jetter[6] as follows:

Group 1. No morphological change is found which can be attributed to the direct chemical action of the agent. Lesions, if present are due to terminal systemic hypoxia, and are dependent on the duration and the severity of the agonal period of circulatory failure. Many poisons are classifiable in this group and particularly those which are rapidly fatal. They include the acute central nervous system depressants, such as alcohol, ether, and hydrocarbons; the chemical 'asphyxiants' such as carbon monoxide and cyanide; and many of the alkaloids. Many poisons which are potentially capable of producing recognizable structural alterations fall in this group when the dose is so great as to cause death before local lesions have had time to develop.

Group 2. Systemic lesions are produced without evidence of injury at the portal of entry. Examples of this group are the acute haemolytic poisons such as arsine and nitrobenzene.

Group 3. Injury is produced at the portal of entry without remote systemic evidence of direct injury. The corrosives and some of the gaseous irritants are the best examples of this group. The local pathological lesion may be the factor immediately responsible for death, e.g. through pulmonary oedema following the inhalation of gaseous irritant, or from acute vasomotor collapse.

Group 4. Both local and systemic evidence of injury is found. The outstanding group of poisons which cause both local and systemic injury are the heavy metals, although numerous other chemicals may be included in this category.

External examination

The colour of the patches of post-mortem lividity may be of value in raising a suspicion of poisoning, e.g. in carbon monoxide poisoning the patches of lividity are pink or red in colour (p. 129) and in potassium chlorate or aniline poisoning the patches of lividity are brown in colour (p. 35).

In cases of death from drug abuse, the skin should be inspected for recent needle punctures and linear needle track scars and if the skin shows tattoo marks, these should be examined for fresh injection sites or scars.[7]

In all cases the skin should be examined for lesions, e.g. hyperkeratosis and pigmentation may be found in chronic arsenical poisoning. The presence of jaundice raises the possibility of liver necrosis, which may occur in senecio and phosphorus poisoning. Jaundice may also arise, in susceptible persons, from acute haemolytic anaemia following the use of certain drugs such as potassium chlorate.

In poisoning by corrosives, areas of discoloration and sloughing may be found in the region of the lips and mouth.

Internal examination

The brain

It is always advisable to open the skull at the commencement of an autopsy in order to detect unusual odours in the brain tissues, before such odours become masked by the opening of the body cavities. This testing by smell is of particular value in cyanide poisoning, as a characteristic odour of bitter almonds may be detected. Other substances which may be recognized at autopsy by their odour are alcohol, phenol, cresols, ether, chloroform and camphor.

The alimentary system

The pharynx. Areas of necrosis of the pharynx may be observed in deaths associated with agranulocytosis caused by drugs such as amido-pyrine, thiouracil, dinitrophenol, sulphonamides and barbiturates.

The oesophagus, stomach and intestines. The corrosive effects of strong acids and some metallic salts on the mucous membrane of the oesophagus and stomach may be readily recognized. This corrosive action may extend through the stomach wall and affect neighbouring viscera such as the liver and pancreas. Corrosive alkalis produce marked softening and desquamation of the mucous membrane of the oesophagus, but they frequently have no effect on the mucous membrane of the stomach, owing to their neutralization by the acid of the gastric juice. Corrosive poisons are rarely used for homicidal purposes.

Auto-digestion of the mucous membrane of the lower part of the oesophagus and of the stomach must not be mistaken for the corrosive action of acids or alkalis.

There are often no characteristic changes in the mucous membrane of the stomach in irritant metal poisoning, as some of the salts of the metals are highly soluble and are rapidly absorbed, e.g. arsenites may be readily absorbed without causing any signs of congestion of the mucous membrane of the stomach. Haemorrhages of varying size may be found in the mucous membrane in acute arsenical poisoning, but this change is frequently seen in other forms of death, including deaths from natural causes.

In acute cantharidin poisoning, which is relatively common in parts of Africa, changes may be observed in the oesophagus and stomach. The mucous membrane of the oesophagus is often swollen and engorged, and may show patches of ulceration. The gastric mucous membrane is almost invariably markedly congested and usually shows petechial haemorrhages with foci of superficial erosion in its substance. These changes may extend to the upper portion of the small intestine. Close examination of the contents and the surface of the mucous membrane of the stomach and intestines, with a hand lens if necessary, may reveal particles of the coloured wing cases of the beetles responsible for cantharidin poisoning. Medical practitioners should be able to recognize these coloured particles.

A characteristic change in the intestines is seen in mercury poisoning. This change, which usually involves the ascending and transverse colons, is a diphtheritic colitis which may resemble the enteritis of acute bacillary dysentery.

The liver. Senecio poisoning and poisoning by substances such as phosphorus, chloroform, trinitrotoluene, and carbon tetrachloride may produce liver necrosis. In senecio poisoning, the seeds and other portions of the senecio plants are gathered with the wheat, and through ineffective sieving and winnowing become incorporated in the flour. Chronic senecio poisoning may give rise to cirrhosis of the liver with ascites.

The kidneys

Parenchymatous degenerative changes are often demonstrable in the kidneys in cases of acute poisoning. Such changes are commonly found in irritant metal poisoning and in cantharidin poisoning. Extensive necrosis of the proximal convoluted tubules may be found in deaths from poisoning by mercuric chloride, phenol, lysol and carbon tetrachloride.[8] Precipitation of crystals of the sulpha group of drugs may cause death by blockage of the tubules or ureters. In one of our cases a combination of sulphathiazole and sulphapyridine caused fatal uraemia through extensive kidney lesions resulting from the precipitation of crystals of the drugs in the tubules.

The respiratory system

The larynx, trachea and bronchi. Oedema of the glottis and congestion and desquamation of the mucous membrane of the trachea and bronchi may be seen in corrosive poisoning when the corrosive acid or alkali has entered the respiratory tract. These changes are seen most commonly in corrosive poisoning in young children.

The lungs. As a general rule the lungs show the non-specific signs of congestion and oedema but marked congestion and massive oedema may be produced by the inhalation of irritant gases such as chlorine.

A terminal hypostatic pneumonia often develops in cases of narcotic poisoning, where the unconsciousness has persisted for 24–36 hours or longer.

The heart

The most common finding in the heart, apart from parenchymatous degenerative changes, are subendocardial haemorrhages in the left ventricle. These haemorrhages occur in most cases of acute arsenical poisoning, and are most commonly situated under the endocardium lining the posterior wall of the left ventricle. Subendocardial haemorrhages are highly characteristic of acute arsenical poisoning, but they are not pathognomic of this condition. Similar haemorrhages occur in other forms of poisoning and in many types of violent death and in deaths from natural causes.

Non-specific changes

Non-specific general pathological changes, as described in Chapter 3, are present.

THE SUBMISSION OF SPECIMENS FOR CHEMICAL ANALYSIS

Medical practitioners should be thoroughly familiar with the procedure that must be adopted in the submission of viscera for toxicological analysis.

As a general rule the only specimens that need be sent for toxicological analysis are the stomach and its contents, the liver, and both kidneys. The ligatured stomach must never be sent to an analyst without being opened, as putrefaction may not only obscure changes in the mucous membrane but the gases evolved may result in the lid of the jar being forced off in transit. The stomach must be opened along its lesser curvature in a clean porcelain dish. In this way the stomach contents can be examined and the mucous membrane of the organ inspected. In most magisterial and administrative districts in all countries, a toxicological box is allotted to a district. A medical practitioner, responsible for autopsy work in the district, should see that a toxicological box is always available in his district. A toxicological box usually contains two stoneware jars.

The medical practitioner responsible for an autopsy in these circumstances, should break the seals of the toxicological box and remove the stoneware jars. The stomach and its contents should be transferred into the smaller of the two jars provided, and the whole liver and both kidneys should be placed in the larger of the two jars.

The chemical examination of specimens for toxicological analysis is usually carried out at a State Chemical Laboratory established in the capital city of the country or in corresponding cities in county or provincial administrations. If the specimens can reach the laboratory within 48 hours no preservative need be added to the viscera. In all other cases, spirits of wine (rectified spirit) must be added as a preservative to each jar. Methylated spirits must not be used as a preservative.

After the preservative has been added the jars are closed, sealed and labelled. The label should set out the nature of the contents, the name of the deceased, the date, and the signature of the medical practitioner. The jars and a labelled and sealed bottle containing a sample of the preservative should be placed in the toxicological box, and the box should be handed over to the police.

In certain circumstances, it may be necessary to submit specimens for analysis from other parts of the body. For instance, poisons may be absorbed from the uterus and in cases of criminal abortion it may be necessary to send the vagina and the uterus for analysis. Additional jars should be procured from the central or regional chemical laboratory for this purpose. In addition, poisons may be injected into the tissues. In one of our cases it was suspected that an overdose of adrenaline had been injected during treatment for asthma, and it became necessary to submit a portion of the soft tissues of the arm for analysis.

In arsenical poisoning the arsenic is excreted into the epidermal tissues, and in cases of intermittent chronic poisoning there will be successive deposits of arsenic in the hairs. With the first administration, the arsenic is initially excreted into the root of the hair, and as the hair grows the deposit of arsenic is moved distally with the hair. If, after a few weeks or months, a further quantity of arsenic is ingested, arsenic is again excreted into the root of the hair. As the hair continues to grow, the fresh deposit of arsenic is moved distally with the hair and the two deposits are separated by a portion of hair containing a relatively small amount of the substance. By analysing the different sections of a hair it is possible to determine the probable number of doses of arsenic ingested by the deceased. Further, from the approximate rate of growth of hair,* it may be possible to determine the times when the arsenic was administered. This method of analysis was of particular value in the case of Rex v. Lee[5] as the Crown sought to establish that in addition to the fatal administration the accused had administered a dose of arsenic to her reputed husband several months before his death.

In cases of suspected chronic arsenical poisoning, several complete nails

---

* Smith[9] states that hair grows at the rate of about half an inch per month.

and a tuft of hair should be sent for toxicological analysis. A large tuft of hair from the head should be selected and the hairs should be tied together before they are removed. The hairs should then be removed by their roots and should be so labelled as to enable the analyst to identify the proximal and distal portions of the hairs. No preservative should be added to the hairs or nails.

All specimens submitted to the central or regional chemical laboratory should be accompanied by a copy of the post-mortem report, together with a statement setting out all the details that are known about the alleged poisoning.

THE INTERPRETATION OF TOXICOLOGICAL FINDINGS

As a general rule, toxicologists' reports are handed into Court in affidavit form. The medical practitioner or pathologist who conducted the autopsy is usually required to interpret the toxicological findings. Such interpretation may be extremely difficult and depends upon knowledge of the following factors: the known properties and pharmacological action of the poison; the chemical stability of the poison; the mode of absorption, distribution, metabolism and elimination of the poison by the body; the age, development and physical condition of the deceased; the character of the clinical features of the illness preceding death and the autopsy findings.

The chemical stability of poisons is variable. Certain inorganic poisons cannot be destroyed by the tissue. When a substance such as arsenic is ingested in the form of a salt, chemical action may convert the salt into some other derivative of arsenic, but if the period of time that has elapsed between the ingestion and the death has not been sufficiently long for the arsenic to be excreted, the element can always be recovered from the viscera or tissues. Arsenic may be recovered from the body many years after burial.

Poisoning may be caused by the toxic salts of certain elements. Non-toxic salts of such elements may be present normally in the tissues of the body (e.g. potassium chlorate is poisonous but several potassium salts are normally found in the tissues). The rate at which toxic salts of this nature are converted by the tissues into non-toxic derivatives is variable. Unless such toxic salts are recovered from the stomach contents before absorption, or are recovered from the viscera before their conversion into non-toxic derivatives, there may be no means of establishing by toxicological analysis that poisoning has taken place.

Many organic poisons, e.g. strychnine, are relatively stable and are only destroyed gradually during metabolic activity. Significant amounts of such poisons may therefore be recovered from the tissues even if death has been delayed after the ingestion of the poison. Other organic poisons, however, are unstable and are rapidly destroyed during metabolic activity. In cases of fatal poisoning by such organic substances, the toxicologist may fail to recover the poison in the viscera, or he may recover an amount of the poison which is less than the commonly accepted 'fatal dose'.

THE CONCEPT OF THE FATAL DOSE

It is widely held that every poison regularly kills at a certain dose—the fatal dose so commonly referred to in cases of criminal poisoning. This common-sense approach has led to strongly held and divergent views among the experts. For example, Glaister,[10] in referring to arsenic, stated: 'The smallest recorded fatal dose is 2 grains. Recovery has, however, occurred after large doses.'

Sir Sydney Smith[11] (an equally recognized authority) wrote of the same poison:

> *Toxic dose.* It is generally stated that 2 grains (0.13 gramme) is a fatal dose of arsenic, but there appears to be little or no authority for such a general statement. In my experience recovery after much larger doses is common, and I have not seen a death from a dose as small as 2 grains.

Although these authors differ from each other, both are probably right; they have merely formulated the problem in a manner which engenders unnecessary forensic speculation.

Glaister's statement incorporates a fallacy, namely, the attempt to meet the problem by quoting the least amount known to kill, i.e. the minimum lethal dose or MLD (see below). This may lead to vague and contradictory generalizations, especially if they are based on inadequate individual case reports.

Every medical practitioner is aware that different patients react differently to the same dose of a drug and that the same patient may react differently to the same dose of the same drug at different times. In pharmocology, the factors influencing the response are listed routinely, e.g. age, sex, weight, nutrition, etc. This variability in response is a fundamental biological principle and should occasion no surprise.

In practice, and even in animal experiments, it is seldom simple to define precisely the lethal dose of a drug. In man, the problem is further complicated by a paucity of adequate information, due partly to the fact that the data must necessarily be based on the investigation of discovered crime or accident. There is clearly ample cause for lack of clarity in this field of inquiry.

To investigate even in animals one clear-cut, all-or-none end point, such as that provided by the death from a poison, requires rigid control of the variable factors. Such a procedure is an elementary requirement, recognized and observed as routine in all methods of biological standardization. A closer look at the way these matters are conducted under laboratory conditions may throw much light on the matter and illustrate an important biological principle.

The strength of digitalis is measured by its effect on various animals. One of the most satisfactory tests for this purpose is based on the capacity of digitalis to kill frogs. The death of the animal is an unequivocal end point which can be observed in sufficiently large numbers of frogs to produce statistically reliable results. In the frog test for the assay of the potency of digitalis preparations, animals in the different groups are sexed, weighed, starved for the same period before the experiment, etc. They are then distributed throughout the test as wholly comparable groups. The digitalis preparations being tested are adjusted for constant volume of each injection, and the size of the dose is related to the body weight of each animal.

The results of such a rigidly controlled experiment show that the lethal effect of the drug is not directly proportional to the increase in the size of the dose administered. The fatal results, when plotted graphically against the dose given, demonstrate that the relation between the dose administered and the effect observed follows an unusual pattern, thus bringing to light a novel biological relation between the two events under investigation. The results form an S-shaped (sigmoid) curve of the general type illustrated in Figure 10.1.

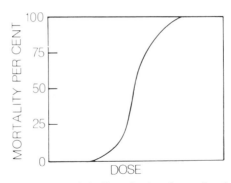

Fig. 10.1 Graph showing that the lethal effect of a drug is not directly proportional to an increase in the size of the dose administered (see text).

There is a range within which no animals are killed. In addition, although all the animals are similar in all respects, a particular dose kills only a definite proportion of the animals injected, until very large doses are reached. Even then, in some experiments, this result may not always be consistent. The curve is seen to rise most steeply in the region of the dose that is lethal to 50 per cent of the animals injected (LD50), and provides one of the convenient and reliable points for assay purposes. In this zone, dose and response are more nearly directly proportional.

Another interesting feature disclosed by animal experiments is the behaviour of the survivors. If these frogs are rested, fed and used subsequently for other assays, those which lived through previous experiments will succumb in later tests.

Experimental data also show how misleading attempts may be to measure a minimum lethal dose. Burns,[12] in reviewing the fundamental contributions made by Trevan, demonstrated the fallacies inherent in an attempt to express the minimum lethal dose, unless there is an appreciation of the overall statistical context in which the matter must be viewed. He wrote:

> The attempts usually made to determine a minimum lethal dose are exposed to great inaccuracy. Let us consider for a moment a definition of a minimum lethal dose as that dose which kills 2 out of 3 rats. If there are 99 rats in a large cage and every one of the rats is injected with this dose, two-thirds will die and one-third will survive. But let us take them from the cage 3 at a time. Is it possible to be sure that 2 will die and 1 will survive out of the first 3 we inject? Of course, there is no certainty. There are 33 rats in the cage which will survive the injection, and it is easily possible that 3 of these may be chosen. Only in a certain proportion of groups taken out 'of the cage will 2 rats die and 1 survive. In other groups, death will occur in 3 out of 3, or in 1 out of 3, or in 0 out of 3.

All these facts have an interesting bearing on the problem in man. Individual lethal effects cannot be predicted with any certainty. The lethal probabilities for a particular dose can be calculated if adequate data are available. A non-fatal dose on one occasion may be lethal to the same animal on another occasion. Moreover, as the relation of the dose to its response is not directly proportional, the true relation can be appreciated only by a statistically satisfactory analysis which, in animals, will fit either an S-shaped or some other characteristic curve.

The sigmoid relation between dose and response applies to many biological phenomena, including the dissociation of oxyhaemoglobin, the induction of convulsions in mice by insulin, the increase in the weight of rat ovaries induced by anterior pituitary extracts, the cure of neck retraction in vitamin B_1-deficient pigeons by vitamin B_1, etc.

It is against this background that contemporary contradictions in standard textbooks must be viewed. Indeed, this approach resolves the difficulties. What appear to be conflicting opinions are, in fact, wholly compatible views. When the statistical nature of the issue is realized, the problem involved in a single particular case is better appreciated. For the individual, death lurks somewhere along the sigmoid.

REFERENCES

1 Fourie H O. Poisoning by chemicals in agriculture and public health, 1st ed. Pretoria: Eng Enterprises. 1984: p xiii.
2 Gleason M N, Gosselin R E, Hodge H C. Clinical toxicology of commercial products, 1st ed. Baltimore: Williams & Wilkins. 1957.
3 Gosselin R E, Smith R P, Hodge H C, with the assistance of Braddock J E. Clinical toxicology of commercial products. 5th ed. Baltimore: Williams & Wilkins. 1984: pp v–viii.
4 Reg. v. Pritchard, Edinburgh, July 1865.
5 Rex v. Lee C P D. March 1948: (A. D.), 949, (1) S.A.L.R., 1134.
6 Jetter W W. Chemical injury. In: Anderson W A D. ed. Pathology. St. Louis: Mosby. 1948: p 153.

7 Baden M M. Investigation of death from drug abuse. In: Spitz W U, Fisher R S. eds. Medical legal investigation of deaths. Springfield: Charles C. Thomas. 1973: pp 485–509.

8 Bell E T. Renal diseases. 2nd ed. London: Kimpton. 1950: pp 266, 270 and 271.

9 Smith S. Forensic medicine. 8th ed. London: Churchill. 1945: p 67.

10 Glaister J L. Medical jurisprudence and toxicology. 10th ed. Edinburgh: Livingstone. 1957: p 515.

11 Smith S. Forensic medicine. 10th ed. London: Churchill. 1957: p 449.

12 Burns J H. Biological standardization. Oxford University Press. 1937: pp 10–11.

11

Wounds

A wound is a disruption of the normal structure of tissues caused by the application of force to the body.

Wounds resulting from thermal and electrical sources have been dealt with in Chapter 6.

MECHANISM OF WOUND PRODUCTION

Medical practitioners should have a broad understanding of the mechanical principles involved in the production of wounds. Some of these principles have been described by Moritz.[1]

General principles: mechanical forces

The mechanical force which causes a wound may be supplied by a moving instrument or object, or by the movement of the body itself (as in a fall)—the counter force in the first instance is provided by the inertia of the body, and in the second instance by the rigidity of some stationary object against which the body falls. In many cases a combination of these events occurs. As a result of the impact between the propelling force and the counter force, energy is transferred to the body tissues and there is a change in their state of rest or motion. As the human body is not a uniform rigid mass but is composed of numerous complex tissues which vary greatly in their physical properties (state of solidity, fluidity, density and elasticity), a change in the state of rest or motion of the body, as caused by a forceful impact, does not affect the tissues uniformly. Some of the transferred energy may be expended in causing the body to move as a whole, but much of the energy may cause non-uniform motion of localized portions of the body tissues. As a result of such non-uniform motion, the affected tissues will be subjected to compression or to traction strains or to a combination of such strains. All the tissues of the body, except those which contain gas, are resistant to compression (i.e. they resist forces tending to reduce their volumes), e.g. it has been estimated that a force of 10 000 tons pressure is necessary to reduce the human brain to half of its normal volume.[2] The application of mechanical force to the body does not lead to a true compression of the tissues but to their displacement and deformation in shape, and traction strains are set up in the affected tissues. Such strains may be due to forces causing simple elongation of tissues, but they may be due to more complex mechanisms such as bending, torsion or shearing.* Because there is a great variation in the resistance of the different tissues to traction forces, they rupture with varying ease as their tenacity is exceeded. The rigid tissues of the body, e.g. the bones, resist forceful attempts at deformation by reacting stresses, but fractures occur if the limits of their elasticity are exceeded by traction forces. The soft tissues of the body (mainly because of their semi-fluid nature) are plastic and readily change their shape when subjected to deforming forces. The extent to which these changes in shape can occur is limited by the cohesion between the tissue cells, by the connective and vascular tissue frameworks of the various organs, and by their limiting membranous capsules. When these structures are stretched beyond the limits of their tensile strength, they rupture and wounds are produced.

Factors governing the nature and extent of wounds

The factors which govern the nature and extent of wounds may be considered under the following headings:
1. The nature of the object or instrument causing the wound.
2. The amount of energy discharged during the impact.
3. The conditions under which the energy is discharged.
4. The nature of the affected tissues.

1. The nature of the object or instrument causing the wound

With blows from pointed or sharp-edged objects or instruments the area of primary impact is virtually limited to a point or a line. This extreme concentration of the force to such a very limited area can cause deep penetration or clear division of the tissues. The passage of the object or instrument through the tissues is resisted by the hardness of the tissues (e.g. cartilage or bone) and by the friction of the divided tissues against the sides of the instrument.

With a blow from a blunt instrument, the area of body surface subjected to impact may be relatively large. When energy is dissipated over a relatively large area, the amount of damage inflicted on a unit mass of tissue within that area is less than when the energy is distributed over a smaller

---

* A shear strain is a strain which is produced in a body by the forceful alteration of its shape but not its volume. Shear strain causes or tends to cause two contiguous parts of a body to slide relatively to each other in a direction parallel to their plane of contact. Holbourn has described shear strain as 'the type of deformation which occurs in a pack of cards when it is deformed from a neat rectangular pile into an oblique-angled pile.'

area, e.g. a blow struck with the edge of a plank will cause more localized damage than a blow struck with the flat of the same plank with the same force to the same region. Irregularities in the shape of the instrument, or curvature of the part of the body struck, may limit the area of actual impact to a small size and concentrate the damage. A fall against a projection, or the hard corner of an object, may have a more serious effect than a similar fall against a flat surface.

When the instrument is plastic, some of the energy liberated by the impact will be expended in deforming the instrument. The change in shape of the instrument at the moment of impact increases the size of the area of impact and prolongs the period over which the energy is discharged. For this reason a plastic instrument causes less damage than a rigid instrument. This fact is illustrated by the difference in effects caused by blows from rubber truncheons and blows from wooden truncheons. When an instrument breaks on impact, much of its kinetic energy may be lost.

2. The amount of energy discharged during the impact

The amount of kinetic energy present in a moving object is measured by the formula $\frac{1}{2}mv^2$, where m = the mass and v = the velocity of the instrument. An instrument of definite mass moving at a definite speed harnesses a definite amount of energy. When the mass of the instrument alone is doubled, the kinetic energy is doubled, but if the velocity only is doubled, this energy is quadrupled. The velocity with which an instrument moves is more important than the mass of the instrument. A light bullet has a relatively great destructive power because of its high velocity.

When a moving instrument is brought to rest on impact with the tissues all the kinetic energy of the instrument is discharged. If, however, a glancing blow is struck, or the tissues are perforated, only that energy commensurate with the decrease in velocity of the instrument caused by the impact or the perforation is discharged to the tissues.

3. The conditions under which the energy is discharged

Much of the energy liberated in an impact may be expended in causing generalized movement of the body and not in causing localized deformation. In such circumstances, although the local injury may be minimal the force may have been sufficient to have knocked a person down. On the other hand, if the body or the part of the body struck is immobilized, the greater part of the striking force may be expended in causing localized tissue damage. A blow to a head which is free to move may cause little damage, but a similar blow to a head resting on a pavement may cause marked injury to the skull.

Any factor which increases the period of time over which the energy is discharged will also decrease the destructive effects of a blow, e.g. when a cricketer catches a hard swift ball, he moves his hand backwards as he grasps it and so prolongs the period and thereby diminishes the 'sting' of the impact.

4. The nature of the affected tissues

The skin. As the skin is very pliable and somewhat elastic it readily changes shape when it is struck. Owing to the firm coherence of its tough layers of keratinized cells it is also strongly resistant to traction forces. For this reason the skin is often not damaged when it is struck with a blunt instrument although the underlying structures may be severely injured. The skin may, however, be readily split when crushed against rigid bone.

The subcutaneous tissues. Because of their fat content and the pliability of their supporting connective tissue fibres, the subcutaneous tissues are very plastic. These tissues protect the body by the cushioning effects which they have on blows. With severe blows from blunt instruments the incompressible fat of the subcutaneous tissues may be crushed and be displaced between the tough outer skin and underlying structures such as bone. In this way, extensive tearing of the fragile supporting connective and vascular tissue framework of the subcutaneous tissue may occur and bruises may develop. Such damage from blunt force is often very extensive in these tissues and may be confined to them.

The muscles. Because of their great plasticity and elasticity and their strong encapsulating sheaths, the muscles frequently escape damage from blows, but they may be crushed or torn against bone or be lacerated by fragments of displaced and broken bone.

If the muscles are unduly stretched they may rupture. By meeting blows, with gradually decreasing resistance and so increasing the period of discharge of energy, the muscles may play an important role in protecting the body from injury, e.g. a boxer is taught to protect himself by rolling his body with the blow of his opponent.

The bones. Bones are relatively rigid, but when a force is applied to a bone it may bend without breaking, and then, by virtue of its elasticity, recoil to its normal shape, e.g. when force is applied to the chest, particularly in children, the ribs may bend without fracturing, even though the thoracic organs are damaged by the same force.

If a bone is bent beyond the limits of its elasticity, it fractures. Such a fracture commences at the point of maximum convexity caused by the bending, in the region where the traction strains are most developed. Sometimes, as in green-stick fractures of the long bones in children, the damage is limited to the convexity of the bend. When a force is applied to a wide area of bone and causes extensive bending strains, multiple fractures may develop with a resultant shattering of the bone. When a twisting force is applied to a bone the fracture has a spiral pattern.

Because of their rigidity, bones may act as levers so that extensive fractures or fracture–dislocations may follow upon relatively small forces appropriately applied.

When a force is applied to a bone the energy may be conducted away from the site of impact and be dispersed gradually and widely to the attached tissues. In these circumstances the bone may escape local damage. Occasionally, when a force is applied to a bone the energy may be conducted away from the site of impact, and be concentrated at some distant point at a mechanical disadvantage. In this way a distal indirect fracture may be caused, e.g. fracture of the clavicle may result from a fall on the outstretched hand.

The joints. Movements of the limbs depend upon the flexibility of the joints and these movements are controlled by muscular action. By offering gradually decreasing resistance to applied force, as described at page 224 the muscles convert the limbs into 'springs' which protect the body.

The spine is extremely flexible because of the structure of the vertebral joints, the elastic nature of the intervertebral discs, and the elasticity of its attached muscles. Because of this flexibility, the spine is able to absorb forces which might otherwise be transmitted from the pelvis to the skull and its contents.

Effects on body fluids and gases. Fluid is virtually incompressible but as it has no shape it may be readily displaced. A blow over a hollow organ which contains fluid may set up powerful hydrostatic forces in that fluid which are transmitted equally and uniformly in all directions. Such transmitted forces may lead to the rupture of anatomically distant and mechanically weak tissues, e.g. a sudden compression of the chest may cause a retrograde displacement of blood in the great thoracic veins which results in the rupture of distal venules and capillaries, producing petechial haemorrhages over the face, neck and shoulders—this condition is often referred to as 'traumatic asphyxia'.

The violent displacement of fluid in the gastrointestinal tract or in the urinary tract may cause distant ruptures of portions of these tracts.

Gases are readily compressible, and their volume varies inversely with their pressure. Organs containing gas, e.g. the lungs, may therefore be extensively compressed without the occurrence of structural damage. When, however, these organs are suddenly and violently compressed, sufficiently powerful pneumostatic forces may be set up to cause damage to anatomically distant tissues, e.g. in blast injuries, widespread rupture of pulmonary alveoli may occur from violent displacement of the air in the respiratory passages.

The mechanics of head injuries are dealt with in Chapter 12. Some aspects of the mechanics of lung and cardiac injuries are dealt with at pages 304–306. The mechanics of 'closed' abdominal injuries is considered at pages 312–316.

Application

It has been shown that the mechanism of wound production is complex and depends upon many variable factors which to a large extent cannot be accurately assessed. Different wounds may result from equal forces when applied to the same region of the body in different circumstances. Sometimes severe wounds may follow upon apparently trivial forces, and sometimes relatively large forces may cause minor wounds. For these reasons, it is often impossible on scientific grounds to express an opinion as to the amount of force which must have been used to cause a particular wound, and conversely it may be impossible to predict the amount of damage which could follow upon the application of a certain force. Questions of this nature often arise in the course of medico-legal investigations, but the medical practitioner should only express an opinion in these matters on the probabilities, and his opinion should be given in broad and qualified terms.

When a force is applied to the body, wounds may or may not be produced at the site of application of the force. Injuries of internal organs or injuries of tissues anatomically distant from the site of application of an external force are often unaccompanied by any sign of external damage.

ABRASIONS

An abrasion is a destruction of the skin which usually involves the superficial layers of the epidermis only.

Abrasions are caused by friction of the skin against some rough or sharp surface resulting in the scraping away of superficial portions of the epidermis. Abrasions often take the form of parallel furrows in the skin surface. These furrows may be broad at one end and tail away in the opposite direction. This appearance is usually indicative of the direction in which the force was applied. When the furrows extend deeply enough into the skin to involve part of the corium there is slight capillary bleeding. When the exuded serum or blood coagulates on the surface, a scab is formed.

Abrasions are of medico-legal importance as they indicate that some force has been applied to the body. Under certain conditions, the characters of abrasions may suggest the nature, direction and cause of the force and, possibly, the purpose for which it was applied. Abrasions are frequently caused by blows from blunt instruments and from falls. Such abrasions are commonly found on the head and the face and over bony prominences. Abrasions, when caused by falls, are often contaminated with gravel. Abrasions are often accompanied by other injuries such as bruises, fractures or internal injuries.

When abrasions are caused by finger nails they may appear either as crescentic marks (when the nails have been dug into the skin) or as relatively broad parallel grooves which tail away at their ends (when the nails have scraped away the epidermis). Abrasions caused by finger nails are commonly found on the front and sides of the neck in cases of throttling (p. 100) and on the front of the neck, the thighs, the vulva and the wrists in cases of rape (p. 359).*

Abrasions may be produced after death when a body is dragged away from the scene of a crime. The distribution of such abrasions depends upon the position of the body while it is being dragged. If the body was dragged face downwards, linear abrasions may be found on the front of the face, trunk, thighs or legs. If there is doubt as to whether an abrasion is ante-mortem or post-mortem in origin, it is advisable to excise the abrasion and submit the tissue for histological examination. On microscopic examination, ante-mortem or post-mortem abrasions may show underlying bruising of the corium, but if the period of survival after the injury has been sufficiently long, evidence of tissue reaction may be found.

Ant erosions of the skin may resemble abrasions. The differentiation of abrasions from ant erosions is dealt with at page 55.

Abrasions heal rapidly, and provided there are no complications such as infection, they do not leave permanent scars.

After death abraded surfaces dry out and acquire a parchment-like appearance. Such abrasions have been mistaken for burns.

BRUISES OR CONTUSIONS

Bruises, contusions or ecchymoses are wounds which are characterized by the effusion of blood into the tissue spaces. Bruises vary in size and shape. They are usually caused by blunt weapons but they can be produced in other ways, e.g. by the pressure of the fingers in throttling.

The extent and the degree of bruising depend upon the amount of force applied to the body, and upon other factors such as the structure and vascularity of the affected tissues. The thickness of the skin, the texture of the subcutaneous tissues, and the relationship of these structures to the deeper tissues vary in different parts of the body. Bruises occur more readily in lax tissues such as the eyelids,† than in dense tissues such as the palms of the hands. Bruising is usually more extensive in fatty tissue, and obese persons tend to bruise more readily than thin subjects. Bruising is relatively more marked in tissues overlying bones than in tissues which are able to yield under pressure, such as the tissues of the abdominal wall. Constitutional factors may predispose towards extensive bruising. This

---

* The debris removed from under the finger-nails of an assailant may contain particles of dried human blood. If this blood belongs to a blood group different from that of the assailant, but the same as the victim, this fact may help in the identification of the assailant.

† In fractures of the anterior portion of the base of the skull blood may be extravasated into the eyelids. Eyelid contusion, therefore, does not necessarily indicate the direct application of force to that region.

predisposition has been specially noticed in many apparently healthy women. In persons with nutritional deficiencies such as scurvy (which can occur in chronic alcoholics), or in persons suffering from blood disorders such as haemophilia, essential thrombocytopenia or other forms of purpura, extensive bruises may be caused by slight injuries.

Because of all these factors, it is not possible to determine the amount of force used from the extent and the degree of bruising.

The shape and size of a bruise may bear no relationship to the shape or size of the weapon or object which caused the bruise e.g. when a bruise is caused by a long rigid weapon such as a stick, the edges of the bruise may be irregular, while the width of the bruise may be greater than the width of the stick because of the infiltration of blood into the surrounding tissues along the edges of the bruise. In certain circumstances, however, the external pattern of a bruise may correspond to the form of the object or weapon with which it was produced. This condition may be of medico-legal importance and was noted in two of our cases of murder. In the one instance the deceased received numerous blows on her head and face with the head of an axe. At autopsy, a rectangular bruise measuring 35 mm from above downwards was observed over the right eye and the right cheek. An axe was found in the possession of the accused when he was arrested. The width of the head of this axe corresponded closely to the width of the rectangular bruise. In the other instance the deceased was severely assaulted by her reputed husband. Numerous external injuries were found on her body. The pattern of one bruise on the right breast above and to the inner side of the nipple had an unusual appearance and its exact dimensions were noted. When the accused was arrested he was wearing a pair of riding boots, and the heel of one of these boots corresponded in form and dimensions to this bruise.

When a rigid weapon such as a stick strikes a curved surface of the body in a region where the soft tissues are particularly pliable, e.g. the buttocks, the tissues may be compressed under the force of the impact. In these circumstances the bruise is not confined to the maximum convexity of the affected part, but it may extend over the whole of the curved surface. A similar appearance may be produced when a plastic weapon, such as a strap, becomes wrapped around the body or the limbs.

When the body is struck by a broad flat weapon such as a plank, the edges of the plank may cause parallel bruises in the skin, separated by apparently normal tissue.

Bruises may appear in the skin at a variable period after an injury to the deeper tissues. Such bruises may appear at some distance from the site of application of the force, as blood in the deeper tissues tends to be extravasated in all directions along the lines of the fascial and muscular planes before coming to the surface. Deep bruises may never appear on the surface of the body.

On external examination during life, bruises appear as swollen, tender, discoloured areas. The colours of bruises change as the extravasated blood undergoes haemolysis, but these changes are not constant and cannot be relied upon as an indication of their age. Bruises are often difficult to detect on external examination in dark-skinned persons.

Pulmonary and cardiac contusions and contusions of the abdominal and pelvic viscera are described in Chapter 12. Internal contusions of this nature are not necessarily accompanied by external evidence of injury.

When a person dies very rapidly, e.g. from parasympathetic inhibition of the circulation (p. 154), the extent of bruising which accompanies a tissue injury may be very slight.

Bruises may not be readily detected at autopsy or they may be obscured by patches of post-mortem lividity or by the colour of the skin in dark-skinned persons. Bruises of the head can best be demonstrated by reflecting the scalp and making incisions into the scalp from the aponeurotic surface. Bruises in the cervical tissues can only be satisfactorily demonstrated by reflecting the various structures of the neck in layers as described at page 66. Bruises in the subcutaneous tissues of the trunk and limbs may be detected by making parallel strip incisions through the skin in the manner described at page 124.

Ante-mortem bruises must be differentiated from post-mortem dissection artefacts (p. 104). Bruises may become visible externally some hours or days after death. This is seen most commonly in putrefied bodies. The pressure of the gases of putrefaction may cause the extravasated blood to extend along the tissue spaces and give rise to a false impression of the extent of ante-mortem bruising. Such apparent post-mortem extensions of bruises may also be due to the haemolysis of extravasated red blood cells and the diffusion of pigment into the surrounding tissues. A similar diffusion of haemoglobin may result from the haemolysis of intravascular collections of blood (p. 52). For this reason particular care should be exercised before regarding as a bruise an extravasation of blood which has only appeared after death.

It may be of medico-legal importance to distinguish between bruises and patches of post-mortem lividity. This subject has been dealt with at page 38.

INCISED WOUNDS

Incised wounds are caused by sharp weapons or objects such as knives, jagged portions of metal or pieces of broken glass. The general features of incised wounds are set out in Table 11.1 below.

An incised wound caused by a sharp cutting weapon is usually linear in shape but it may have a curved or V-shaped appearance if the direction of movement of the weapon is changed during the infliction of the wound. The shape of an incised wound may depend upon the shape of the blade of a weapon, e.g. in one of our cases a curved incised wound of the front of the

Table 11.1 General features of incised wounds, lacerated wounds and punctured wounds

Description of wound	Incised	Lacerated	Punctured
Production	By sharp objects or weapons	By blunt objects or weapons	By pointed weapons which may be sharp or blunt
Shape	Linear or spindle-shaped	Varies; usually irregular	Linear or irregular, according to nature of weapon
Edges	Clean-cut and everted	Ragged and often undermined	Varies according to nature of weapon, but edges often everted from withdrawal of weapon
Dimensions	Usually longer than deep, but often gaping	Depth varies, but hand-lens examination reveals bridges of tissue joining the edges	Depth greater than length and width
Haemorrhage from wound	Usually profuse, especially if vessels incompletely cut	Not pronounced	Varies, profuse if vessels are cut in depth of wound
Condition of skin surrounding wound edges	Bruising may or may not be present	Bruising usually present	Bruising rarely present

neck was caused by a curved pruning knife. Incised wounds caused by jagged portions of metal or pieces of broken glass may appear to be irregular in shape but the close examination of such wounds shows that the edges are characteristically clean-cut and everted.

As incised wounds usually gape, the breadth of the cutting edge of a sharp weapon cannot be determined from the width of the wound. In deep incised wounds, the degree of gaping is greater when the muscles are cut transversely than when they are cut in the longitudinal plane of their fibres. In a deep incised wound, blood vessels, nerves and tendons may be severed. Bleeding from an incised wound may be profuse, e.g. when a vessel is partially cut. Paralysis, deformity and loss of function may follow the cutting of nerves and tendons.

Infection of incised wounds is relatively uncommon and if the edges are approximated by surgical suture, and incised wound usually heals by first intention with minimal scar formation.

As there is a limited destruction of tissue, an uncomplicated incised wound is usually unaccompanied by traumatic shock, but shock may be a prominent feature if the wound extends into one of the body cavities and involves an internal organ.

A single movement of a sharp weapon over the skin surface usually produces a single incised wound. When the skin becomes folded under the cutting edge of the weapon a single movement of this nature may produce a series of incised wounds separated one from another by bridges of normal skin.

Incised wounds are commonly seen in cases of assault and homicide. Homicidal incised wounds are usually multiple and can occur in any region of the body. If, in a case of homicidal wounding, the victim tried to defend himself by warding off blows or by grasping the weapon, multiple incisions may be found on his forearms and in the palms of his hands.

Accidental incised wounds are seen in traffic injuries when they are usually caused by pieces of broken glass and involve exposed parts of the body such as the face and the hands. Fragments of glass may be found in such wounds and it is important to retain such fragments or any other foreign bodies which may be found in the wounds.

Suicidal incised wounds are commonly seen in the region of the wrists and the neck (p. 300). Incised wounds are sometimes self-inflicted for the purpose of bringing false charges against other persons. According to Smith[3] these fabricated wounds are usually superficial and they often consist of a series of parallel or crossing incisions. Although these injuries may be found in any region they are seen most commonly over the top of the head, the outer side of the left arm, the front of the left forearm, the front and outer side of the thighs, and the front of the abdomen and chest. Smith has stressed the need for an examination of the clothing in these cases as the fabricator seldom injures himself through his clothes.

Incised wounds may be produced after death. Haemorrhage from such post-mortem wounds and their differentiation from ante-mortem wounds is dealt with at pages 245–246.

LACERATED WOUNDS

Lacerated wounds are wounds in which the tissues are torn as a result of the application of blunt force to the body. The force may be produced by some moving weapon or object or by a fall. Localized portions of tissue are displaced by the impact of the blunt force. This displacement sets up traction forces and tearing or rupture of the tissues results (p. 221). Displacement of tissues is prone to occur when soft tissues are crushed against bone. Bruises are produced by the same mechanism as lacerated wounds, and these two types of tissue injury are often associated. Both types of injury are commonly complicated by fractures and dislocations and by injuries to internal viscera.

The general features of lacerated wounds are set out in Table 11.1.

An external lacerated wound caused by the splitting of soft tissues against underlying bone (in regions such as the head, the face and the shins) is often linear in shape and may resemble an incised wound. A hand-lens examination, however, will show that the edges of the wounds are irregular and often bruised while there is an incomplete separation of the tissues between the edges of the wound. If hair-bulbs are present in the area involved, they will be seen to be crushed instead of cut. The shape and size of a lacerated wound usually bears no relationship to the shape or size of the weapon or object which produced it. A lacerated wound, e.g. from a single blow with a rod-shaped instrument, may have a Y-shaped termination.

The depth of a lacerated wound is variable and a hand-lens examination may show intact vessels, nerves or tendons stretching across the wound.

A single blow with a blunt weapon may produce more than one lacerated wound, e.g. a single blow over the side of the head may produce lacerated wounds over the lower jaw, the ear and the parietal prominence.

As the blood vessels are usually crushed, external haemorrhage from lacerated wounds is not pronounced, but internal haemorrhage from ruptured viscera may be severe and lead to death. The clinical manifestations of internal haemorrhage may be delayed for several hours (see p. 316). Lacerated wounds are often contaminated with particles of sand and gravel and infection of such wounds is relatively common (see p. 238). The healing of a lacerated wound usually results in well-marked scar formation.

Lacerated wounds of the skin are seen most frequently in cases of assault and murder and in traffic injuries and other accidents. Self-inflicted lacerated wounds are uncommon. A combination of incised and lacerated wounds may be seen in cases of assault when a bottle has been used by the assailant.

In certain circumstances, even though the skin may not be damaged by a blunt force, widespread lacerations of the underlying soft tissues and viscera may occur.

Lacerations of internal viscera may be caused by the direct injury of the viscera by fragments of fractured bone; by the development of traction strains or shear strains in the viscera; by the stretching of visceral attachments; and by hydrostatic forces. These injuries are dealt with in Chapter 12. Lacerated wounds may be produced after death. Such wounds are commonly caused by animals, and their differentiation from ante-mortem wounds is dealt with at page 242.

PUNCTURED WOUNDS

Punctured wounds are caused by long narrow instruments with blunt or pointed ends. Punctured wounds are described as 'penetrating' when they pierce deeply into tissues and as 'perforating' when they transfix tissues and cause exit wounds. Glaister[4] has suggested that the terms 'penetrating–incised' or 'perforating–lacerated', etc., should be used in the description of 'stab' wounds so as to indicate the nature of the weapon which caused them.

The general features of punctured wounds are set out in Table 11.1. Bullet wounds are described in Chapter 13.

The shape and dimensions of a pointed weapon cannot be determined from the shape and dimensions of the external opening of a punctured wound. When a sharp weapon such as a knife has been used, the external wound almost invariably takes the form of a slit having two pointed extremities. The mechanism whereby such a wound is produced has been described in detail by Gross.[5] Gross states that

> . . . when the point of a knife penetrates into the body to a depth of half an inch more or less, it forms at first a wound with a sharp or pointed angle at each end; as the knife proceeds farther in, the end in contact with the cutting side of the knife naturally remains sharp and pointed; but the other end which is in contact with the back of the knife remains so also. This is because the back of the knife does not give its shape to the skin, but only causes further separation, so that the skin continues to be torn in the original direction and still forms a sharp and pointed angle. . . When a wound has each end sharp and pointed, it must not be concluded that the wound has been inflicted by a dagger or other double-edged instrument; more frequently the wound has been caused by a knife with a round or square back.

When a knife is twisted as it is withdrawn from the tissues, the external wound may have a cruciate appearance.

An external wound caused by a rounded sharp weapon such as a skewer is not necessarily circular in shape as the skin may be split during the process of penetration. The external opening of a punctured wound may have a triangular or cruciate shape if it is caused by a weapon such as a file or a bayonet, or by a square-sectioned instrument such as a spike.

The dimensions of the external opening of a punctured wound may be smaller than the diameter or transverse dimensions of the weapon, as the elastic skin is often stretched during the process of penetration. On the other hand, the opening may be larger in cases where the weapon is withdrawn obliquely after penetration.

The depth of a punctured wound may be greater than the total length of the penetrating object or weapon because the tissues deep to the skin are often compressed during the process of penetration.

A single wound track is usually found in relation to a single external opening in a punctured wound. In certain cases, however, where the weapon is partially withdrawn and then reinserted in another direction, two or more tracks may be found in relation to a single external opening.

External haemorrhage from punctured wounds is usually limited in amount but serious internal haemorrhage may result from penetrating wounds of the thorax and abdomen. The clinical signs of such internal haemorrhage may be delayed (pp 236, 316).

When a weapon such as a knife or a dagger is thrust into the tissues with considerable force the skin surrounding the wound may be bruised by the shaft of the weapon.

As a weapon such as a knife or a dagger is usually held with the point downward, most such wounds are directed downwards through the tissues of the body. When such a weapon is held with the point upward (in the so-called 'continental' manner), the wound is directed upwards through the tissues of the body. These factors should be borne in mind when an attempt is made to determine the positions of an assailant and his victim at the time of an assault.

Punctured wounds occur most commonly in cases of assault and homicide, but they are also seen in traffic injuries and accidental falls on projecting objects. Self-inflicted punctured wounds are uncommon.

Penetrating wounds of the viscera are dealt with in Chapter 12.

COMPLICATIONS OF WOUNDS

Neurogenic or primary shock

Neurogenic or primary shock is a reflex neurovascular disturbance which follows immediately after an injury. The disorder may result from parasympathetic inhibition of the circulation or from sympathetico-adrenal stimulation of the circulation (Chapter 7). Parasympathetic inhibition results in syncope and in exceptional circumstances such syncope may be fatal (p. 155). As the exciting stimuli in neurogenic shock are usually of a painful nature, however, and are accompanied by the emotion of fright, sympathetico-adrenal effects are more commonly found in primary shock than parasympathetic effects. The main clinical features of sympathetico-adrenal stimulation are anxiety, tremor, abdominal discomfort, dilatation of the pupils, sweating, tachycardia and an elevation of blood pressure. As indicated at page 152, sympathetico-adrenal stimulation may result in rapid death, particularly in persons with chronic cardiac lesions.

Although the stimulus which gives rise to sympathetico-adrenal stimulation may be of a momentary nature, the systemic effects of the stimulation may persist for as long as half an hour.

The sudden rise in blood pressure which may occur in neurogenic shock can precipitate a serious complication such as an intracerebral haemorrhage (resulting from the rupture of an arteriosclerotic vessel or from the rupture of a congenital aneurysm of a cerebral vessel) or a dissecting aneurysm of the aorta (resulting from a rupture of the vasa vasorum into a zone of medial necrosis of the aorta). In such cases, if death occurs and if there is evidence that the deceased received some minor trauma, it is important to emphasize to the investigating officers that the essential cause of death was the underlying disease process.

Traumatic, haematogenic or secondary shock

Traumatic, haematogenic or secondary shock is a constitutional disturbance which develops gradually after injury. In a detailed review of the pathology of this form of shock Wilson[6] has observed that it is difficult to give an adequate definition of shock or to place its aetiology under one causative factor. Traumatic shock is a progressive phenomenon affecting most of the physiological systems of the body. Wilson states that the essential feature of traumatic shock appears to be a reduction of the total circulating blood volume, with a secondary decline in venous return, cardiac output, and blood pressure. This is generally referred to as hypovolaemic shock.

Pathogenesis

Two main theories have been advanced to explain the reduction of circulating blood volume in shock, namely, (1) that the reduction is due to a local loss of fluid (blood or plasma) at the site of injury, and (2) that the reduction is due either to capillary dilatation with a loss of effective circulating blood volume or to increased capillary permeability with a loss of actual circulating blood volume.

Wilson considers that it is probable that a local loss of fluid at the site of injury is an important initiating factor in the aetiology of shock. The maintenance of shock depends upon the development of generalized capillary atony. Moon[7] believes that this change is due to the absorption of toxic substances from the injured tissues. Other workers consider that nervous impulses from the area of trauma play a dominant role in perpetuating the condition.

Whatever the mechanism is whereby capillary atony is brought about, this change produces a series of pathological effects which ultimately result in a vicious cycle of circulatory failure and death. (Fig. 3.1, p. 86.)

Clinical features

The onset of traumatic shock may be insidious and the early signs may be indefinite. There is progressive prostration and muscular weakness. Apathy and depression are common. Perspiration is often profuse and the patient complains of feeling cold. The pupils are commonly dilated. The respiratory rate is increased and the patient may complain of thirst. The skin is pale, cold and clammy. The pulse rate is increased and there is a fall in arterial blood pressure. There is a tendency for the systolic pressure to fall before the diastolic pressure so that there is a progressively diminishing pulse pressure.

Autopsy findings

The pathological changes of traumatic shock are of a non-specific nature and consist mainly of generalized capillovenous engorgement which may be associated with widespread petechiae in the tissues and serous membranes. Some degree of oedema, which is often only discernible in the lungs, may occur. In severe and prolonged shock there may be slight effusions into serous cavities, and parenchymatous visceral degenerative changes and bronchopneumonia may develop.

The pathological changes of secondary shock are essentially similar to the general pathological changes found in hypoxic and anoxic deaths (p. 93).

Haemorrhage

Haemorrhage is a common and often serious complication of wounds. Haemorrhage may arise from injured arteries, capillaries or veins. Arterial haemorrhage may be severe, e.g. in incised wounds when a vessel is partially cut, or slight, e.g. in lacerated wounds when the vessels are crushed and there is effective contraction and retraction of the ruptured ends of the vessels.

As a general rule, capillary haemorrhage is limited as the flow from the capillaries is controlled by coagulation of the blood at the site of injury. In certain blood disorders, however, e.g. haemophilia, there may be defective blood coagulation and serious haemorrhage may result from continuous oozing from capillaries.

Venous haemorrhage is seldom serious unless one of the great veins of the neck, thorax or abdomen is injured.

Primary, reactionary and secondary haemorrhage

Haemorrhage is often described as being Primary, Reactionary or Secondary. Primary haemorrhage follows immediately after an injury. Reactionary haemorrhage occurs from the same site as primary haemorrhage but is usually delayed for several hours up to twenty-four hours after the injury. It is believed to depend upon a rise in blood pressure (which accompanies the recovery from shock) and muscular movements (which result in a loosening of the blood clot at the site of coagulation in the vessel). Secondary haemorrhage is due to infection of a wound which results in the disintegration of formed blood clot and the erosion of vessel walls. Wilson[8] states that there is often a history of severe bleeding at the time of injury and that the secondary haemorrhage usually occurs between the 10th and 16th day after the injury. In certain circumstances, however, secondary haemorrhages may be delayed as long as three months after the original injury.

External and internal haemorrhage

Haemorrhage may be described as external or internal, depending upon whether the blood flows away from the body surface or passes into a body cavity or into the lumen of a hollow organ.

External haemorrhage. Best and Taylor[9] state that the total volume of whole blood present in the body amounts to about one-ninth of the body mass. On the basis of this estimation the average healthy adult has about 6 litres of whole blood in his body. Such persons may lose up to 500 ml of blood, e.g. in giving a blood transfusion, without showing any ill-effects.*

In the healthy adult, symptoms of acute haemorrhage become manifest when the loss amounts to about 1 litre of blood. An acute loss of 2 litres of blood in a healthy adult constitutes a danger to life.

Internal haemorrhage. The effects of an internal haemorrhage are only partially dependent upon the amount of blood lost. The accumulation of blood in a body cavity often gives rise to the compression of organs, with fatal results, e.g. cerebral compression from extradural or subdural haemorrhage, cardiac tamponade from haemorrhage into the pericardial sac; and collapse of the lung and displacement of the mediastinum from a haemothorax.

Internal haemorrhage into the peritoneal cavity is relatively common in penetrating wounds and blunt injuries of the abdomen.

Owing to the accumulation of blood between the coils of intestine and the gravitation of blood into the pelvis or subphrenic spaces, estimations of the amount of blood present in a peritoneal cavity are often misleading. For this reason it is essential at autopsy to carry out an actual measurement of the amount of blood found in a peritoneal cavity. Haemorrhage into a peritoneal cavity often takes place slowly and several hours may elapse from the time of injury until symptoms of acute haemorrhage or peritoneal irritation become manifest.

Internal haemorrhage is often associated with traumatic shock.

Pathogenesis

Although many workers have claimed that the effects of traumatic shock and haemorrhage are essentially similar, Moon[10] states that there are certain pathological and biochemical changes which differentiate traumatic shock from haemorrhage. These changes, such as haemodilution (in contrast to haemoconcentration which occurs in traumatic shock) may serve to distinguish an acute massive haemorrhage from shock in the early stages, but the terminal effects of both conditions are similar (Fig. 3.1, p. 86).

Clinical features

The clinical features of acute haemorrhage are similar to those of traumatic

* After the donation of blood for a blood transfusion the circulating blood volume is restored to normal within 24 hours by the passage of tissue fluids into the blood stream. The restoration of the blood protein to its pretransfusion level may take several days, while the red cells and haemoglobin are only restored to normal after 3 to 6 weeks.[11]

shock. Some clinicians claim that, unlike a person who is shocked, a person suffering from acute haemorrhage is anxious and restless, and shows signs of 'air-hunger'. In practice, however, acute haemorrhage and traumatic shock are usually combined.

Autopsy findings

In deaths due to massive haemorrhage, post-mortem lividity is very limited in extent and generalized venous congestion is absent. The great veins appear abnormally empty, the lungs are unduly pale and light, and the spleen is contracted. According to Moon, petechiae are poorly developed and tissue oedema does not occur in cases of uncomplicated massive haemorrhage. Although the general autopsy findings may indicate considerable acute blood loss, the findings do not allow of an accurate estimation of the amount of that blood loss.*

Infection of wounds

A common and important complication of wounds is the occurrence of infection. Wound infection may be caused by organisms which are normally present on the body surfaces or by organisms which invade the tissues from the environment.

Causative organisms

The more important types of organisms which cause wound infection are:
1. Organisms normally present on the body surfaces:
      (a) Skin: Gram-positive cocci, e.g. staphylococci; and Gram-negative bacteria, e.g. coliform organisms, *B. proteus* and *B. pyocyaneus*.
      (b) Respiratory mucosa: Gram-positive cocci, e.g. streptococci, pneumococci and staphylococci; and Gram-negative bacilli, e.g. Friedländer's bacillus.
      (c) Gastrointestinal mucosa: Gram-positive cocci; e.g. streptococci, including anaerobic types; Gram-negative bacteria, e.g. coliform organisms, *B. proteus* and *B. pyocyaneus*; and anaerobic spore-bearing organisms, e.g. *B. welchii*.
2. Organisms invading the tissues from the environment:
      (a) Organisms present in the air through 'droplet' infection or contaminated dust: Gram-positive cocci, e.g. streptococci; *C. diphtheriae* and related organisms; and Gram-negative bacteria, e.g. coliform organisms.

---

  * Cases of severe but non-massive haemorrhage are often associated with severe shock. In such cases sufficient blood may remain in the body to cause some degree of capillovenous congestion and the general signs indicative of serious blood loss may not be noticeable at autopsy.

(b) Organisms present on contaminated instruments, dressings, and the hands of attendants: Gram-positive cocci, e.g. streptococci and staphylococci; and Gram-negative bacteria e.g. coliform organisms.

(c) Organisms present in street dirt and debris: anaerobic spore-bearing organisms, e.g. *B. welchii* and *B. tetani*; and Gram-negative bacteria, e.g. coliform organisms.

(d) Organisms present in the saliva of animals (in cases of wounds caused by bites): Gram-positive cocci, e.g. streptococci; anaerobic spore-bearing organisms, e.g. *B. tetani*; and viruses, e.g. the virus of rabies (p. 172).

Primary and secondary infection

Infection of wounds may be primary or secondary. Primary wound infection is caused by organisms which are carried into the wounds at the time of the injury, e.g. from the skin, clothing or street dirt. Secondary wound infection is caused by organisms which invade the wound after the injury, e.g. by air-borne droplet infection, contaminated dressings, etc. Primary infection often cannot be avoided but secondary infection can usually be prevented by adequate aseptic surgical measures.

The nature of the inflammatory lesion produced by a primary or secondary infection of a wound depends upon the nature of the wound and the type of infecting organism.

Pyogenic infections

Pyogenic cocci may produce a localized abscess (usually in staphylococcal infections) or a diffuse spreading cellulitis (usually in streptococcal infections). Coliform organisms, *B. proteus* and *B. pyocyaneus*, may also give rise to suppurative lesions in association with pyogenic cocci.

The main complications of pyogenic infections are suppurative lymphadenitis, pyaemia and septicaemia.

Infections by anaerobic spore-bearing organisms

The anaerobic spore-bearing organisms elaborate highly toxic exotoxins but their power of invasiveness is poor. Anaerobic spore-bearing organisms develop in wounds in which there is much devitalized or necrotic tissue. These infections are more likely to occur in extensive lacerated wounds which have been heavily contaminated with street dirt or debris, e.g. in traffic accidents. Two main types of lesion are produced by these organisms, namely Clostridium cellulitis and gas gangrene.

In Clostridium cellulitis the infection is confined to the connective tissues. Gas is produced in these tissues but the muscles are unaffected. In gas gangrene there is a massive and rapid necrosis of muscle tissue accompanied by profound toxaemia. The types of organisms causing these infections may be established by anaerobic culture methods.

Tetanus infection

Tetanus infection is likely to occur only in a person who has no artificially induced immunity to the disease. As a general rule the infection only develops in deep wounds containing necrotic tissue, but it may become established in relatively slight and superficial wounds, particularly in malnourished children. The organisms do not invade the tissues but produce a powerful exotoxin which gives rise to the convulsions which characterize the disease. Tetanus usually develops within 5–14 days of the infection, but the onset of symptoms may be delayed for weeks or months. This delay is seen when the organisms have remained dormant at the site of injury, and in these cases the original wound has usually healed by the time the tetanus develops.

Predisposition of injured tissue to blood-borne infections

In cases where the original injury has not been directly responsible for the introduction of the infection it is often difficult to establish a cause and effect relationship between the injury and the subsequent infection. This difficulty was well illustrated in a death investigated by one of us:

> It was alleged that a workman received a head injury 6 days before his death. He resumed work immediately after the injury and became ill with cerebral symptoms on the following day. Three days later he was admitted to hospital, and although there was no external evidence of head injury the symptoms were such that it was necessary to trephine the skull. At the operation the openings were made at the usual sites on the sides of the skull. The surgeon found no evidence of intracranial haemorrhage. The patient died on the following day, and at autopsy a diffuse purulent meningitis and a bilateral subarachnoid haemorrhage distributed over the vertex were observed. There were no fractures of the skull or dural tears. Culture of the pus revealed a mixed growth of organisms but no meningococci or pneumococci were isolated.

In a case of this nature it becomes necessary to establish that the injury predisposed the tissues to infection. In dealing with this problem in general, Moritz[12] refers to a series of experiments which tend to show that an injury, by producing a local increase in capillary permeability, facilitates the passage of circulating organisms into the site of tissue damage. In addition, dead tissue and extravasated blood provide an environment which is favourable to bacterial growth. Tissue damage may be of submacroscopic dimensions, and Moritz states that the susceptibility of a previously injured tissue to secondary infection does not necessarily bear any direct relationship to the severity of the original injury. It is apparent that each case has to be considered on its own merits. In the case under consideration, the possibility of the injury having predisposed the meninges to infection could not be excluded.

Complications due to healing

Wounds heal through the development of granulation tissue, and although complete healing may take place, the resulting fibrous scar tissue is usually weaker in structure than the original tissue. If fibrous scar tissue is not subjected to tension it may contract, and such contraction may give rise to complications, e.g. a fibrous scar in a hollow muscular organ may lead to a stricture and obstruction. On the other hand, if a fibrous scar is subjected to continuous tension it may stretch, and such stretching may give rise to complications, e.g. a fibrous scar in the wall of an artery may bulge into a traumatic aneurysm.

Death may result indirectly from healing, either through the contraction or the stretching of a fibrous tissue scar.

This condition was seen in one of our cases. A youth received a bullet wound of the neck and died nine months later from a ruptured false aneurysm of the subclavian artery. Although the aneurysm could be regarded as a new lesion, it arose as a complication of the original injury through a process of healing in the vessel wall. The death could therefore be attributed indirectly to the original bullet wound. In this case the person responsible for the shooting was charged with culpable homicide.

THE DESCRIPTION OF WOUNDS FOR MEDICO-LEGAL PURPOSES

In reporting on the examination of accused persons or complainants, the nature, exact position, direction and dimensions of every injury found should be described. The alleged manner in which the injury was produced and the probable time of its occurrence may be recorded, if this information is available.

Autopsy reports on wounds should contain a description of their nature, direction and exact situation. The dimensions of the wounds as measured with a ruler should also be recorded. Numbers should be assigned to each of the wounds that are described.

Records of diagrams to chart the approximate situation of injuries found on examination during life or at autopsy are often of value.

Photographs (including colour photographs) are also of assistance, but they do not replace anatomical description in the report.

In all cases (whether the report deals with the living or the dead) the appearance of the wound must be described in objective terms, excluding any nomenclature implying the manner in which the wound was inflicted.

THE AGE OF A WOUND IN THE LIVING

A medical practitioner may be required to estimate the period that has elapsed between the infliction of a wound and the time of examination of a complaint or an accused, on the basis of the naked-eye appearances of the wound. An exact determination of the age of a wound by this method is not possible as the intensity of the local inflammatory reaction varies. Under average conditions, however, the edges of a wound are red and swollen after a lapse of about 12 hours. A small wound may show scab formation after approximately 24 hours, and when a wound has become infected, pus may be seen after a period of about 36 hours.

Epithelium begins to grow at the edges of a wound after about 24 hours and epithelialization of small clean wounds may be complete in 4 to 5 days.

The naked-eye appearances of a wound depend to a large extent upon whether healing is proceeding with or without infection. Once infection has supervened, healing may be delayed and it is usually impossible to determine the age of the wound with any degree of accuracy.

DISTINCTION BETWEEN ANTE-MORTEM AND POST-MORTEM WOUNDS AND THE ESTIMATION OF THE APPROXIMATE AGE OF AN ANTE-MORTEM WOUND[12,13]

It may be possible on naked-eye examination to state that a wound is ante-mortem in origin if it shows evidence of a marked inflammatory reaction. In cases of doubt an ante-mortem wound must be distinguished from a post-mortem wound by a microscopic examination for evidence of tissue reaction. Although margination and a limited emigration of leucocytes may occur in tissues in response to injury after somatic death, marked cellular exudation and reactive changes in the tissue cells are seen in ante-mortem wounds only. The absence of tissue reaction, however, does not necessarily indicate that a wound was post-mortem in origin. There may have been insufficient time before death for the development of tissue reaction, or, in the case of small wounds, the reaction may have terminated in resolution. In small wounds such as small contusions, the degree of cellular injury may have been insufficient to elicit an appreciable leucocytic exudation, while in severe injuries the associated circulatory failure may have interfered with the normal reaction.

The intensity of the local reaction to an injury depends upon many factors, such as the severity of the injury, the vascularity of the injured tissue, and the presence or absence of infection or foreign bodies. The course of tissue reaction is therefore variable. For this reason it is never possible to determine the age of an ante-mortem wound within narrow limits, but an estimate of its approximate age may be made by comparing the microscopic reactive changes in the wound with the course of tissue reaction as it has been observed experimentally. When the age of an ante-mortem wound has to be determined for medico-legal purposes, medical practitioners should submit portions of the excised wound, preserved in formol-saline, to a pathologist for histological examination.

According to Moritz the time of occurrence of the reactive changes of inflammation to an aseptic mechanical injury under experimental conditions is as follows: dilatation of the capillaries and margination of the leucocytes may be seen within a few minutes of the injury. Emigration of leucocytes is usually observed within an hour of the injury; the first leucocytes to pass into the tissues are the polymorphonuclear neutrophils. Monocytes appear at a later stage and are seldom seen in the exudate before the lapse of about 12 hours. In traumatic aseptic inflammation the exudation usually reached its maximum intensity within 48 hours of the injury. Reactive changes in the tissue histiocytes and swelling of the vascular endothelium may be observed within an hour of the injury. The fibroblasts at the site of injury show reactive changes within a few hours and these cells begin to undergo mitotic division about 15 hours after the injury. The rate of proliferation of the fibroblasts and the formation of new capillaries varies, but it usually takes at least 72 hours for vascularized granulation tissue to develop. The time taken for the formation of collagen varies, but new fibrils may be seen in the injured tissue within 4 to 5 days of the injury. In small wounds a fibrous tissue scar may be apparent at the end of one week. The presence of infection leads to considerable modification in the time of occurrence and the duration of the changes which have been described. Once infection has supervened it may be maintained for days or weeks and the age of a wound cannot be determined reliably in these circumstances.

The microscopic evidence relied upon for the determination of the age of a wound includes histochemical as well as conventional histological techniques.

Raekallio,[14–26] in a study of human autopsy material, claims that the microscopic demonstration of enzyme reactions in wounds provides evidence that they were sustained before death. Robertson and Hodge,[27] using conventional histological techniques, classified the various stages in the healing of ante-mortem abrasions into four stages as shown in Table 11.2.

This classification provides reasonable confidence limits within which the ante-mortem age of an abrasion can be determined. Their work confirms the earlier observations by Robertson and Mansfield[28] demonstrating the difficulty of determining the age of an ante-mortem bruise with any accuracy.

Distinction between ante-mortem and post-mortem bruises

It is usually accepted that small bruises resembling ante-mortem bruises can be produced if marked force is applied to a body within a few hours of death. If the force applied after death is sufficiently great, the capillaries

Table 11.2 Histological changes which occur in ante-mortem abrasions

Stage	Survival period
1. Scab formation	Dead on arrival at hospital or survival less than 4 hours. 4–12 hours.
2. Epithelial regeneration	12–48 hours 2–4 days
3. Subepithelial granulation tissue formation and epithelial hyperplasia	4–8 days 8–12 days
4. Regression of both the epithelial hyperplasia and granulation tissue formation.	over 12 days (weeks to months)

in the affected area may be ruptured and blood may be extravasated into the tissue spaces, with the production of a bruise which is similar in structure to an ante-mortem bruise.

It may be impossible to distinguish an ante-mortem bruise from a post-mortem bruise if the death occurs rapidly after the injury, but if the death is delayed, these bruises may be differentiated on microscopic examination. Moritz has described the microscopic changes which a bruise undergoes during life, and has drawn attention to the criteria upon which an estimate of the approximate age of a bruise may be based. These criteria include the rate of disintegration of the red cells and the extent and character of the tissue reaction. If the red cells have lost their shape and staining characteristics, and if iron-containing pigment is demonstrable either at the site of injury or in the regional lymph nodes, it is probable that at least 12 hours have elapsed since the injury. The presence of tissue reaction of a degree beyond a margination and limited emigration of the white cells would indicate that the bruise was probably ante-mortem in origin.

Robertson and Mansfield[28] have, however, emphasized the difficulty of determining the age of an ante-mortem bruise with any accuracy. The microscopical examination of skin contusions does, therefore, not give as much assistance as does the microscopical examination of abrasions. As the two are, however, often closely associated, as examination of any overlying abrasion may assist with the ageing of an injury.

The differentiation between ante-mortem bruises and post-mortem dissection artefacts of the neck has been dealt with at page 104.

In his studies, Raekallio[19,20,24,26] claims that the microscopical demonstration of enzyme reaction in wounds precede morphological alterations, thus providing evidence of the ante-mortem nature of wounds, since enzymes and other substances are essential in the inflammatory response to injury.

Haemorrhage from ante-mortem and post-mortem wounds

Evidence of profuse haemorrhage from a wound usually indicates that it was received before death. The absence of haemorrhage, however, even when a relatively large blood vessel has been injured, does not necessarily indicate that the wound was post-mortem in origin. This condition may be seen in ante-mortem wounds where shock has been a major factor in causing the death.

External haemorrhage may occur from post-mortem wounds, but such bleeding is usually slight in amount unless a large blood vessel or a vein in a dependent portion of the body has been injured. It should be noted that ante-mortem wounds may continue to bleed externally after death, particularly if they are situated in a dependent portion of the body.

Problems which arise in determining the amount of bleeding which can occur into a pleural cavity before death and after death may be illustrated by the findings in a case reported by one of us:[29]

> In a murder trial an unmeasured volume of blood (estimated at 1–1½ pints for the first time by the medical practitioner concerned 4 months after he had performed the autopsy) was found in the right pleural cavity of the deceased, who had been shot in the back of the chest and the back of the head.
>
> The bullet wound in the chest shattered the 5th rib posteriorly. The intercostal vessels were torn across and the bullet wound traversed the upper lobe of the right lung. It made its exit through the second intercostal space in front.
>
> At the preparatory examination medical experts for the Crown expressed the view that it would have taken at least half an hour for 1–1½ pints of blood to accumulate in the pleural cavity as a result of the bullet wound in the chest. They regarded the head wound as almost immediately fatal and drew the inference that the deceased had been shot in the chest in another part of the city and then brought to the place where he was ultimately found and where the fatal head wound was administered.
>
> On this basis two accused persons were indicted with murder.
>
> The Crown's medical hypothesis raised several interesting points for consideration:
>
> 1. How rapidly during life can 1 to 1½ pints of blood accumulate in the chest cavity following a bullet wound of the type described?
>
> 2. To what extent can post-mortem bleeding account for the quantity of blood found at autopsy?
>
> It was submitted that the Crown's contention that it would have taken at least half an hour for 1 to 1½ pints of blood to accumulate in these circumstances, was unacceptable and provided no basis for the view that the chest wound was inflicted before the head wound.
>
> The impropriety of guessing the volume of blood in the chest cavity from inspection, instead of measuring the amount, was a matter for criticism, especially in view of the grave inferences which the Crown sought to draw on the basis of this observation.

During life bleeding will continue until arrested by the usual processes of clotting and contraction of the vessels; but death may occur before this happens. The amount of bleeding may be considerable within the short space of three or four minutes. This depends, amongst other things, on the size of the vessels injured.

It is often overlooked that vessels of substantial calibre take a course close to the periphery of the lung and that they may be a source of considerable bleeding from lung wounds.

The absence of clots in cases of intrapleural bleeding does not assist in determining whether the bleeding occurred *ante mortem* or *post mortem*. Sellors[30] has pointed out that blood shed in the pleural cavity in most cases does not appear to have clotted. He attributes this phenomenon to the rapid defibrination of the blood as it is being shed. The blood is subjected to violent agitation; the collapsed lung splashes about in the blood, bouncing with each transmitted cardiac pulsation. There is little chance for any firm clot to form. Fibrin shreds may be deposited in the course of this process.

The possibility that the autopsy dissection has contributed to the quantity of blood found in the chest cavity must be excluded. This source of contamination may be considerable and rapid. We have demonstrated that when clear fluid is aspirated out of the chest cavity (for measurement of the quantity) bleeding from divided vessels can colour the pleural fluid within a matter of seconds. In cases of this nature, therefore, the dissection technique described by Gonzales et al[31] is to be commended. They state:

> The sternoclavicular joint is disarticulated by cutting downward from the top of the joint and then cutting outward at right angles; these joints and the first costal cartilages are not cut until the pleural cavities are inspected, for fear of contaminating them with blood from severed innominate vessels.

The extent of bleeding after death depends basically on the fact that in almost all circumstances the blood is liquid *post mortem* in most parts of the body. This applies particularly to the peripheral vessels and the capillaries.[32]

Other factors include the patency of the divided vessels, e.g. the lack of obstruction to the lumen by firm clot, the influence of gravity and the size and nature of the vessels concerned, i.e. the importance of veins as opposed to arteries, which are generally almost empty.

In the chest cavity, damage to the intercostal vessels may have a special significance.[33] The right intercostal vessels drain into the vena azygos, which receives the superior and inferior hemiazygos veins from the left side. The vena azygos itself forms an anastomosis between the superior vena cava and the inferior vena cava.

If, therefore, the blood is liquid and if gravity assists drainage, for purely anatomical reasons there will be a vast reservoir of liquid blood which may be drained through even a small incision.

In view of the absence in the literature of quantitative data on the amount of post-mortem bleeding from lung wounds, experiments were conducted by Shapiro and Robertson[29] on recently dead bodies. The results are shown in Table 11.3.

Table 11.3 Results of experiments on post-mortem bleeding of lung wounds (after Shapiro and Robertson[29]).

Case no.	Case history	State of body	Time between infliction of wound and opening of body (minutes)	Cause of death and main findings	Amount of blood in right pleural cavity (ml)
59/60	Female, aged 35 years Sudden collapse	Warm to the touch Tissues appear fresh	20	Hypertensive cardiac disease; left ventricular hypertrophy; left lung slightly congested; no fluid	375
40/60	Male, aged 22 years Collapsed at work; died in ambulance *en route* to hospital	Warm to the touch Tissues appear fresh	15	Cerebral haemorrhage; old head injury with cortical scarring	50
87/60	Male, aged 16 years Knocked down by motor-car	Slightly warm to the touch Tissues appear fresh	15	Multiple fractures involving all the bones of the vault of the skull with cerebral contusion; no thoracic injury	50
98/60	Male, aged 35 years Drowned in car which drove over the jetty	Slightly warm to the touch Post-mortem interval 6 hours	30	Drowning; lungs oedematous but not markedly congested; no injuries present	800 (clots present)
192/60	Male, aged 28 years Collapsed at work	Post-mortem interval 5 hours	7	Subendocardial fibrosis; pyelonephritis with marked scarring and contraction of the kidneys	175
149/60	Male, aged 62 years Collapsed whilst sitting at home; died *en route* to hospital	Post-mortem interval 6 hours	30	Slight emphysema of upper lobes only; vascular atherosclerotic disease marked; no injury	1000

Procedure: A scalpel was passed through the rib interspace 6.3 cm (2½ in.) to the right and 7.6 cm (3 in.) below the spine of the seventh cervical vertebra. The body was opened in the usual way, after lying recumbent for an interval. The blood in the right pleural cavity was measured with precautions to avoid contamination by the dissection technique.

These experiments indicate the very considerable amount of bleeding which may occur after death from wounds of the lung tissue.

DISTINCTION BETWEEN SUICIDAL, ACCIDENTAL AND HOMICIDAL WOUNDS

In most deaths the circumstances are such that it is usually possible to state whether the fatal injury was of accidental, suicidal or homicidal origin. Difficulties may arise, however, when bodies are found in places such as fields or on the roadside or in deserted dwellings. In such cases medical practitioners are usually called to the scene before the body is moved and they should carefully note the position of the body, the state of the clothing, the position of blood stains and the condition of the surroundings. As a general rule the police take a photograph of the body in the position in which it was found. The nature of the injury in these cases must be determined from the character of the wounds taken in conjunction with a knowledge of the circumstances of the injury.

The character of the wounds

The presence of a large number of wounds is usually suggestive of homicide if an accident can be excluded, but multiple wounds may occasionally be self-inflicted. Suicidal wounds may be found in any part of the body which can be reached by the person concerned, but certain sites such as the front of the neck, the front of the left wrist, the upper portion of the left thigh and the front of the chest are commonly selected for these injuries. Wounds of the back and the back of the neck are generally homicidal in origin, but suicidal wounds in these regions have been described. Wounds of the front, back and sides of the head may be accidental or homicidal, but wounds on the top of the head are usually of homicidal origin. Suicidal and homicidal wounds of the neck are considered at page 300. Multiple incised wounds of the forearms, palms and fingers are suggestive of an assault in which the victim has attempted to defend himself. The recognition of self-inflicted fabricated wounds has been dealt with at page 231.

A combination of fractures of the bones of the legs and lumbar and head injuries is suggestive of a pedestrian traffic injury (p. 335).

The circumstances of the injury

A weapon found firmly grasped in the hand of the deceased is strong presumptive evidence of suicide. The finding of hair or a portion of clothing in the hands of the deceased, and not belonging to him, may be indicative of homicide (p. 33). The finding of a weapon beside the body is not necessarily indicative of suicide as a murderer may leave a weapon at the scene of the crime to simulate suicide. Conversely, a person committing suicide may have had sufficient time to dispose of the weapon.

Evidence of a struggle or the presence of drag marks at the scene is suggestive of homicide. As it is unusual for a person committing suicide to injure himself through his clothes, the presence of a wound in a region ordinarily covered by clothing without any corresponding damage to the overlying clothes is suggestive of suicide. Recent tears in clothing and the loss of buttons may be indicative of a struggle and homicide.

A weapon is often produced as an exhibit at an inquest or criminal trial and a medical witness may be asked whether the injuries found could have been caused by that particular weapon. In certain circumstances it may be possible to show that the pattern of an injury corresponds to the form of the weapon with which it has been produced, but this is exceptional (p. 228). As a general rule it is impossible to show that a particular wound has been caused by a specific weapon, and the medical witness should therefore confine himself to an opinion as to whether the injuries could or could not have been produced by the exhibit weapon.

It will be apparent that the manner in which an injury is produced cannot be determined on the basis of any general rules; every case has to be considered on its own merits in relation to the particular circumstances obtaining at the time of the injury.

PERIOD OF SURVIVAL AFTER INJURY

In cases where death has occurred from haemorrhage, a medical witness may be asked to estimate the length of time that the deceased could have lived after the infliction of the injury. This period will depend upon the nature of the injury, the degree of associated shock and the rate of bleeding. The degree of shock and the rate of bleeding cannot be determined from the autopsy findings. Wounds of the heart, the lungs and the great blood vessels often lead to death within a few minutes of the injury, but cases have been recorded where persons have lived for many hours with large wounds of these structures. A medical witness should be cautious before expressing an opinion in this type of case.

VOLUNTARY ACTIVITY BEFORE DEATH IN RAPIDLY FATAL INJURIES

In cases where the injuries are presumed to have caused rapid death, a medical witness may be asked whether it would have been possible for the deceased to have performed some voluntary act, such as walking, after the infliction of the injury. Individuals vary in their reaction to injuries. A punctured wound of the heart, for instance, may lead to instantaneous death in one person, while another person with a similar wound may be capable of walking or running a considerable distance before collapsing. In the same way, although it is unusual, a person may remain conscious for several minutes before dying from a severe intracranial injury. Unless it can be shown that an injury would have been immediately incompatible with life, it is seldom possible to state that a deceased person could not have performed some activity before his death.

REFERENCES

1 Moritz A R. The Pathology of Trauma. Philadelphia: Lea & Febiger. 1942: pp 13–19.
2 Holbourn A H S. Mechanics of head injuries. Lancet 1943; 145: 438–441.
3 Smith S. Forensic Medicine. 9th ed. London: Churchill. 1949: pp 168–173.
4 Glaister J. Medical Jurisprudence and Toxicology. 9th ed. Edinburgh: Livingstone. 1950: p 244.
5 Gross H. Criminal Investigation. 3rd ed. London: Sweet & Maxwell. 1934: pp 418–419.
6 Wilson J V. The Pathology of Traumatic Injury. Edinburgh: Livingstone. 1946: pp 1–23.
7 Moon V H. Shock: its Diagnosis, Occurrence and Management. Philadelphia: Lea & Febiger. 1942.
8 Wilson J V. The Pathology of Traumatic Injury. Edinburgh: Livingstone. 1946: p 92.
9 Best C H, Taylor N B. The Physiological Basis of Medical Practice. 4th ed. Baltimore: Williams & Wilkins. 1945: p 16.
10 Moon V H. Shock: its Diagnosis, Occurrence and Management. Philadelphia: Lea & Febiger. 1942: pp 97–109.
11 Wright S. Applied Physiology. 8th ed. Oxford University Press. 1945: pp 354–355.
12 Moritz A R. The Pathology of Trauma. Philadelphia: Lea & Febiger. 1942: pp 93–99.
13 Some of the data in this section have been obtained from Moritz A R. The Pathology of Trauma. Philadelphia: Lea & Febiger. 1942: pp 19–35.
14 Raekallio J. Enzymes histochemically demonstrable in the earliest phase of wound healing. Nature (Lond) 1960; 188: 234–235.
15 Raekallio J. Histochemical studies on vital and post-mostem skin wounds. Ann Med Exp Biol Fenn 1961; 39 (Suppl. 6): 1–105.
16 Raekallio J. Die Altersbestimmung Mechanisch Bedingter Hautwunden mit Enzymhistochemischen Methoden. Lübeck: Verlag Max Schmidt-Römhild. 1965.
17 Raekallio J. Enzyme Histochemistry of Wound Healing. Stuttgart: Gustav Fischer Verlag. 1970.
18 Raekallio J. Determination of the age of wounds by histochemical and biochemical methods. Forens Sci 1972; 1: 3–16.
19 Raekallio J. Estimation of the age of injuries by histochemical and biochemical methods. Z Rechtsmed 1973; 73: 83–102.
20 Raekallio J, Kovacs M, Mäkinen P L. The appearance of oxidoreductases in healing fractures. Acta Pathol Microbiol Scand [A], 1970; 78: 658–664.
21 Raekallio J, Mäkinen P L. Histamine content as vital reaction I. Experimental investigation. Zacchia 1966; 41: 273–284.
22 Raekallio J, Mäkinen P L. Aminopeptidases in serum and skin of rats during early wound healing. Ann Med Exp Biol Fenn 1967; 45: 224–229.
23 Raekallio J, Mäkinen P L. Alkaline and acid phosphatase activity in the initial phase of fracture healing. Acta Pathol Microbiol Scand [A] 1969; 75: 415–422.
24 Raekallio J, Mäkinen P L. Serotonin content as vital reaction I. Experimental investigation. Zacchia 1969; 44: 587–594.
25 Raekallio J, Mäkinen P L. Serotonin and histamine contents as vital reactions II. Autopsy studies. Zacchia 1970; 45: 403–414.
26 Raekallio J, Mäkinen P L. Biochemical distinction between ante-mortem and post-mortem skin wounds by isoelectric focusing in polyacrylamide gel. I. Experimental investigation on arylaminopeptidases. Zacchia 1971; 46: 281–293.
27 Robertson I, Hodge P R. Histopathology of healing abrasions, Forens Sci 1972; 1: 17–25.
28 Robertson I, Mansfield R A. Ante-mortem and post-mortem bruises of the skin, their differentiation. J Forens Med 1957; 4: 2–10.
29 Shapiro H A, Robertson I. The significance of blood in the pleural cavity observed after death. J Forens Med 1962; 9: 5–9.

30 Sellors T H. Haemothorax. Lancet 1945; 1: 143–144.
31 Gonzales T A, Vance M, Helpern M, Umberger C J. Legal Medicine: Pathology and Toxicology. 2nd ed. New York: Appleton-Century-Crofts. 1954: p 86.
32 Mole R H. Fibrinolysin and fluidity of blood post-mortem. J Path Bact 1948; 60: 413–427.
33 Johnston T B, Whillis J. Gray's Anatomy 28th ed. London: Longmans, Green. 1942: Figs 780, 781, pp 826–827.

12

Regional injuries of medico-legal importance

HEAD INJURIES

The head consists of concentric planes of different tissues; these tissues are made up of contrasting substances and textures; soft tissue, bone, air and fluid. Their anatomical relations and their own consistency determines their reaction to the application of force.

Head injuries may be caused by sharp-edged or sharp-pointed weapons but most head injuries are due to the application of a blunt force.

Sharp objects and missiles can produce penetrating injuries and may be defined as a type of *so-called* 'open head injury'.

The application of blunt force to the head may result in injury to the contents of the skull, either alone or in combination with a fracture of the skull; it is exceptional for the skull to be fractured without some intracranial injury. Injury to the contents of the skull may affect the brain or the meninges and their related vessels.

The extent and degree of an injury to the skull and its contents is not necessarily proportional to the amount of force applied to the head. The application of a moderate force to the head may cause a severe intracranial haemorrhage while a greater force may produce no injury.

The skull and/or its contents may be severely injured without any external evidence of the injury. (The hat or the hair of the victim often affords protection to the surface of the underlying scalp.)

The position has been summed up by Munro[1] as follows:

Any type of cranio-cerebral injury can be caused by any kind of blow on any sort of head.

Wounds of the scalp

Wounds of the scalp may or may not be associated with fractures of the skull and/or injuries to the intracranial contents. Most wounds of the scalp are caused by the application of blunt force to the head, e.g. from falls or blows. Such wounds of the scalp take the form of contusions or lacerations.

Bleeding from scalp wounds produced by sharp-edged weapons may result in considerable blood loss.

Contusions of the scalp

Contusions of the scalp often result from the crushing of the soft tissues against the underlying bone. When the vault of the skull is fractured, blood may extravasate into the scalp tissues from ruptured diploic veins. Contusions may occur in the superficial fascia, in the temporalis muscles, or in the loose areolar tissue between the galea aponeurotica and the periosteum (Fig. 12.1). Contusions in the superficial fascia appear as localized swellings (or haematomata) and tend to be limited in size because of the dense nature of the fibro-fatty tissue of the fascia. Contusions deep to the galea aponeurotica, however, are usually of an extensive nature because the extravasated blood can diffuse in the loose subaponeurotic tissues. Deep bruises of this nature may not be recognizable clinically.

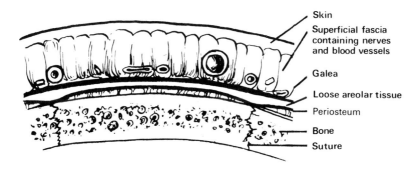

Skin

Superficial fascia containing nerves and blood vessels

Galea

Loose areolar tissue

Periosteum

Bone

Suture

Fig. 12.1 Cross-section of the scalp.

As multiple contusions of the scalp may coalesce, it is often difficult to determine the number of blows which were inflicted from the area of contusion found in the scalp tissue.

Lacerated wounds of the scalp

Lacerated wounds of the scalp may result from the splitting of the soft tissues against the underlying bone or from the tearing of the tissues by fragments of fractured bone. Lacerated wounds of the scalp are often linear in shape and may resemble incised wounds. The criteria which differentiate lacerated wounds from incised wounds are set out in Table 11.1 (p. 230).

A lacerated wound may extend through the galea aponeurotica and if the wound becomes infected the infection may spread widely in the subaponeurotic space. The veins of the scalp and the face are connected with the parasagittal, lateral and cavernous sinuses through emissary veins which pass through foramina in the skull. Infected wounds of the scalp and the face may be complicated by thrombophlebitis of scalp veins and facial veins and this process may extend through the emissary veins to the intracranial sinuses (p. 268).

Fractures of the skull

(a) Rowbotham's hypothesis

Fractures of the skull are caused (1) by the direct application of force to the skull, or (2) by indirect violence.

Fractures of the skull caused by the direct application of force. According to Rowbotham[2] the direct application of force to the head may result in (1) a local deformation of a segment of the skull at the site of impact, and/or (2) a general deformation of the skull.

Fractures of the skull due to local deformation. The bones of the skull have a limited amount of elasticity,* and if a force is applied to the vault of the skull the bone may bend without the occurrence of a fracture. If the bending is sufficiently great a fracture occurs.

The sequence of events in a fracture of the skull by local deformation is shown in Figure 12.2. At the site of impact the bone is indented in the form of a shallow cone. At the apex of the cone, the inner table is stretched and the outer table is compressed, but at the periphery of the cone the convexity of the bend is directed outwards. If the limits of elasticity are not exceeded, the bone will recoil to its normal shape and no fracture will result (Fig. 12.2B).† If the deformation is of short duration and results in maximal distortion at the apex of the cone, a fracture confined to the inner table may result (Fig. 12.2C).‡ With the application of greater force, both the inner and outer tables of the skull may be fractured (Fig. 12.2D). The figure illustrates how, at the apex, the inner table fractures before the outer table, while at the periphery the outer table fractures first. In fractures of this nature, by an extension of the 'break' in the inner table at the apex through to the outer table, and by an extension of the 'break' in the outer table at the periphery through to the inner table, a depressed–comminuted fracture

---

* The bones of the skull of an infant are more elastic than the bones of the skull of an adult. In old age the bones of the skull are relatively brittle.

† A transient deformation of this nature may be sufficiently marked to produce a localized superficial contusion of the underlying brain tissue or a rupture of a meningeal vessel.

‡ In a fracture of the inner table, the sharp edges of bone may penetrate the dura and lacerate the underlying brain tissue. As the deformation is transient, the bone fragments may recoil to the positions which they occupied before the fracture. There may be no clinical signs or radiological evidence of such a fracture. Subsequent healing of the lesions in the dura and brain tissue, however, may result in the development of adhesions between the dura and the brain. Adhesions of this nature may result in so-called 'traumatic epilepsy' within months or years of the injury.

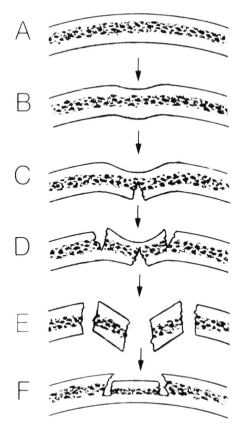

Fig. 12.2 The sequence of events in fracture by local deformity. (After Rowbotham.)
A, Normal skull; B, Indentation of skull without fracture; C, Fracture of inner table;
D, Fractures of outer and inner tables; E, Localized comminuted depressed fracture;
F, Outer table crushed into diploë.

is produced (Fig. 12.2E). The fracture lines in a depressed–comminuted
fracture tend to run radially from the central point at the apex, and at the
periphery the fracture lines tend to run in a circular manner (Fig. 12.3).
Localized depressed–comminuted fractures of the skull may occur in association with fissured fractures due to general deformation from the same
injury.

Moritz[3] states that if the spongiosa between the inner and outer tables
is fragile, a circumscribed segment of the outer table may be driven into
the diploë without in any way disturbing the inner table (Fig. 12.2F). This
type of fracture is relatively uncommon.

Fractures of the skull due to general deformation. Rowbotham[4] states that
the skull behaves like an elastic sphere, so that when it is compressed in
one plane it bulges in other directions, e.g. if the skull is compressed
laterally the vertical and longitudinal diameters are increased and fractures

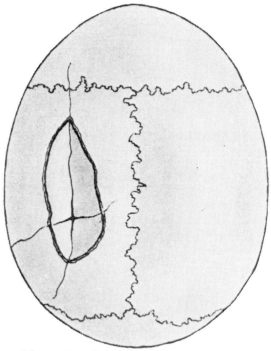

Fig. 12.3 The lines of fracture in a depressed-comminuted fracture of the skull. (After Moritz.)

may occur in these planes if the bone is stretched beyond the limits of its elasticity. The head may be compressed between two external objects or between an external object and the spinal column. Compression of the head between an external object and the spinal column is the more common of the two methods.

Fractures due to general deformation are usually fissured and they occur in parts of the skull distant from the site of application of the force.

Fracture patterns. The bones of the skull vary in thickness and strength. Relatively weak panels of bone are enclosed within strong ridges and buttresses of bone. The general disposition of the various bands of thickening and areas of relative thinness are shown in Figures 12.4 and 12.5 which have been taken from Rowbotham.[5] In the vault there are vertical thickenings at the glabella, the external angular processes, the mastoid processes and the external occipital protuberance. These vertical ridges are united by three arches on each side, namely, the supra-orbital ridge in front, the curved lines of the occiput behind, and the temporal crests at the side. In addition, there is a strong anteroposterior arch of bone in the midline over the vertex of the skull. The thin plates of bone in the base are enclosed within strong buttresses of bone. One buttress runs anteroposteriorly in the midline. The petrous portions of the temporal bones form

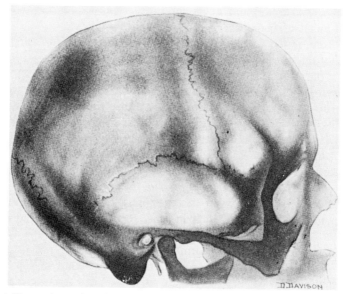

Fig. 12.4 The weak panels and strong buttresses of the vault.

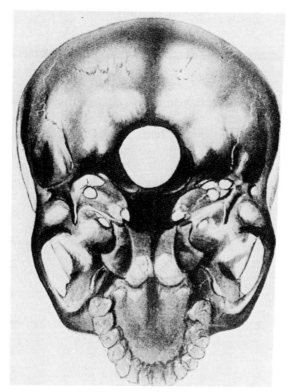

Fig. 12.5 The weak panels and strong buttresses of the base.

buttresses on each side and more anteriorly a buttress is formed by the thickened edges of the wings of the sphenoid.

Apart from the influence of the anatomical structure of the skull in determining fracture patterns, the lines of a fracture may depend upon the mode of application of the force, e.g. a force applied to the glabella region in an upward direction may lift off a dome of bone and cause extensive horizontal fractures radiating backwards in a direction parallel to the base.

Fractures of the skull due to indirect violence. Fractures of the vault and base of the skull due to indirect violence may be caused by forces applied to the face or chin or by forces applied upwards through the spinal column, e.g. in falls from heights on to the feet or buttocks. Blows on the chin may result in fractures of the glenoid fossae, but it is exceptional for the mandibular condyle to be driven into the cranial cavity. The force of a blow on the mandible, e.g. an uppercut in boxing, may be transmitted through the maxilla and its internal angular processes to the base of the skull and result in a fracture of the cribriform plate of the ethmoid.

Forces transmitted upwards through the spinal column may produce a ring fracture around the basiocciput. A similar type of fracture may result from a severe blow on the vertex which drives the skull downwards on to the spinal column.

(b) The hypothesis of Gurdjian et al

1. Adult skull fracture: the magnitude of the forces and the mechanism involved. The vulnerability of the head and that artifacts can be used to inflict fatal injuries on it, goes back to the beginning of man's existence; but the distinction between skull fracture and injury to the intracranial contents may only have come much later.

A primary distinction has long been made between depressed fractures and fissured or linear skull fractures. Rowbotham sums up a fairly widely held view in his statement that local deformation of the skull produces a depressed fracture and general deformation produces a linear fracture.[2] The accuracy of such hypotheses has been tested in recent years by the production of skull fractures under controlled laboratory conditions. These experiments[6] have thrown considerable light on how and why the skull fractures. They have also made necessary considerable modification of previous theories.

The damage done to the bone is due to the way in which it absorbs energy applied to it. Although the size and shape of the traumatizing object as well as the thickness of the skull are of some importance, the over-riding factor is probably the velocity with which the object strikes the head (or the head strikes the object).

The magnitude of the forces involved. Information about the magnitude of the forces involved may be important in the design of vehicles and protective head and seat gear.

This is equivalent to dropping a 10 lb weight through a distance of 7 feet.

(c) What happens when a baseball pitcher pitches a fast ball?

The baseball weighs about 5 oz ($\frac{5}{16}$ lb).

The velocity of the pitch is about 100 feet per second.
The energy involved is calculated from the formula

$$E_k = \frac{1}{2} mv^2,$$

$$= \frac{1}{2} \times \frac{5}{16} \times 100 \times 100 \text{ foot-poundals,}$$

$$= \frac{5}{32} \times \frac{100 \times 100}{32} \text{ foot-pounds,}$$

$$= \pm 50 \text{ foot-pounds.}$$

This is equivalent to dropping a 10 lb weight through a distance of about 5 feet.

Experimental studies. The principles involved in the mechanism of skull fracture are convincingly illustrated by the experimental work of Gurdjian et al[6], who dropped cadaver heads of known weight through known distances onto a flat steel plate weighing 160 lb. Therefore the energies involved can be calculated for each head.

The weight of the isolated heads (including all coverings and contents) ranged from 7.3 to 14.6 lb.

The distance dropped in one set of experiments was about $3\frac{1}{2}$ feet, the head being dropped onto the mid-frontal region, sustaining a deceleration impact (Table 12.1).

In the case of a head weighing 10 lb, dropped through a vertical distance of 3.5 feet, the energy involved on deceleration impact is 35 foot-pounds.

This is 7 times as much energy as is involved in walking into an obstruction in the dark. It involves half the energy with which the 4-minute miler runs head-on into an obstruction; and it is seven-tenths of the energy absorbed by a batter's head when it is hit by the ball in a fast pitch.

The calculated and the observed energies correspond, are not of a very considerable magnitude, and indicate that the energy required to produce a fracture of the skull under experimental conditions in the laboratory matches the amount of energy required to fracture the skull of a living head.

How does the skull fracture?
How does the bone actually break? If we know this, we may be able to predict where fractures are likely to occur or, in reconstructing how a fracture happened, we may be able to deduce where the force producing it was likely to have been applied.

We are not here concerned with the varying effects produced by high velocity missiles but with blunt forces and relatively low velocities.

Very instructive data were obtained from the experiments (already referred to) carried out by Gurdjian et al.[6] They coated skulls inside and out with a brittle lacquer. Under the stress of impact when the skulls were alowed to fall measured distances onto a heavy polished steel slab, the deformation was indicated by the cracks which appeared in the lacquer.

The following physical facts were established:

Table 12.1 Experimental skull fracture (mid-frontal deceleration impact)

No.	Weight of head (pounds)	Distance dropped (feet)	Energy (foot-pounds) (approximate)	Fractures*
1	10.38	$3\frac{1}{3}$	34.6	II
2	10.63	$3\frac{1}{3}$	35.4	I
3	11.00	$3\frac{2}{3}$	40.3	I
4	12.63	$3\frac{2}{3}$	46.3	II
5	14.38	$4\frac{2}{3}$	67.0	I
6	12.38	$3\frac{1}{3}$	41.3	III
7	10.00	$3\frac{1}{2}$	35.0	III
8	11.00	$3\frac{1}{3}$	36.7	III
9	11.63	$3\frac{1}{3}$	38.7	III
10	14.63	$2\frac{5}{6}$	41.4	III

* Fractures:

I: A single linear fracture; II: Two linear fractures; III: Stellate fractures.

Based on Table I from Gurdjian E S, Webster J E, Lissner H R (1949): *Studies on Skull Fractures with Particular Reference to Engineering Factors.* Am J Surg 78: 736–742.

All impacts produce deformation of varying intensity if the energy expenditure be adequate. Occasionally a *contre coup* outbending was observed diagonally opposite the point of impact.

The skull bends inwards under the direct point of impact (Fig. 12.6A). Cracks appear in the stress-coat lacquer on the inner surface of the skull immediately under the point of impact and radiate outwards from the point of impact (Fig. 12.6B).

This area of inbending can rebound (the skull bone is quite remarkably elastic) or fail, in which case a depressed fracture results.

The depressed fracture will be determined partly by the thickness of the skull and the shape of the weapon but mainly by the velocity of the injuring object (brick, baseball, hammer, axe, bullet).

If the blow is sufficiently severe, cracks also appear in the lacquer on the outer surface of the skull, at a distance from the area of inbending (Fig. 12.6C). This indicates an outbending of the bone peripheral to the area of inbending but running towards it.

The tearing-apart forces in the area of outbending may result in a linear fracture which starts at a considerable distance from the point of impact and runs towards it, but it also extends in the opposite direction

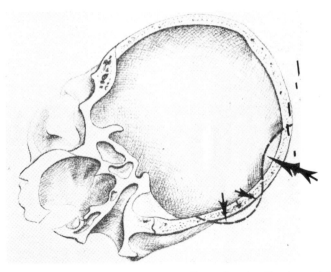

Fig. 12.6A Diagramatic representation of the inbending and outbending (arrows) following an impact in the posterior parietal region. If the area of inbending rebounds, the fracture initiated in the temporal region from outbending of the bone in that area extends towards the point of impact and in the opposite direction.
From Gurdjian E S, Webster J E, Lissner H R (1950): *The Mechanism of Skull Fracture*, J Neurosurg 7:109, (Fig. 4).

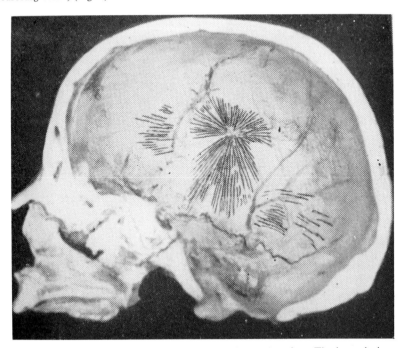

Fig. 12.6B A dry human skull was dropped on to a flat steel surface. The low-velocity deceleration impact in the parietal region produced the stress-coat pattern depicted on the inner surface of the skull. These cracks of the brittle lacquer coating the inner surface of the skull result from inbending of the skull bone.
From Gurdjian E S, Webster J E (1958): *Head Injuries: Mechanisms, Diagnosis and Management.* p. 64, Fig. 6b. London: J. and A. Churchill.

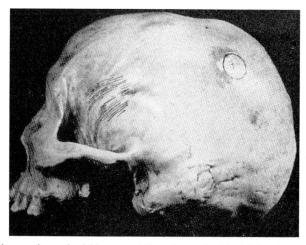

Fig. 12.6C A posterior parietal blow was delivered on a freshly dried cadaver skull coated with brittle lacquer. The resultant stress-coat pattern developed in the temporal region due to tearing apart forces from outbending of the bone in that area. Immediately around the point of the blow there would be radially arranged cracks in the lacquer on the inner surface of the skull, denoting the extent of the inbending from the blow.
From Gurdjian E S, Webster J E, Lissner H R (1950): *The Mechanism of Skull Fracture.* J Neurosurg 7:109 (Fig. 3)

(Fig. 12.6D). This is the primary stress area for that particular point of impact.

The fracture line generally reaches the impact area; but if the energy is insufficient, the fracture may remain limited and not reach the impact area.

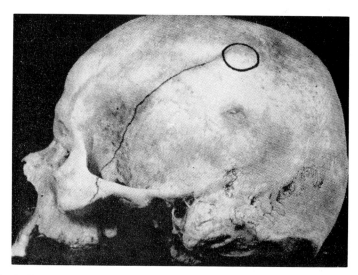

Fig. 12.6D The fracture resulting when an intact cadaver head received a posterior parietal blow. The presence of hair, scalp and skull contents did not alter the position of the resulting fracture. The site of fracture corresponds to the stress-coat pattern illustrated in Fig. 12.6C.
From Gurdjian E S, Webster J E, Lissner H R (1949): *Studies on Skull Fracture with Particular Reference to Engineering Factors.* Am J Surg 78:738 (Fig. 6).

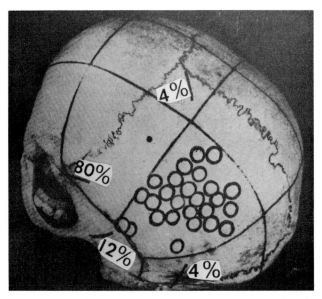

Fig. 12.6E Composite diagram representing the effect of blows in the left parieto-occipital region delivered to 25 skulls, showing the percentage variation in position where the fracture line was initiated. Fractures extend to the point of the blow from the regions indicated. 80% of the linear fractures are initiated in the temporal region when the blow is delivered to the parieto-occipital region.
From Gurdjian E S, Webster J E, Lissner H R (1949): *Studies on Skull Fracture with Particular Reference to Engineering Factors, Am J Surg* 78:741 (Fig. 9).

The variation in position of the initial site of fracture is slight (Fig. 12.6E).

With increasing amounts of energy, outbending occurs in additional regions of the skull (Table 12.1).

The basic pattern is as follows:

A primary stress area, resulting in a single linear fracture (Figs. 12.6F (A, B)).

A secondary stress area, resulting in additional linear fractures (Figs 12.6F (C, D)).

A tertiary stress area, resulting in multiple linear fractures, stellate and even circular in shape and virtually shattering the skull bone (Figs 12.6F (E, F)).

Different regions of the skull, when struck, produce their own characteristic fracture patterns. A comprehensive summary of this experimental work on skull fracture has been published by Gurdjian and Webster[6].

The experiments of Gurdjian *et al* demonstrate that when intact heads are dropped, the fractures that result conform to the pattern indicated by the cracks in the stress-coat lacquer experiments.

The studies further demonstrated (in respect of linear fractures) that:

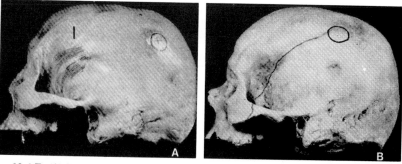

Fig. 12.6 F. (A) Region of primary stress (1) in the temporal area resulting from outbending of the bone in that region and producing cracks in the lacquered surface of the skull at the site of outbending.

Fig. 12.6 F. (B) A moderate blow in the posterior parietal region resulting in a single linear fracture, initiated in the temporal region and corresponding to the primary stress-coat pattern in Fig. 12.6 F (A).

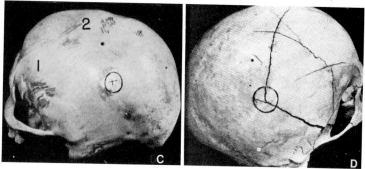

Fig. 12.6 F. (C) A heavier blow with primary (1) and secondary (2) stress areas, illustrated by cracks in the lacquered surface of the skull.

Fig. 12.6 F. (D) A moderately heavy blow resulting in fractures corresponding to the stress-coat patterns in Fig. 12.6 F (C).

(i) Hair, scalp and intracranial contents did not alter the position of the fractures that resulted;

(ii) Fractures in the dry skull (i.e. without coverings or contents) could be produced by as little as 3.3 foot-pounds;

(iii) In the cadaver head weighing 10 lb (i.e. with coverings and intracranial contents) about 35.0 foot-pounds were required to produce a linear fracture of the skull.

Therefore the energy-absorbing capacity of the scalp shows its importance as a protection against fracture and emphasizes the value of helmets for motor cyclists.

(iv) More or less the same amount of energy can produce different numbers of fractures in different skulls (Table 12.1: Heads 1, 2 and 7).

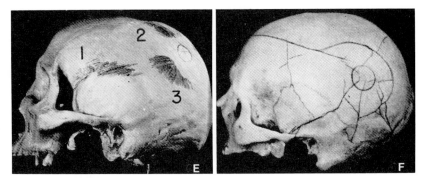

Fig. 12.6 F. (E) Areas of primary (1) secondary (2) and tertiary (3) stress produced by a more severe blow.

Fig. 12.6 F. (F) A severe blow in the posterior parietal region resulting in multiple linear fractures, indicated by the stress-coat patterns in Fig. 12.6. F (E). The comminution of the skull roughly follows the inbent area and depression occurs at the point of impact.
From Gurdjian, E S Webster, J E. (1958): *Head Injuries: Mechanisms, Diagnosis and Management.* London: J. and A. Churchill p. 67 (Fig. 8).

Fig. 12.6 F. (A–F) The stress-coat pattern and the corresponding fractures resulting from posterior parietal blows inflicted on cadaver skulls.

(v) After enough energy has been absorbed to produce a single linear fracture, very little more is required for multiple fractures and even complete destruction of the skull (Fig. 12.6F (F); Table 12.1).

(vi) Although fractures may be produced with as little as 33.3 foot-pounds, they may fail to be produced with as much as over 90 foot-pounds.

(vii) The average energy necessary to produce a single linear fracture varies with the area of skull involved, its shape and thickness, the thickness of its coverings, etc. (Table 12.2).

Table 12.2 Skull region and energy required for linear fractures

Region of impact	Energy required (in foot-pounds)
Frontal Midline	47.6
Occipital Midline	43.0
Vertex Midline	59.0
Temple (Above Ear)	51.3

From Gurdjian *et al*. Am J Surg 1949; 78: 738–739.

The variation for the midfrontal region ranges from 34.6 to 67 foot-pounds. It is least with blows in the posterior parietal area. But this variation really overshadows everything else.

(viii) Radiological observations on cases with linear fractures where the position of the blow was definitely known, confirm the experimental observations. Radiological confirmation was noted in the fracture shown in Figure 12.6G.

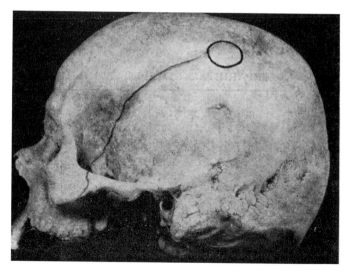

Fig. 12.6 G A fracture obtained in an experiment with an intact cadaver head which received a blow in the posterior parietal region.

It may, therefore, be possible, in a limited way, to predict where a linear fracture is likely to occur or, in the reconstruction of a case, to suggest the likely site of application of the blunt force which produced the linear fracture.

Gurdjian and Webster[6] have plotted the likely sites of fracture for deceleration forces acting on different parts of the human skull.

Clinical experience as well as experimental observations, however, confirm that considerable variations in the extent of the fractures may result from the application of sometimes only slightly differing amounts of blunt force to the cranium.

Summary

1. The skull may sustain a linear fracture from comparatively slight violence, e.g. when a person walks into an obstruction in the dark, when his head is hit on the side by a stone weighing 3–4 oz, thrown without great force, or by a golf ball or a baseball.

2. The human adult head weighs about 10 lb on the average, and the forces involved in fracturing the skull can therefore be calculated from standard formulae.

3. These calculations demonstrate that 5 foot-pounds may be enough to produce a linear fracture of the skull, i.e. the kinetic energy involved is no more than that produced when a weight of 5 lb is dropped through a distance of 1 foot.

4. If Roger Bannister ran into an obstruction while doing the 4-minute mile, his head would hit the obstruction at 15 miles per hour and the energy

involved when his head hits the obstruction would amount to about 70 foot-pounds.

5. When a head is hit by a baseball in a fast pitch (about 100 feet per second) the energy involved is about 50 foot-pounds.

6. Gurdjian et al[6] dropped cadaver heads of known weight through known distances on to a flat steel plate.

7. The calculated and the observed energies corresponded, were not of a very considerable magnitude and indicated that the energy required to produce a linear fracture of the skull under experimental conditions matched the amount of energy required to fracture the skull of a living head.

8. The energy-absorbing capacity of the scalp lessens the risk of fracture and emphasizes the value of helmets for motor cyclists.

9. After enough energy has been absorbed by the scalp to produce a single linear fracture, little more is required for multiple fractures or even extensive comminution of the skull.

10. Radiologically demonstrable linear fractures due to blows on the head occur at sites predicted by the experiments carried out by Gurdjian et al.

11. Within limits, therefore, it can be predicted where a linear fracture is likely to occur as the result of the application of a blunt force or the likely site of application of the blunt force which produced the linear fracture may be deduced.

Complications of fractures of the skull

Intracranial infections. Fractures of the floor of the anterior and middle cranial fossae of the base of the skull may involve the roof of the nose, the walls of the paranasal sinuses or the middle ear and mastoid antrum cavities. In these cases the overlying dura and arachnoid may be torn and an intracranial abscess or a meningitis may arise by a direct spread of infection from the nose or ears to the meninges. The basal fracture should be demonstrated at autopsy to establish the traumatic origin of such a meningitis. As a general rule the site of a basal fracture can be readily recognized, but there may be difficulty in cases where the fracture is limited in extent. In all cases it is essential to strip the dura completely from the underlying bone (p. 64).

Meningitis may arise in other ways after head injuries. The dura and arachnoid may be torn in compound fractures of the vault and organisms may reach the meninges directly from the skin. Meningitis may develop in the absence of a skull fracture by the spread of infection from a septic scalp wound to the meninges through the diploic veins. It is also possible for head injuries to predispose the meninges to infection even in the absence of skull fractures or external wounds (pp 240–241).

In all forms of intracranial infections, symptoms may not develop until days or weeks have elapsed after the head injury.

Cranial nerve injuries. Cranial nerve injuries may arise through stretching or bruising of the affected nerves. It is uncommon for cranial nerves to be severed even when the lines of a fracture involve foramina through which the nerves enter or leave the skull.

Injuries of the brain

The brain may be injured in penetrating wounds of the head, but most brain injuries result from the application of blunt force.

The mechanical force which produces a brain injury often causes—at the same time—wounds of the scalp, fractures of the skull and intracranial haemorrhages. A fatal cerebral injury, however, may be unaccompanied by such associated injuries.

The occurrence of brain injury

Rowbotham[8] states that injuries of the brain may be caused (1) by distortions of the skull, or (2) by movements of the brain in relation to the skull.

Injuries of the brain from distortions of the skull. When a localized segment of the skull undergoes deformation, shear strains may develop in the brain tissue underlying the indentation, and a zone of contusion may be produced in the surface layers of the brain tissue. If the local deformation results in a fracture, fragments of bone may penetrate the dura and lacerate the underlying brain tissue.

Brain injuries due to local distortions of the skull are less common than the injuries which result from movements of the brain in relation to the skull.

Injuries of the brain due to movements of the brain in relation to the skull. The cranial cavity is divided into three compartments by the falx cerebri, situated between the cerebral hemispheres, and the tentorium cerebelli, overlying the cerebellar hemispheres (Fig 12.24, p. 297). The falx cerebri and the tentorium cerebelli are relatively rigid structures and by virtue of their attachments to the bone act in the same way as the skull in resisting the movements of the brain. The three compartments of the cranial cavity communicate with one another and the shape and size of the portions of brain which they contain conform to the shape and size of the compartments. The brain does not completely fill the cranial cavity, the extra space being occupied by the cerebrospinal fluid in the subarachnoid space.

The mechanism of brain damage and intracranial haemorrhage: Holbourn's hypothesis

The mechanism of brain injury. Speculative theories about how brain damage occurs have largely been eliminated by the simple and convincing experiments reported by Holbourn.[9] The main features of the Holbourn hypothesis are as follows:

> Brain tissue, blood and cerebrospinal fluid have a comparatively uniform density. Like water, brain tissue is extremely incompressible. It requires a force of about 10,000 tons to compress the brain to half its volume. But it offers very small resistance to changes in shape, e.g. only a small force on a retractor can produce a large deformation of the brain. By contrast, the rigidity of the skull is very considerable.

The shape of the skull and the brain is important in determining the location of injuries when the head is subjected to a blow.

Holbourn postulates that brain tissue is injured when its constituent particles are pulled so far apart that they do not join up again properly when the blow is over. In the case of brain tissue which is virtually incompressible, the amount of this pulling apart is proportional to the shear strain. As stated at page 273, shear strain, or slide, is the type of deformation produced when a pack of cards is deformed from a neat rectangular pile into an oblique-angle pile. The shear strain (or slide) at any point in the brain is a rough measure of the probability of injury at that point.

In other words, because brain tissue is incompressible but easily deformed, shear strains are the cause of injury, whereas compression and rarefaction strains are not.

A pure hydrostatic (i.e. compression) pressure of 10 000 lb per in^2 (which is vastly greater than what arises in a head injury) does not impair conduction of impulses along a nerve.[10] But the slightest degree of shear, e.g. crushing the nerve with forceps or stretching it, produces considerable injury.

The forces which are transmitted from the rotating skull to the brain act chiefly upon the surface of the latter. These forces are not evenly applied to the brain surface, but are maximally developed in those regions where, owing to the projection of bony ridges or dural septa from the internal surface of the skull, the latter obtains its best purchase on the brain surface, e.g. the projecting wings of the sphenoid over the temporal poles drag upon these poles when the head is rotated. The lesions are usually bilateral but are not necessarily symmetrical.

The strains will be maximally developed where the greatest forces are applied to the brain, i.e. chiefly on the brain surface and usually most markedly at the poles. The effect of these strains will be to cause the superficial layers of the brain to slide on the deeper (Fig. 12.7). By using gelatine models, Holbourn demonstrated that the intensities of the strains may vary in different portions of the brain according to the planes in which the head is rotated. Figure 12.8 illustrates diagrammatically the relative intensities of the strains which are produced in various parts of the brain from rotatory movements from blows to certain parts of the head.

As there are innumerable different planes in which the head may rotate, innumerable different patterns of strains caused by rotatory movements of

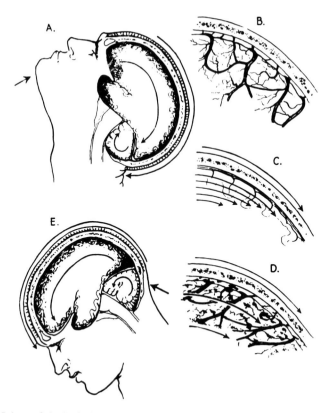

Fig. 12.7 Injury of the brain by rotation. Whenever the head is struck by a force not directed along that line which passes through the centre of gravity of the head and the occipito-atlantal joint (the fulcrum), it is set into rotation. The skull necessarily takes the first impact of the blow and moves before the brain. Then the brain is secondarily set into motion by the skull and particularly by projecting bony prominences and dural septa. Since the brain is soft and not rigid, it rapidly becomes deformed. In closed injuries it is the shearing forces associated with deformity that cause the maximum damage to the cerebral tissues and tear the cerebral arteries and veins.

A. When a patient is struck on the chin the head is thrown backwards; B, C, D, show the resulting deformity of the brain in relation to the vault of the skull; E, If a patient falls backwards and strikes his head on the ground, the head will be knocked forwards into an anterior rotation, the shearing forces in this case being in the opposite direction. Probably, in most accidents, the head is set into violent rotation about different axes at different phases of the infliction of the violence.

the head are possible in the brain tissues.

Because the cerebellum is smaller and lighter than the cerebral hemispheres, it is less liable to damage from rotatory movements of the head.

Rowbotham[11] has explained that in rotational head injuries, as there are no projecting ridges from the vault of the skull, the brain surface in this region slips backwards in relation to the skull at the pia-arachnoid dural interface, and that this movement may result in the tearing of vessels which traverse the subdural and subarachnoid space.

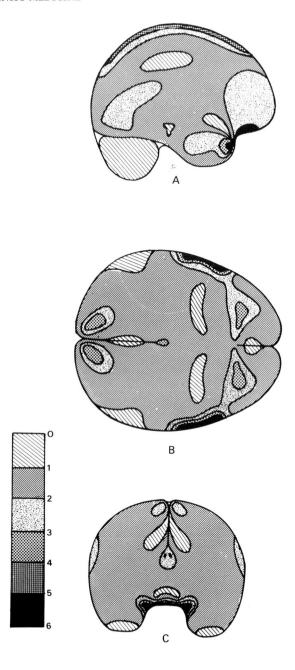

Fig. 12.8 Shear strains in gelatine models. A, Intensity of the shear-strains resulting from a forwards rotation caused by a blow on the occiput; B, Intensity of the shear-strains due to a rotation in the horizontal plane caused by a blow near the upper jaw or temples; C, Intensity of the shear-strains due to a rotation in the coronal plane caused by a blow above the ear.

Key: Scale of maximum shear-strain (= distortion) in arbitrary units of shear. The units differ in the three diagrams.

How are shear strains produced in brain tissue by a blow on the head?
When a head receives a blow, it can undergo linear change in velocity or a rotational change in velocity about some axis. The forces involved are linear acceleration (or deceleration) forces due to the change in linear velocity and centrifugal and rotational velocity. Linear acceleration forces tend to produce compressional or rarefactional strains. Waves of compression and rarefaction (sound waves) start from this point and travel back and forth through the brain. But as only shear strains can cause injury, these sound waves do not cause any damage. Indeed, this is why sound waves can be used safely to produce echograms of the brains. According to Holbourn, compressional and rarefactional strains can be neglected as a cause of intracranial injury. The shear strains mainly near the small foramina are small and can therefore also be neglected. They cannot explain damage remote from the foramina. The foramen magnum may, in certain circumstances, be an exception.

The innocuous effects of linear acceleration (or deceleration) on brain tissue are demonstrated by Holbourn's model, which admittedly is an oversimplification of the problem. But it demonstrates the fallacy that the brain lies loose in the skull and when the head is struck 'it rattles about like a die in a box, thereby causing coup and contrecoup injuries'. The rotational shear strains, however, are substantial and produce considerable damage, as demonstrated with Holbourn's gelatine models of the brain (Fig. 12.8).

With blows on the occiput, damage occurs in the very regions seen *post mortem* in a brain after a severe occipital injury which produces forward rotation.

The same comparable results are found for the effects of rotation produced by a lateral (sideways) blow above the ear or on the upper jaw.

The pathology of brain injuries

According to Rowbotham[12] only three types of primary brain damage can occur at the time of a head injury, namely, diffuse neuronal injury, contusion and laceration. Any one or any combination of these lesions may occur. Rowbotham regards all other phenomena such as oedema and massive intracerebral haemorrhages as secondary phenomena, even though they may develop soon after the injury. In addition, increasing attention is given at present to diffuse axonal injury as described at page 278.

Diffuse neuronal injury. In some deaths from head injuries, no naked-eye lesions are found in the brain at autopsy. In these cases, examination of the brain by routine histological methods may reveal microscopic haemorrhages in the tissues, but such an examination may fail to show any visible disruption of tissue. The experimental work of Denny-Brown and Russell[13] suggests that such deaths are caused by diffuse neuronal damage of submicroscopic dimensions. The exact nature of the neuronal damage is knot known, but Rowbotham[14] suggests that it probably depends on widespread intracellular disturbances and damage to synaptic junctions between neurones.*

Denny-Brown and Russell believe that diffuse neuronal injury is the essential cause of concussion, provided the head is free to move, and they regard concussion as a transient reversible neural paralysis which is produced by physical stress on the neurones themselves.[†] These workers have shown experimentally that concussion may be intensified by repeated blows and death may occur without the appearance of any visible lesions at autopsy.

It is possible that the fundamental effect of any head injury which results in concussion or some disturbance of consciousness is the production of diffuse neuronal injury or injury involving the midbrain and brain-stem systems. Diffuse neuronal injury may be wholly or partially reversible or it may prove fatal.[19] Keen has pointed out that, at autopsy, lesions resulting from the original injury which are distinct from diffuse neuronal injury are often found, e.g. intracranial haemorrhages or zones of contusions and laceration. Death may be due to these 'added' injuries, but when the gross lesions are limited in extent or degree it is probable that diffuse neuronal injury is the primary cause of death. This view is supported by Jefferson,[20] who stresses the importance of distinguishing between the fundamental functional disturbance of neuronal injury and the effect of the epiphenomena of head injury such as intracranial and intracerebral haemorrhages.

In a case of fatal diffuse neuronal injury which is unaccompanied by any gross lesions, it is impossible to establish on the basis of the autopsy findings alone that death was due to head injury. If a clinical history is available the diagnosis will have to depend upon clinical information that the deceased sustained a head injury which was followed by concussion or some disturbance of consciousness and was then succeeded by a progressive failure of the central nervous system.

Cerebral contusions. Cerebral contusions are circumscribed areas of brain tissue destruction which are accompanied by extravasations of blood into the affected tissues. Contusions are often multiple and vary in size.

---

* There is evidence to suggest that although most head injuries affect the brain by direct action on the neurones themselves the tissues can be injured indirectly through vascular mechanisms.

Rand[15] has described the occurrence of disseminated non-haemorrhagic focal degenerative and necrotic lesions in the brain in cases of fatal head injury. The lesions, which consist of small ill-defined foci of degeneration and necrosis, occur most commonly in the cerebral cortex (particularly in the Sommer's sector of Ammon's Horn—a region which is believed to be supplied by a single end artery). These lesions are also found in the Purkinje layer of the cerebellum and in the thalamus[16] Moritz[17] states that the lesions, which usually require about twenty-four hours to develop, are of ischaemic origin and are probably caused by reflex vasospasm. The lesions may be reversible, but in non-fatal cases they may undergo healing and give rise to a disseminated focal gliosis. It is possible that disseminated gliosis of this nature accounts for the progressive mental deterioration which occurs in some pugilists.[18]

† The work of Holbourn and Denny-Brown and Russell suggests that diffuse neuronal injury and concussion are caused by rotational movements of the head.

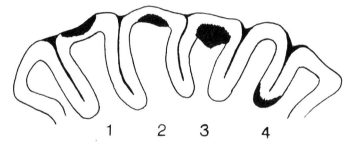

Fig. 12.9 Sites of focal cortical contusions. 1. Predominantly over cortical crest; 2. Deeper zone of cortical crest; 3. More severe injury with extension to underlying white matter; 4. Site for watershed ischaemic changes.

Contusions are found most commonly in the cortex of the brain, but they occur also in the deeper tissues. In the cortex they are often covered by a narrow zone of intact cerebral tissue; they are frequently wedge-shaped, and are surrounded by numerous petechiae.

Cerebral contusions may be produced by distortions of the skull or by rotational movements of the brain in relation to the skull (p. 269).

The possible sites of focal contusions are shown in Figure 12.9. It will be noted that the contusions are found on the surface and in the depth of cortical crests. Neurones in the depth of the sulci are often spared.

Cerebral lacerations. Cerebral contusions and cerebral lacerations are fundamentally similar types of disruptive injuries. Lacerations are larger lesions than contusions. Unlike cortical contusions which are subpial, surface lacerations are accompanied by ruptures of the pia mater. Lacerations are usually surrounded by groups of contusions.

Lacerations are caused by the same mechanisms as contusions, namely, by distortions of the skull and by movements of the brain in relation to the skull. Lacerations are particularly prominent in regions where the brain is in contact with projecting buttresses and ridges on the inner surface of the skull, e.g. the temporal poles and the orbital surfaces of the frontal lobes. Extensive lacerations may result from the penetration of brain tissue by fragments of fractured bone. Because of the rupture of the overlying pia, lacerations are often accompanied by extensive subarachnoid haemorrhages.

The general appearance of contusions and lacerations of the brain is shown in Figure 12.10.

The healing of surface lacerations may result in the development of adhesions between the brain and the overlying dura mater. Such adhesions may give rise to secondary epilepsy—a condition which may only become manifest months or years after the head injury which caused the original lesions.

When deep lacerations involve the ventricles, healing may result in the formation of large glial cysts filled with cerebrospinal fluid. These cysts are known as traumatic porencephalic cysts and must be distinguished from

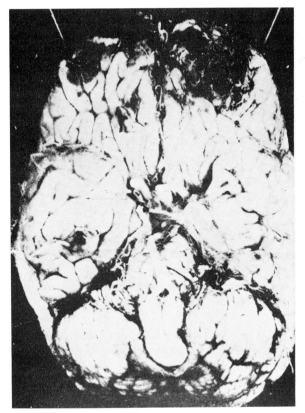

Fig. 12.10 Contusion and laceration of the orbital surfaces of both frontal lobes of the brain.

cysts which develop in zones of contusion and haemorrhage. The walls of haemorrhagic cysts usually show well-marked blood pigment staining.

Intracerebral haemorrhages. Haemorrhages into the brain arising directly from trauma usually occur near the surface. Relatively large deep-seated traumatic haemorrhages may occur, however, in the cerebrum, cerebellum or brain stem (Fig. 12.11). Such haemorrhages are usually accompanied by other types of brain injury, e.g. cortical contusions. It is exceptional for a large intracerebral haemorrhage to be the only manifestation of a head injury.

A single deep-seated haemorrhage is usually due to some disease process. Emotional excitement or physical exertion may precipitate an intracerebral haemorrhage in an arteriosclerotic and hypertensive subject, and if such a person falls and sustains a scalp wound before death, the haemorrhage may appear to be of traumatic origin. Factors which assist in the differentiation of such haemorrhages from traumatic haemorrhages are: the age of the subject; the site and the extent of the haemorrhage; the presence of vascular

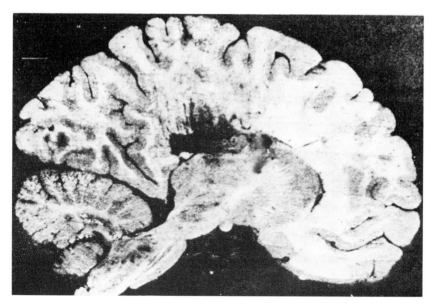

Fig. 12.11 A deeply placed intracerebral haemorrhage resulting from trauma.

lesions in the cerebral vessels; signs of cardiac hypertrophy and generalized arteriosclerosis.

Symonds[21] has drawn attention to the occurrence of delayed intracerebral haemorrhage some time after a head injury.* It is believed that such haemorrhages occur into regions of the brain which were damaged at the time of the trauma. Moritz[22] states that a haemorrhage may be attributed to the late effects of trauma only if it can be shown that the haemorrhage occurred at or near the site of mechanically damaged brain tissue.

Intraventricular haemorrhages usually arise from the extension of a non-traumatic intracerebral haemorrhage through the ventricles, but traumatic intraventricular haemorrhages can occur (particularly in children) from tearing of the choroid plexuses.

Cerebral oedema. Cerebral oedema or cerebral swelling represents an increase in brain volume, due to a localized or diffuse abnormal accumulation of water and sodium. The causes of cerebral oedema include an increase in the intravascular pressure, damage and increased permeability of the cerebral vascular wall and/or a decrease in plasma colloid osmotic pressure.

Increased fluid in the extravascular compartments of the brain may be focal, and is almost invariably associated with and secondary to contusions and lacerations of the brain. Focal areas of cerebral oedema are almost

* This is the so-called traumatic delayed apoplexy (*traumatische Spätapoplexie*) of Bollinger.[23]

invariably found surrounding contusions and lacerations of the brain. The focal oedema associated with small areas of contusions or haemorrhage is frequently fatal when occurring in the physiologically important though comparatively small area of the brain-stem. Mid-brain or pontine injuries are very common, and form a clinically distinct syndrome. The damage to the brain-stem may be the only evidence of trauma to the head.

Generalized cerebral oedema occurs with diffuse brain injury and is an important cause of death due to the difficulty in reversing the oedema clinically.

The macroscopic criteria upon which a diagnosis of generalized oedema is usually based include flattening of the cerebral convolutions with obliteration of the sulci and a herniation of the inner portions of the temporal poles through the tentorial hiatus and of portions of the cerebellar lobes in addition to the cerebellar tonsils through the foramen magnum (p. 290). Shapiro and Jackson[24] have attributed this swollen appearance of the brain to ventricular dilatation and increased blood content rather than to oedema. Evans and Scheinker,[25] however, consider that the escape of fluid into the brain tissues, from paralysed vessels, is a common event after head injuries and occurs most prominently in the deep tissues of the brain. This view is supported by White et al[26] who claim that generalized oedema may succeed a diffuse neuronal injury.

Although certain microscopic criteria, such as an apparent dilatation of perivascular spaces, have been regarded as evidence of cerebral oedema, it is often difficult to distinguish these appearances from post-mortem artefacts.

Diffuse axonal injury

When the force applied to the head is sufficiently great, the deforming effect produces shearing strains with damage to axones and vessels. If a sufficient number of axones are damaged, specific changes will be noted clinically and pathologically. Strich[27,28] demonstrated axonal loss in patients with severe head injuries who survived long enough for the clinical picture of dementia to occur.

The same mechanism concentrated in the hypothalamus accounts for the catabolic state that commonly accompanies severe head injuries and the less common salt-losing nephropathy, and inappropriate ADH secretion. Accumulative minor episodes of axonal injury give rise to the punch-drunk syndrome of boxers, in which the microscopic appearance of the brain may be indistinguishable from that in senility. Pathologically, a triad of focal lesions is described in diffuse axonal injury, involving the corpus callosum, rostral brain-stem and diffuse damage to white matter.[29,30]

Intracranial haemorrhages

Injuries to the meninges and their related vessels often result in intracranial haemorrhages. These haemorrhages are described as extradural, subdural, subarachnoid or subpial* haemorrhages according to their situation in relation to the membranes.

Extradural haemorrhages

Extradural or epidural haemorrhages occur between the inner surface of the skull and the outer surface of the dura mater. Extradural haemorrhages of significant size are relatively uncommon. Rowbotham[31] states that extradural haemorrhages large enough to be of surgical significance occur in about 3% of acute head injuries.

Extradural haemorrhages may result from torn diploic veins or from ruptured venous sinuses or meningeal arteries. Diploic bleeding accompanies fractures of the skull, but such bleeding is usually limited in extent and does not give rise to symptoms of cerebral compression. Extradural haemorrhage from a venous sinus is rare, and when it does occur it is usually caused by the penetration of a wall of the sinus by spicules of bone from a fracture.

Although it is stated that the mechanism of extradural haemorrhage is invariably caused by rupture of the middle meningeal artery or one of its branches, in fact this is uncommon. It is more common to see an extradural haemorrhage underlying a linear fracture, or a compound fracture in any area of the skull, and not involving one of the branches of the middle meningeal artery. Certainly, arterial disruption does occur, but occurs rarely in comparison with the diploic vein bleeding as a primary mechanism of the extradural haemorrhage. If the mechanism of the haematoma is that of a ruptured artery (Fig. 12.12), then the vessel which is most commonly ruptured is the middle meningeal artery, or one of its branches. The proximal part of the middle meningeal artery is invariably embedded in a deep bony groove within the skull. From the Sylvian point onwards, vessels are firmly attached to the dura and may break at this point of junction whenever the skull is separated from the dura. In this situation, the mechanism of the haematoma formation would be that of separation of the skull from the dura, tearing the artery as it leaves the bony groove. Fracture of the skull across the groove in which the artery lies will also invariably disrupt the vessel.

A large haemorrhage can accumulate in the extradural space within a few hours of the head injury and give rise to a rapid compression of the brain (Figs 12.13, 12.14 and 12.15).

Extradural haemorrhage in infancy and in young children is rare despite the marked vascularity of the skull in these age groups. The reason for this is that the dura is functionally the periosteum of the inner surface of the

---

* Subpial haemorrhages cannot be distinguished from cerebral contusions by naked-eye examination.

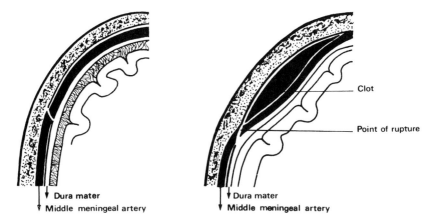

Fig. 12.12 Rupture of the meningeal vessels by stretching at the point where they leave a bony tunnel or groove to become attached to the dura.

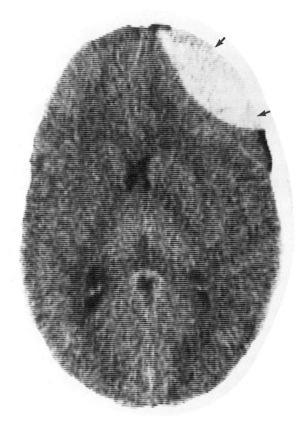

Fig. 12.13 Extradural haemorrhage. CT scan showing typical lens-shaped frontal haematoma.

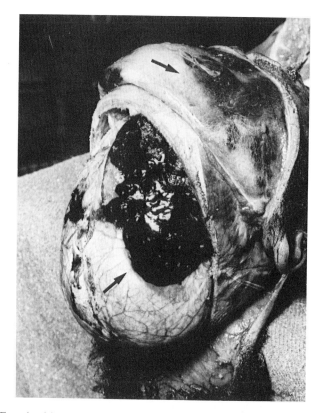

Fig. 12.14 Extradural haemorrhage. Post-mortem appearance of brain. Subaponeurotic haemorrhage also indicated.

skull and therefore is firmly attached to bone (Figs 12.16, 12.17 and 12.18).

Extradural haemorrhage still carries a high mortality rate. This may have been reduced in recent years with earlier diagnosis by CT scanning (Fig. 12.13). However, extradural haematoma must still be considered as a very dangerous clinical condition and an important cause of death.[32-38]

Subdural haemorrhages

Subdural haemorrhages occur between the inner surface of the dura mater and the outer surface of the arachnoid (Fig. 12.19).

Subdural haemorrhages may be the only manifestation of a head injury, but they usually occur in association with other intracranial haemorrhages, with brain injuries and with skull fractures.

Subdural haemorrhages may arise from tears in the dural venous sinuses or cortical veins, but the commonest cause of subdural bleeding is the rupture of bridging or communicating veins. The bridging veins are small unsupported thin vessels which traverse the subarachnoid and subdural

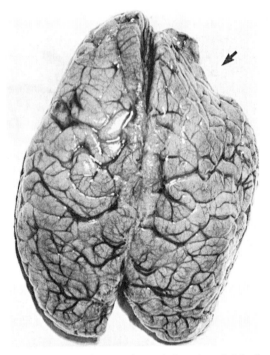

Fig. 12.15 Extradural haemorrhage. Compression and distortion of right frontal lobe of brain.

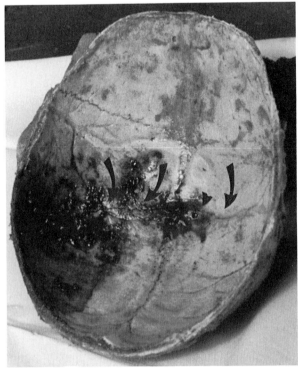

Fig. 12.16 Extradural haemorrhage in a 7-year-old child. Removal of vault of skull after dissection.

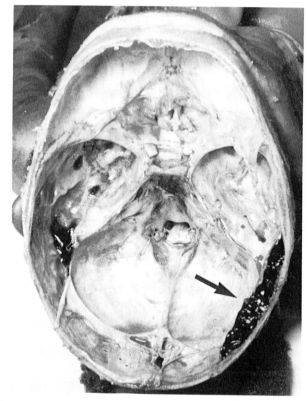

Fig. 12.17 Extradural haemorrhage. Same case as in Fig. 12.16. After removal of brain.

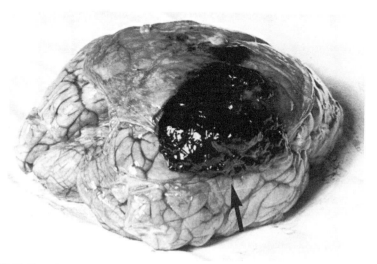

Fig. 12.18 Extradural haemorrhage. Same case as Fig. 12.16. Haematoma located over temperoparietal region of right cerebral hemisphere.

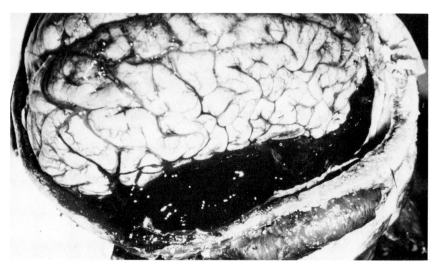

Fig. 12.19 Subdural haemorrhage. (Prof. L. S. Smith's case.)

spaces and drain the cortical veins into the sinuses. They are most numerous over the vertex where they drain into the superior sagittal sinus, but they are also found over the inferior surface of the brain. The bridging veins are commonly ruptured when the brain moves in relation to the dura (Fig. 12.20). The veins may be ruptured in rotational movements of the brain in relation to the skull. In rotational movements there is a sliding of the pia relative to the arachnoid, and of the arachnoid relative to the dura, and in this manner the bridging veins are stretched and ruptured (Fig. 12.7 p. 271). See also pages 270, 392.

Surface cortical arteries are not infrequently ruptured and give rise to an arterial subdural haematoma.

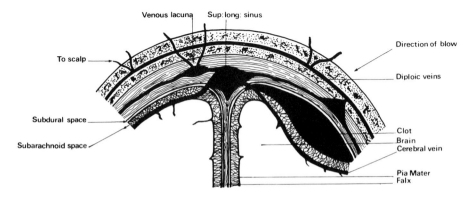

Fig. 12.20. The tributaries of the superior sagittal sinus. The communicating veins which run from the cortical vessels into the sinus are commonly ruptured when the brain moves across the face of the dura. In this case a unilateral subdural haematoma is shown.

In various rotational movements of the head different communicating veins are subjected to different degrees of stretching, and for this reason the site of distribution of a subdural haemorrhage may bear no relationship to the site of application of a force. Subdural haemorrhages may be found on the side of the head where the force was applied, or they may occur on the contralateral side, or they may be bilateral.

There are basically three types of subdural haemorrhage. The first type is the acute subdural haemorrhage in which either a large bridging vein has been ruptured and so a haematoma accumulates rapidly; but more frequently, a rapidly collecting subdural haematoma is caused by rupture of one of the cortical arteries. These injuries are frequently accompanied by very severe cerebral oedema. Acute subdural haematomas are an important cause of death and approximately 90% of patients with acute subdural haematomas die. The reason for this is that unless treatment can be instituted quickly, irreversible brain damage occurs, leading to death within a few hours. Even after surgical intervention, the malignant oedema which accompanies this injury makes the outlook poor.

There is an entity of sub-acute subdural haematoma which occurs when the bleeding is from smaller bridging veins. As this bleeding is relatively slow, it usually takes several days for sufficient blood to accumulate to give rise to cerebral compression. The mortality rate of this type of haematoma is much less, because the acute nature of the injury is reduced.

Greenfield[39] dealing with acute subdural haematomas, states:

> Although the layer of blood may be thin, often less than 5 mm thick, it may cover a large area of the cerebral cortex and its total bulk may be such that it makes an important contribution to an increase of intracranial pressure. Especially when unilateral, it is likely to produce herniation of the uncus and hippocampal gyrus through the tentorium cerebelli and so to be the cause of the haemorrhages, or foci of ischaemia, in the midbrain which are common sequelae of this . . . Clinically many such cases remain unconscious from the time of the accident until death or have at best a period of semi-stupor; but in the writer's experience a thin unilateral subdural layer of blood associated with secondary haemorrhages in the midbrain may be the only evident cause of death in patients who, after minor head injuries with transient loss of consciousness, relapse within a few hours into coma.

The amount of blood which collects in a subdural space is often insufficient to produce cerebral compression in the early period after the formation of the haematoma, but secondary changes in the haematoma may lead to a considerable expansion in its size. These changes are brought about during the process of healing. (See also p. 286.)

Chronic subdural haematoma. The blood which accumulates in a subdural space cannot be reabsorbed, but within a few hours of the haemorrhage reactive changes occur in the overlying dura. A thin membrane composed of granulation tissue develops on the dural surface of the haematoma and gradually extends over the arachnoid surface to completely envelop the haematoma (12.21). The outer part of the membrane becomes thickened and attached to the dura but the inner part remains thin and non-adherent. If the haematoma is stripped off the dura at this stage, numerous small blood vessels which have extended into the haematoma from the dura will be ruptured. The membrane on the arachnoid surface is gradually thickened and at the end of 3 to 4 weeks the haematoma is usually completely encapsulated.[40]

Perper and Wecht[41] have tabulated histological features of subdural haematomas for the period 24 hours to beyond one year.

A small haematoma may be replaced by fibrous tissue, but the central part of a large haematoma often remains fluid. Such haematomata may undergo considerable expansion and give rise to compression of the brain several months after a head injury (p. 294). Various theories have been advanced to explain the expansion of subdural haematomata. Rowbotham[42] states that it has been suggested that the expansion is caused by small repeated haemorrhages from the highly vascular membrane which envelops the haematoma. Such haemorrhages may be caused by repeated trivial head injuries (below). Gardner[43] states that the membrane of the haematoma has semipermeable properties. He believes that as the haematoma disintegrates, its molecular concentration increases. This results in a rise in the osmotic pressure within the haematoma and cerebrospinal fluid is drawn from the subarachnoid space through the semipermeable membrane into the haematoma.

The appearance of the fluid in the haematoma changes with time. Initially it is reddish-brown and clearly blood-stained, often with fibrin clots within it. As the haematoma breaks down and becomes more fluid, the contents of the haematoma take on a much darker colour and looks not unlike old machine oil. As the haematoma ages, the dark colour alters to that of a mildly brownish discoloured fluid.

The original trauma responsible for a subdural haemorrhage may be of a trivial nature and may be overlooked. This fact explains why the analogous condition of chronic pachymeningitis haemorrhagica interna was for many years regarded as a separate pathological entity.

Chronic pachymeningitis haemorrhagica interna was originally described as an incidental finding in the deaths of chronic alcoholics, elderly persons with cerebral arteriosclerosis, and persons suffering from general paralysis of the insane. Leary[44] considers that certain pathological changes which occur in these conditions render such persons particularly liable to subdural haemorrhage after relatively trivial head injuries. In cerebral arteriosclerosis and general paralysis of the insane, the marked atrophy of the brain increases its mobility within the skull. In chronic alcoholics it is possible that subarachnoid oedema favours the rupture of bridging veins. All three classes of persons are particularly liable to sustain repeated head injuries of a trivial nature.

Although most subdural haematomata are of traumatic origin, subdural haemorrhages may be secondary to disease processes, e.g. in cerebral

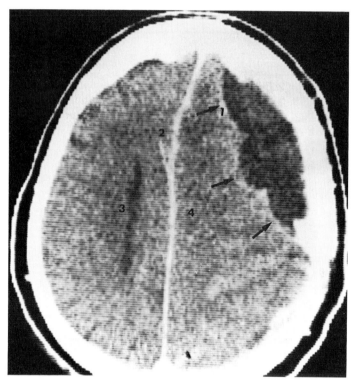

Fig. 12.21 Chronic subdural haematoma. Contrast study revealing: 1. Enhancing membrane encapsulating non-lens-shaped haematoma; 2. Shift of lower part of falx cerebri; 3. Compression of contralateral lateral ventricle; 4. Obliteration of ipsilateral lateral ventricle.

neoplasms, from ruptured cerebral aneurysms, during anticoagulant therapy and from blood disorders.[45]

Chronic subdural haematomas are probably far more common than is realized. It is only with the advent of modern techniques, such as the CT scanner (Fig. 12.21) that the frequency can generally be appreciated. Many subdural haematomas do not present with sufficient neurological deficit to warrant further neurological investigation and, therefore, are not recognized clinically. However, calcified subdural haematomas may be found at autopsy as a legacy of a previous incident.

Subdural hygroma. When the arachnoid is torn, cerebrospinal fluid may pass from the subarachnoid space into the subdural space. In this manner a large collection of fluid may accumulate in the subdural space and give rise to cerebral compression. The term 'subdural hygroma' is applied to this lesion. Rowbotham[46] considers that large collections of cerebrospinal fluid can only accumulate in the subdural space when the tear in the arachnoid acts as a one-way valve and allows fluid into the subdural space but not out of it.

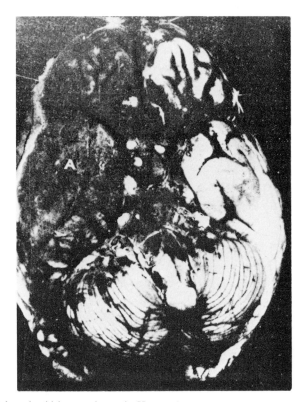

Fig. 12.22 Subarachnoid haemorrhage. A, Haemorrhage.

Subarachnoid haemorrhages

Subarachnoid bleeding is the commonest form of traumatic intracranial haemorrhage. Subarachnoid haemorrhages occur between the arachnoid and the pia mater and usually arise from the rupture of bridging veins. The blood mixes with the cerebrospinal fluid in the subarachnoid space and may be distributed over practically the whole of the brain surface (Fig. 12.22). In other cases the blood collects in the dependent basal cisterns.*

Although a subarachnoid haemorrhage may be the only manifestation of a head injury,[48] it often occurs in association with other intracranial haemorrhages, with brain injuries and with skull fractures. In cases where the haemorrhage is the only manifestation, the possibility of a spontaneous subarachnoid haemorrhage from natural causes has to be excluded. An important cause of spontaneous subarachnoid haemorrhage from natural causes is the rupture of a congenital or 'berry' aneurysm of one of the

---

* Moritz and Wartman[47] have described delayed deaths from internal hydrocephalus in cases where the organization of clots in the basal cisterns has resulted in a closing of the foramina of Magendie and Luschka.

arteries of the circle of Willis. Such ruptures occur most commonly in young adults.

As the rupture of a congenital aneurysm may be precipitated by excitement or physical exertion, e.g. during a fight, the clinical features may be misleading and may suggest the possibility of a traumatic haemorrhage. In order to demonstrate the aneurysm, the brain should be placed in a fixative solution before the vessels are dissected.*

The pathology of cerebral compression

As the cranium is a rigid cavity and cannot be expanded, any increase in the size of the brain, e.g. through generalized swelling, or the development of any space-occupying lesion within the cranial cavity, e.g. an extradural haemorrhage or a subdural haemorrhage, must result in compression of the brain. As the brain tissue itself is incompressible, the first effects of the compression are to diminish the amount of cerebrospinal fluid in the subarachnoid space and in the ventricles, and to diminish the blood content of the brain. The amount of cerebrospinal fluid that can be displaced is limited and a continued rise in intracranial pressure leads to a progressive interference with the blood supply of the brain.

During the development of the compression, processes of brain tissue may be forced through the openings of the tentorum and the foramen magnum. These herniations are known respectively as the tentorial pressure cone and the cerebellar pressure cone. The nature of the tentorial pressure cone is illustrated diagrammatically in Fig. 12.23. As the intracranial pressure above the tentorium rises, a process of brain tissue from the inferior and inner surface of the temporal lobe (the uncus) herniates through the opening of the tentorium. The midbrain is compressed against the opposite free edge of the tentorium or it is compressed between the two processes if the herniation is bilateral. This compression, by interfering with the transmission of impulses from the cerebrum, may give rise to a condition analogous to 'decerebrate rigidity'. Uncal grooving is a common post-mortem finding and frequently occurs in the absence of overt cerebral disease. This sign must not be misinterpreted as evidence of uncinate herniation.[50]

A cerebellar pressure cone is less common than a tentorial pressure cone and is due to a rise of pressure below the tentorium in the posterior cranial fossa. The rise of pressure forces portions of the cerebellar lobes in addition to the tonsils of the cerebellum through the foramen magnum, with a resulting compression of the medulla oblongata. Progressive failure of respiration will follow such compression. The normal post-mortem

---

* The anatomy of the circle of Willis and the locality of congenital aneurysms have been described in detail by Drake.[49]

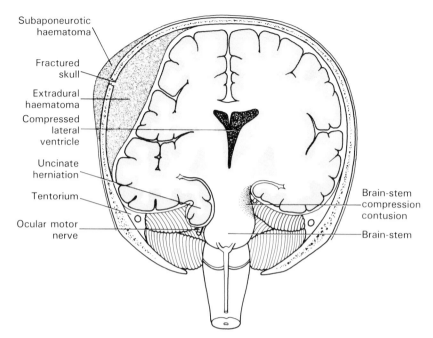

Subaponeurotic
haematoma

Fractured
skull

Extradural
haematoma

Compressed
lateral
ventricle

Uncinate
herniation

Tentorium

Ocular motor
nerve

Brain-stem
compression
contusion

Brain-stem

Fig. 12.23 Diagrammatic representation of tentorial pressure cone in the presence of an extradural haematoma. Note the uncinate herniation, the compressed lateral ventricle and the compression contusion of the brain-stem.

foraminal indentation of the cerebellar tonsils must not be misinterpreted as a sign of cerebellar coning.

The recognition of cerebral compression at autopsy may be difficult. Findings such as flattening of the gyri, narrowing of the sulci, and an apparent diminution of cerebrospinal fluid are not unequivocal signs of compression (p. 278). The presence of a deep grooved marking around the uncus of a temporal lobe, or the presence of a similar marking on the cerebellum lateral to the normal anatomical marking around the cerebellar tonsils, is suggestive evidence of cerebral compression.

CLINICAL FEATURES OF HEAD INJURIES

Concussion, 'cerebral irritation' and compression

The most common clinical manifestation of an acute head injury is concussion. The term 'concussion' is used in various senses, but Wilson[51] has emphasized that the use of the term should be restricted to the disorder of cerebral function which follows immediately upon the impact of a force to the head. Wilson considers that concussion is still best described in the terms of the definition originally given by Trotter as 'an essentially transient state due to head injury which is of instantaneous onset, manifests widespread symptoms of a purely paralytic kind, does not as such comprise any evidence of structural cerebral injury, and is always followed by amnesia from the actual moment of the accident.'

Denny-Brown and Russell[52] believe that concussion is caused by a direct and generalized physical effect on the neurones which results in a diffuse neuronal injury of submicroscopic dimensions (p. 273). This injury is of a reversible nature.

The essential clinical feature of concussion is a loss of consciousness. The disturbance of consciousness may be of such slight degree and of such momentary duration that the patient may not even fall to the ground. In these cases the condition may be overlooked or mistakenly thought to be of no significance. In other cases immediate deep unconsciousness may occur and full consciousness may only be gradually regained after a period of hours. The longer, however, that unsconsiousness, or a disturbance of consciousness, persists after the infliction of a head injury the more likely are 'added' lesions, e.g. zones of cerebral contusion or laceration, or complications, e.g. intracranial haemorrhages, to be present.

Concussion (i.e. loss or impairment of consciousness immediately on receipt of a blow on the head) with immediate recovery and no after-effects must represent the least possible damage to the neurones involved.

Occasionally concussion may be fatal, due to irreversible paralysis of the respiratory and cardiac centres in the brain-stem. Autopsy may fail to reveal any naked-eyed or microscopic evidence of damage to the brain.

One of the first-recorded examples of fatal concussion was described by Littré, the French surgeon and anatomist (1658–1726). The account is reproduced by Courville[53] in his *Commotio Cerebri* in the following words:

> A young, robust criminal who was to be put on the rack wished to escape his punishment and so, with his hands behind his back and his head lowered, he ran about fifteen paces across the dungeon where he was confined, and struck his head with all his might against the opposite wall. He fell dead on the spot without uttering a word or making a single sound.
>
> M. Littré, called to see the body, began by examining the head externally; he was surprised to find no contusion, swelling, wound or fracture. He incised and separated consecutively the various layers of the scalp at the vertex of the head where the blow had been sustained, according to the report of several other criminals in the same dungeon who had witnessed the act. He then examined the layers internally, but found nothing more than he had externally. He noted nothing remarkable about the bones of the cranium after he had exposed them, except for the squamous portion of the temporal bone which lay a third of a line beyond; and this exposure was continued up to two lines in depth at some points and one or more in others. There was no evidence of anything sufficient to cause death, much less such a sudden death, and moreover nothing else of significance appeared.
>
> It was necessary, therefore, to cut away the cranium and examine the cerebrum, but the astonishment of M. Littré increased when it was found entirely in its natural state and, so to speak, in perfect health. Only the cerebrum did not completely occupy the interior capacity of the skull, as it ordinarily does, and its substance, as well as that of the cerebellum and the

medulla, was firmer and more compact than usual both on inspection and palpation. M. Littré was further assured on this point because it was relatively easy to replace the sectioned portions of the brain in the cranial vault which it is often difficult to do in other cadavers.

In short this was the only finding, therefore, which could account for his sudden demise, the cerebrum being considerably depressed by the sudden commotion of the blow and, as it had little inherent elasticity, there had been but little recovery from this state. In conseqeunce, the distribution of the spirits in all the rest of the body, necessary for its various movements, had ceased at this instant. Therefore, M. Littré drew this very natural conclusion since he did not find any contusion of the coverings of the calvarium at the point of the injury. A contusion is formed by the blood which ordinarily circulates through this region, being released from the vessels which are broken and torn, with its consequent coagulation in the tissues. In this case, the blood ceased to circulate at the precise moment in which the vessels of the scalp were ruptured, for the heart immediately lost its movement with consequent failure of the spirits.

Keen[19] has reported a similar case (p. 274).

It is well known that concussion is rarely produced if the head remains fixed and easily produced if the head is movable. Thus the soccer player can 'head' a ball without becoming concussed because his fixed head cannot rotate, so there can be no rotational shear strains.

When a head is crushed between railway buffers in a shunting accident, concussion (i.e. loss of consciousness) may not be produced, because rotational movement of the head is minimal.

These examples are in contrast to the classic knock-out blow in boxing, which is an upper-cut to the point or just to the side of the chin. This suddenly produces rotational shear strains in the brain tissue, temporarily disrupting neuronal function.

In their experiments on cats, dogs and monkeys, Denny-Brown and Russell[13] could not produce concussion by a blow on the head when the head was not free to move.

Failure to lose consciousness following a blow to a head which is not free to move is a matter of ancient record.

In more recent times Pudenz and Shelden[54] replaced the convex part of a monkey skull by a transparent lucite calvarium. They then recorded the effects of blows on various parts of the head by cinematography. They confirmed that blows on the head when it was free to move produced swirling, rotatory movements of the brain within the cranial cavity.

All the evidence therefore indicates that concussion is a rotational brain injury.

How is loss of consciousness produced by a blow which does not result in marked rotation of the head, e.g. blows from a truncheon, the butt of a revolver, an axe, etc.?

The local indentation of the skull beneath the site of impact easily displaces intracranial contents (because brain tissue has very little rigidity). The brain-stem can thus be dislocated momentarily through the foramen magnum and this may distort the brain-stem, disorganizing its function temporarily, thus producing a loss of consciousness.

Summary

1. Intracranial damage can occur without skull fracture and vice versa.

2. Local skull deformation (with or without skull fracture) can damage the related underlying intracranial structures.

3. A blow which produces a sudden rotation of the head (but does not produce a fracture of the skull) can, by the mechanism of shear strain, injure the intracranial contents at a distance remote from the site of application of the force (subdural and subarachnoid haemorrhage, cerebral contusion).

4. Experimental observations confirm the view that concussion results when the brain is subjected to sudden rotational shear strain and that subdural and subarachnoid haemorrhage as well as cerebral contusion can be produced by the same mechanism, although there has been no fracture of the skull.

Following upon concussion the patient may develop the clinical features of 'cerebral irritation' which are characterized by the patient lying curled up in bed with his back to the light and resentful of any interference. When a patient is in this condition it may be difficult to examine him properly and to assess his condition clinically. Such patients may be mistakenly diagnosed as suffering from acute alcoholic intoxication (p. 419).

A loss of consciousness which occurs some time after the infliction of a head injury always suggests the development of the syndrome of cerebral compression. In many of these cases the patient first suffers from immediate loss of consciousness due to concussion, then slowly recovers consciousness only to relapse into unconsciousness gradually, due to the development of compression. A so-called 'lucid interval' thus intervenes between the two stages of unconsciousness. This 'lucid interval' is of great clinical diagnostic importance, but it is by no means an invariable occurrence in patients who develop the compression syndrome. In some caes no lucid interval occurs, but the stage of unconsciousnes due to severe concussion merges imperceptibly into the stage of unconsciousness due to compression which may be caused by a rapidly developing intracranial haemorrhage. In other cases no initial loss of consciousness due to concussion occurs, or is noted, but the patient gradually loses consciousness from compression some time after the infliction of the injury.

A large extradural haemorrhage can give rise to rapid compression and the signs are often apparent within a few hours of the injury. The onset of compression from large subdural harmorrhages is relatively slow as it usually takes several days for sufficient blood to accumulate in the subdural space to produce compression.

A chronic subdural haematoma is occasionally responsible for a 'delayed' death after a head injury. The main clinical evidence of such a haemorrhage may be a progressive mental deterioration of the patient. This condition was seen in one of our cases in which a worker died from bilateral subdural haematomata three months after an assault.

Head injuries and acute alcoholic intoxication

After a head injury a person may be confused and disorientated and the general clinical manifestations may simulate acute alcoholic intoxication.

A person under the influence of alcohol may sustain a head injury and it may be impossible to assess to what degree his condition is due to the head injury or to the alcoholic intoxication.

When a person, arrested on a charge of being under the influence of alcohol, appears to have sustained a head injury, he should not be placed in a police or prison detention cell but should, whenever possible, be sent to a hospital for observation. In cases of this nature it is the primary duty of a medical practitioner to protect the life of the accused; a medical examination to obtain evidence of intoxication is of secondary importance.

The interrogation of persons who have sustained head injuries

A person who has sustained a head injury and been rendered unconscious, is likely to be mentally confused. He usually suffers from amnesia to a varying degree and may have no recollection of sustaining an injury and may be quite unable to give an account of himself. It may be necessary for the purpose of investigation to interrogate such a person in regard to events preceding and following the injury. During such an interrogation particular care must be exercised not to ask the person leading questions or to suggest answers to him. By asking such questions, not only may incorrect information be obtained but the suggestions may become impressed on the mind of the person and may result in his having a 'false memory' in relation to the events.

Whenever possible the police authorities should be advised to delay interrogating an accused person (or a complainant) who has sustained a head injury until he appears to have recovered completely from his initial confusion.

In some instances, amnesia after a head injury may be permanent.

Admission to hospital after head injuries

When a patient who has been concussed is admitted to hospital, it is advisable to obtain a clinical history of the injury from the person, or persons, who brought him to the hospital, as any account given by the patient himself may not be reliable. Patients who have sustained head injuries should be kept in hospital for observation for a period of at least 24 to 36 hours. If a patient refuses to stay in hospital, every effort should be made to persuade him to stay. If any of his relatives or friends accompanied him to the hospital, they should be warned of the danger of allowing him to go home and they should be asked to use their influence to persuade him to remain in hospital.

If the patient finally decides to leave the hospital, he should sign a document to the effect that he is leaving of his own accord and against the advice of the medical attendants. It is of little value advising the patient himself of the symptoms and signs which may develop if a complication of the head injury should occur, but the patient's relatives or friends should be told that they must obtain medical assistance or bring the patient back to hospital if he develops symptoms such as mental confusion or drowsiness.

The most important lesions which may become manifest after a head injury and which are amenable to direct surgical treatment are subdural and extradural haemorrhages. A subdural haemorrhage usually takes days to develop and so may give ample warning for the obtaining of medical assistance. Some acute subdural and most extradural haemorrhages, however, may develop to a critical stage within 24 hours and require prompt surgical treatment. Close medical observation of recent head injuries is therefore esential for at least this period.

The sequelae of head injuries

Rowbotham[55] states that in the recovery from any severe injury of the head, three distinct phases can be recognized. The first phase is the return of consciousness which may take from a few moments to several weeks, the usual period being a matter of days. This phase is followed by a phase of convalescence and gradual recovery before the patient attains his pre-accident state. The third phase is the period of the so-called 'post-concussional syndrome', and Rowbotham states that 'few patients escape without suffering to a lesser or greater extent from one or a combination of the following conditions: pains in the head, dizziness, insomnia, diplopia, changes in disposition or intellectual impairment'. Apart from these disorders, various physical sequelae (such as spastic paralysis, aphasia, epilepsy and cranial nerve paralyses) may result.

A head injury may be succeeded by psychoneurotic symptoms and it may be extremely difficult to differentiate a neurosis of this nature from malingering, particularly when the question of compensation for an injury is in issue. It is rare for psychoses to develop after head injuries. When they do, a latent mental disorder such as schizophrenia is present and the injury merely acts as a precipitating factor of the illness.

Fatal head injuries in newly born infants

Fatal head injuries in newly born infants may be caused during labour or they may be produced after birth by accidental trauma or homicidal violence. Accidental trauma may arise when an infant is allowed to fall either during a precipitate labour or through the carelessness of an attendant.

In cases of alleged infanticide it is necessary to exclude the possibility of birth injury and accidental trauma. This exclusion may be very difficult, but some of the differences between the commoner findings in these three conditions will be considered under the following headings:
1. Injuries of the scalp;
2. Fractures of the skull;
3. Intracranial haemorrhages;
4. Injuries of the brain.

1. Injuries of the scalp

External wounds of the face and head are usually absent in birth injuries but they may be present in accidental falls when they are generally limited in number and extent. In cases of infanticide, however, multiple wounds of the face and head are commonly found. These wounds take the form of abrasions, bruises and lacerated wounds and are often accompanied by injuries to other regions of the body.

The demonstration of areas of bruising in the tissues of the scalp does not serve to differentiate a postnatal trauma from an antenatal injury as widespread bruising of the scalp tissue may be produced during labour. A caput succedaneum usually forms in the scalp tissues during the ordinary process of labour, but it is unusual to find this condition when an infant has been born after a precipitate labour. A large caput succedaneum and well-developed moulding can therefore be regarded as evidence against the occurrence of a precipitate labour.

2. Fractures of the skull

Fractures of the skull are uncommon in birth injuries. When they do occur they usually take the form of limited fissured fractures and depressed fractures which are occasionally described as 'celluloid ball' depressions or 'pond fractures'. These fractures usually affect the frontal and parietal bones only and seldom radiate into the base. Fissured and depressed fractures occur in accidental falls but they are usually localized to the site of impact.

In cases of infanticide, fractures of the skull are often found and commonly occur as extensive comminuted fractures which radiate from the vault of the skull into the base. These fractures are often compound in nature and are found in relation to external injuries on the face and head.

3. Intracranial haemorrhages

Intracranial haemorrhages occur during the process of labour. These haemorrhages are usually unaccompanied by fractures of the skull as the infant's skull may undergo considerable distortion during labour without bony injury. Extradural haemorrhages are unusual but subdural haemorrhages are common. Extradural haemorrhages in infants are limited to single bones because of the adherence of the dura to the skull along the suture lines. The relatively high incidence of subdural haemorrhages at birth has been emphasized by Ingraham and Matson.[56] Subdural haemorrhages are often the only manifestation of a birth injury. They are usually bilateral and are most commonly caused by ruptures of the bridging veins, but they may also arise from tears of the tentorium cerebelli, or less commonly, from tears of the falx cerebri. Tentorial tears may be bilateral and bleeding occurs into the subdural space either above or below the tentorium. The haemorrhages occasionally result from ruptures of the internal or great cerebral veins. The mechanism whereby the tentorium is torn in moulding of the head during birth is shown in Fig. 12.24.

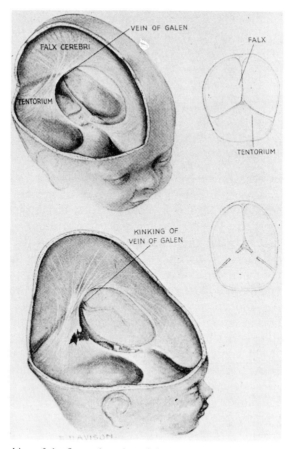

Fig. 12.24 Stretching of the flax and tearing of the tentorium in moulding.

Accidental falls may result in intracranial haemorrhages. These haemorrhages are commmonly subdural in type and are often bilateral.

In cases of infanticide any type of intracranial haemorrhage may occur. Subdural and subarachnoid haemorrhages are common and are usually accompanied by fractures of the skull and contusion and laceration of the brain.

4. Injuries of the brain

Macroscopic injuries of the brain are unusual in birth trauma and accidental falls, but they are of common occurrence in homicidal violence. In cases of infanticide, contusion and laceration of the brain are often found in association with fractures of the skull and intracranial haemorrhages. In certain of these cases portions of brain tissue may be extruded through wounds of the scalp overlying comminuted fractures of the skull.

Summary. Although birth injuries and accidental injuries usually take the form of intracranial haemorrhages only, and homicidal violence is characterized by a combination of fractures with severe intracranial injury, it may be difficult, on pathological grounds, to exclude the possibility of a birth injury or an accidental injury in a particular case of alleged infanticide. Each case must be considered on its own merits in relation to the circumstances of the death.

FRACTURES OF THE SPINE AND INJURIES OF THE SPINAL CORD

Moritz[57] states that fractures of the spine are caused by hyperflexion, hyperextension or vertical compression of the spinal column. Hyperflexion may cause comminution of one or more vertebral bodies with crushing of their anterior portions. Hyperextension may cause crushing of the posterior portions of the vertebral bodies and the vertebral arches. In both types of injury the displacement of portions of the vertebral bodies or the vertebral arches into the spinal canal may result in injury to the spinal cord and meninges. Hyperflexion and hyperextension injuries can produce rupture of the posterior and anterior longitudinal spinal ligaments respectively, without fracture, resulting in instability of the spinal column and possible cord damage. Compression fractures of the spinal column are usually caused by falls from heights and may be unaccompanied by any displacement of the vertebral bodies. Although the spinal cord may not be injured in these types of fractures, damage may occur to the spinal nerves. Most fractures of the spinal column are produced by indirect violence. In compression and hyperflexion fractures the force may be transmitted to the spine by violence applied to the head.

Dislocations of the spinal vertebrae may lead to injury of the spinal cord without any associated gross fracture of the spine. On the other hand, seemingly inconsequential fractures can give rise to very profound effects on the spinal cord, for example, fracture of an articular process may lead to dislocation. The whole spectrum of spinal fracture and cord injury can occur in diving accidents, where the diver dives too deep or the water is too shallow, striking his head on the bottom and producing a hyperflexion or hyperextension injury. The spinal cord can be damaged to a greater or lesser degree indirectly by damage to the vascular supply, either where it enters the spinal column through the intervertebral foramen, or in the thecal canal itself.

As abnormal mobility of the spine and haemorrhage into the surrounding muscles nearly always accompany a significant fracture–dislocation of the spine, it is usually possible to demonstrate such an injury by examination of the anterior aspect of the vertebral bodies after removal of the viscera, but in all cases if such suspected injury it is advisable to expose and dissect the vertebrae and spinal cord posteriorly (p. 75).

Spinal cord injuries are most frequently found in fracture–dislocations at the level of the upper cervical, lower cervical, lower thoracic and upper lumbar vertebrae, and take the form of contusions and lacerations. Spinal contusions may occur without any fracture or dislocation of the vertebrae and are not always accompanied by injuries to the spinal meninges. Spinal cord contusions are recognized by the occurrence of haemorrhages into the substance of the cord. The haemorrhages usually extend in the long axis of the cord and the extent of the lesion must be demonstrated by a series of cross-sections through several segments of the cord. Lacerations of the cord may be produced in cases of gross displacement of the vertebrae and are usually accompanied by injuries to the spinal meninges. Injuries to the meninges often result in haemorrhages which are described as extradural, subdural or subarachnoid haemorrhages, according to their situation.

Punctured wounds of the neck and back may extend to the spine and penetrate the spinal canal, but this is a relatively rare injury. We have seen this type of injury in two of our cases. In both cases the cord was not injured but haemorrhage occurred into the subarachnoid space and extended upwards over the surfaces of the medulla, the pons and the midbrain.

A fracture of the spine which is accompanied by contusions or lacerations of the lower lumbar or sacral segments of the cord, or the cauda equina, or the sacral nerve roots may give rise to a neurogenic disturbance of the bladder resulting in a derangement of the function of micturition. As the bladder becomes overdistended and cannot be emptied completely, cystitis may develop. The cystitis is often followed by pyelonephritis and calculus formation, and death may occur from renal failure.

High velocity gunshot wounds, where the bullet track misses the spinal canal by anything up to several centimetres, can produce profound changes in the cord, including total cessation of function permanently, due to oscillation of the bullet as it passes through the body. The oscillation permanently disrupts cord function.

INJURIES TO THE NECK

Various types of injuries to the neck may result in death, e.g. the injuries caused by throttling, strangulation and hanging, and the injuries caused by incised and punctured wounds. Injuries to the neck caused by throttling, strangulation and hanging are described in Chapter 4.

Incised and punctured wounds of the neck

Incised and punctured wounds of the neck are usually of suicidal or homicidal origin. Suicidal incised wounds are more common than homicidal incised wounds but punctured wounds are usually homicidal.

A suicidal incised wound is usually situated in the upper part of the neck. In a case where the victim is right-handed the wound is generally directed obliquely downwards from left to right. The incision is deepest at its commencement and may extend backwards through the muscles of the neck on to the anterior surfaces of the cervical vertebrae. The common carotid artery and the external and internal jugular veins may be severed. Super-

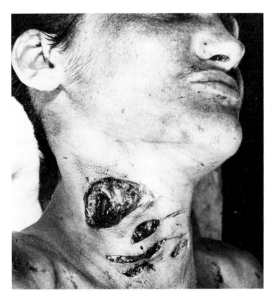

Fig. 12.25 Homicidal incised wounds of the neck.

ficial tentative incisions may often be seen in relation to the main incised wound.

Homicidal incised wounds may be situated in any region of the neck and they vary in their direction and depth (Fig. 12.25).

Homicidal incised wounds are usually deeper than suicidal wounds, but extensive damage to the tissues of the neck does not necessarily exclude the possibility of suicide. This may be illustrated by reference to a remarkable case described by Schuessler,[58] in which a man cut his throat with a single-edge razor blade and then put his fingers into the wound and pulled out and cut off a portion of tissue consisting of the hyoid bone, the larynx, the thyroid gland (including three parathyroids), a section of the trachea, and 5 cm of the anterior part of the oesophagus. The man's life was saved by prompt treatment and the oesophagus was subsequently reconstructed.

Homicidal punctured wounds of the neck are relatively common. They may occur in any region of the neck but they are often situated in the lower part of the neck. The track of a punctured wound in the lower part of the neck is usually directed backwards, medially and downwards. Such a wound may sever the subclavian vessels or it may extend through the apical pleura and penetrate the lung. When the wound is directly medially, the trachea or oesophagus may be severed. An incision of the trachea may give rise to surgical emphysema in the cervical tissues. Air may be aspirated into a severed cervical vein and give rise to pulmonary air embolism (p. 372).

Multiple incised wounds of the forearms, palms and fingers may be observed in association with homicidal incised or punctured wounds of the neck, in cases where the victim has attempted to defend himself.

INJURIES TO THE CHEST

Injuries to the chest may be divided into two groups:

(1) penetrating or 'open' chest injuries; and
(2) non-penetrating or 'closed' chest injuries.

1. Penetrating or 'open' chest injuries

General

Penetrating injuries of the chest may be produced by bullets, but they are caused most commonly by punctures with pointed weapons such as knives, skewers or sharpened sticks. Punctured wounds of the chest may involve the lungs, the heart, the great blood vessels, the trachea or the oesophagus. These structures may be injured alone or in any combination.

Homicidal punctured wounds are usually caused by knives; they may occur in any region of the chest, and may pass in varying directions through the chest cavity. These wounds, however, commonly occur over the front of the left side of the chest and the tracks of such wounds are usually directed downwards, medially and backwards. Punctured wounds in the lower part of the chest may penetrate the diaphragm and injure the abdominal viscera. A punctured wound may pass into the chest cavity through the intercostal muscles between two ribs, or it may sever a costal cartilage or a rib.

The depth of a punctured wound of the chest may be greater than the total length of the blade of a knife which caused the wound, as the tissues are often compressed during the process of penetration.

Penetrating wounds of the lungs and pleura

Penetrating wounds of the lungs and pleura may result in a rapidly fatal haemothorax or pneumothorax (p 307–308). When haemorrhage into the bronchi or trachea prevents inhalation of air into the alveoli, death may result from anoxia.

Leverage of the instrument on the fulcrum of a rib during the act of withdrawal of the instrument may greatly extend the wound. Moritz[59] has also pointed out that the respiratory movements of the lung at the time of penetration may increase the lung injury.

A punctured wound of the lung and pleura may result in infection and delayed death from broncho-pneumonia or empyema.

Penetrating wounds of the heart

A punctured wound of the chest may pass directly into the heart through the anterior chest wall, or it may traverse a pleural cavity or the abdominal cavity before reaching the heart. In traversing a pleural cavity the wound may first pass through the lung.

A punctured wound of the heart may involve the muscle only, it may penetrate into one of the heart chambers, or it may pass through the heart. When the heart is penetrated, a coronary vessel may be injured. The immediate effect of a punctured wound of the heart is haemorrhage. The haemorrhage may be external but more often it is internal, and the blood flows into the pericardial sac or into a pleural cavity. Penetrating wounds of the heart are not invariably fatal but they often result in rapid death. Deaths of this nature may be caused by shock and haemorrhage or cardiac tamponade (p. 309–310).

Moritz[60] states that external penetrating wounds of the pericardium almost invariably become infected. If healing takes place with the formation of adhesions, the contraction of the scar tissue, particularly around the ostia of the great veins and over the surfaces of the atria, may lead to chronic cardiac compression and circulatory failure.

Penetrating wounds of the large blood vessels and the oesophagus

In a punctured wound of the chest the penetration of a large vessel, such as the superior vena cava, the pulmonary artery, or the aorta, may result in profuse haemorrhage. Such haemorrhage is usually internal and occurs into the pericardial sac, a pleural cavity, or the mediastinum.

A punctured wound of the oesophagus is usually accompanied by wounds of the great vessels and the haemorrhage from these vessel is responsible for death. Penetration of the oesophagus may result in the development of mediastinal and cervical surgical emphysema. Punctured wounds of the oesophagus may be followed by fatal mediastinitis.

2. Non-penetrating or 'closed' chest injuries

General

Wilson[61] has defined a closed injury of the chest as 'one in which the skin and subcutaneous tissues are intact, or else, if pierced, the course of the missile (or object) has been such that neither the pleural nor pericardial sacs have been injured and so these spaces have no direct contact with the outside air.' Most 'closed' chest injuries are caused by blunt force. Wilson states that the injuring force may act directly on the chest wall itself or it may act by pressure transmitted through from the abdomen. Pressure transmitted to the chest from the abdomen may be secondary to an abdominal injury or it may arise from a force applied elsewhere to the body, e.g. in falls from heights.

The application of a blunt force directly to the chest may result in injuries to the lungs, the heart, the large blood vessels, or the oesophagus. Such injuries may or may not be accompanied by external wounds of the chest wall or fractures of the ribs or the sternum. The symptoms and signs of an internal chest injury may be clinically latent and may only become manifest several hours after the injury.

Injuries of the chest wall

Abrasions of the skin, bruises of the subcutaneous tissues and simple fractures of the ribs are relatively common. Such fractures are usually caused by indirect violence and arise through compression of the chest. The commonest sites for such fractures are along the mid-axillary line and in the region of the posterior angles of the ribs. Fractures due to indirect violence are usually multiple and are often bilateral. In these fractures the rib fragments usually bend outwards, but should they bend inwards lacerations of the lungs and pleura may occur.

Fractures of the ribs may also be caused by direct violence and the fractured rib-ends are often driven inwards and lacerate the pleura and the lungs. Wilson[62] has drawn attention to the occurrence of the so-called 'stove in' chest injury. In this injury a group of ribs is fractured both anteriorly and posteriorly, and a segment of the chest wall becomes mobile with respiration. This type of injury is particularly liable to lead to laceration of the lung and injury to the intercostal vessels.

Fractures of the sternum are uncommon. They may be caused by direct violence, e.g. in the 'steering wheel impact' type of injury in traffic accidents (pp 336–337), or they may be caused by indirect violence, e.g. during extreme hyperextension of the trunk.

Injuries of the lungs

Injuries of the lungs in 'closed' chest injuries take the form of lacerations and contusions.

Lacerations of the lungs. Lacerations are usually produced by the penetration of lung tissue by fractured rib-ends, but in children lacerations may occur without associated fractures of the ribs (p. 224). Lung lacerations may result in a fatal haemothorax or pneumothorax (pp 307–308). Other complications which may result from lung lacerations include haemorrhage into the tracheo-bronchial 'tree', interstitial emphysema and pulmonary infections.

Pulmonary contusions. A sudden compression of the chest, e.g. from blows or from crushing injuries in traffic accidents, may cause pulmonary contusions. Although these contusions may occur in all parts of the lungs, Osborn[63] has shown that—depending upon their mechanism of production—contusions are often found in certain specific zones of the lungs. Osborn states that pulmonary contusions may be caused by direct violence, by contrecoup injury and by pincer forces.

Contusions caused by direct violence occur in those portions of the lung which are situated immediately deep to the site of impact of the force on the chest wall. The contusions usually appear as single or multiple irregular haemorrhagic zones in the lung tissue, but they may take the form of horizontal bruises corresponding to the rib markings on the lateral surfaces of the lungs.

Contusions of the lungs by contrecoup injury may arise during sudden compression of the chest. These injuries are probably chiefly caused by pneumostatic waves due to violent displacement of air in the lungs. They usually appear over the posterior surfaces of the lungs in a line corresponding with the angles of the ribs. They may extend laterally or forwards into the substance of the lungs.

Pincer forces operating in V-shaped spaces in the chest produce lung contusions in various positions. Osborn regards the phrenicocostal contusion as the commonest example of this type of lung lesion. The phrenicocostal sinus is a V-shaped space and the lung lesion consists of a wedge-shaped contusion, situated in the lateral portion of that part of the base of the lung which enters the phrenicocostal sinus of the pleural cavity in deep inspiration. In full inspiration this part of the lung enters the sinus and may be compressed between an external force transmitted directly to the chest or through the lower part of the arm and elbow and an internal force provided by the resistance of the weight of the liver on the right side and the weight of the spleen and its related organs on the left side.

Injuries of the heart

Lacerations of the heart. Fractures of the ribs or the sternum may cause lacerations of the pericardium and the heart. Such lesions may cause death from shock and haemorrhage, from haemothorax or from cardiac tamponade (pp 309–310). Traumatic ruptures of the heart may occur in the absence of fractures of the ribs or the sternum and such lesions may be unaccompanied by any external evidence of injury.

A rapid increase in intracardiac pressure may be caused by the sudden displacement of blood into the thorax from the abdomen and lower limbs. This displacement may occur in falls from heights and in traffic accidents where the wheels of a vehicle passed over the trunk. The hydrostatic forces set up in the cardiac chambers may be sufficiently powerful to rupture the heart. Moritz[64] states that the common sites of traumatic cardiac rupture listed in order of diminishing frequency are: right atrium, left ventricle, right ventricle, left atrium, interventricular septum and valves.

Cardiac contusions. Cardiac contusions are relatively common and may be caused by blows over the front of the chest, by falls on projecting objects and by compression forces in traffic accidents. Osborn states that cardiac contusions are produced by direct violence, by contrecoup injury, by pincer forces and by a mechanism associated with the heart's contraction. Contusions caused by direct violence are found in any part of the front and margins of the heart, while contrecoup lesions are seen over the posterior wall of the left ventricle. These lesions often occur in cases of the so-called 'steering wheel impact' type of injury in which the driver is thrown forward against the steering wheel and the heart is compressed against the vertebrae. The commonest pincer lesion is a contusion of the right atrium at the entrance of the inferior vena cava. This lesion arises in compression injuries and is produced by an impact between the liver and the heart across the right pericardiophrenic angle. It is frequently accompanied by some injury to the related part of the liver. Pincer lesions of the heart are of importance because they may give rise to sudden and unexpected death several days after the injury. According to Osborn the fourth type of lesion is produced by the heart's contraction at the time of injury. One of these lesions takes the form of a partial rupture of papillary muscles from the endocardium.

Moritz[65] states that although cardiac contusions may result in sudden death or in progressive circulatory failure terminating after a few hours or days in death, there is no evidence that such injuries ever lead to residual cardiac disability.

Sagall[66] has also reviewed the mechanism of production of cardiac contusions and their related medico-legal considerations.

Injuries of the large blood vessels

Traumatic 'asphyxia'. A sudden compression of the chest or abdomen may cause a retrograde displacement of blood from the superior vena cava into the subclavian veins and the veins of the head and neck. Valves in the subclavian veins prevent the spread of the hydrostatic force (set up in the column of blood) to the veins of the upper limbs, but the displacement of blood into the valveless veins of the head and neck results in the rupture of distal venules and capillaries. These ruptures lead to the formation of numerous petechial haemorrhages in the conjunctivae and in the skin and subcutaneous tissues over the face, neck and shoulders. Petechial haemorrhages may also be found over the surface of the cerebral hemispheres. Apart from the haemorrhages, a striking clinical feature of this condition which has become known as 'traumatic asphyxia' is the development of a bluish-black discoloration of the skin in the affected regions. Injuries associated with 'traumatic asphyxia' are often of a serious nature and may lead to rapid death.

Ruptures of the aorta. Although ruptures of the aorta may be caused by direct thoracic trauma most ruptures result from indirect force. Ruptures of the aorta may be complete or partial. The ruptures are usually transverse and occur in the ascending aorta. Partial ruptures usually involve the intima only. A possible explanation of the mechanism of traumatic aortic rupture has been given by Fiddler, quoted by Wilson.[67] In a series of deaths from trauma, Fiddler found seven instances of aortic rupture. In all seven cases the lesions had a constant situation about 1.5 cm distal to the aortic attachment of the ligamentum arteriosum. Four cases were cases of suicide where the deceased persons had jumped from heights. The other cases were road and air accidents. Fiddler considered that in all the cases a sharp deceleration strain applied to the caudal end of the body caused the abdominal and thoracic viscera to be forced caudalwards and in this manner the aorta was ruptured. He suggested that the constancy of the site of rupture may depend on fixation of the aortic arch by the great vessels arising from the convexity of the arch and by the attachment of the arch to the pulmonary artery by the ligamentum arteriosum.

An alternative explanation for these injuries has been suggested by Tannenbaum and Ferguson.[68] These authors consider that rapid deceleration strains cause a sudden great elevation in the intravascular pressure of the aorta and that this elevation is responsible for aortic ruptures.

Lasky[69] has reviewed (with illustrative cases) the biomechanics of human aortic laceration secondary to impact.

Complications and sequelae of chest injuries

Pneumothorax

There are two types of pneumothorax, namely, 'open' pneumothorax and 'closed' pneumothorax. In an 'open' pneumothorax, air enters the pleural cavity through an open wound in the chest wall. In a 'closed' pneumothorax air passes into the pleural cavity through a wound in the lung and visceral pleura. A combination of these types of pneumothorax may be present in penetrating wounds of the lung.

The immediate effect of a pneumothorax is to cause a collapse of the lung. In an 'open' pneumothorax, if less air enters the pleural cavity through the aperture in the chest wall than through the trachea and bronchi, expansion of the lung can occur on inspiration, and there may be relatively little interference with pulmonary ventilation. On the other hand, if more air enters the pleural cavity through the opening in the chest wall than through the trachea and bronchi, the mediastinum will be forced towards the normal side on inspiration and back towards the injured side on expiration. This condition is known as 'mediastinal flutter', and it may give rise to severe circulatory embarrassment.[70] In another form of pneumothorax—the so-called 'compressive' or 'tension' pneumothorax—defects in the injured visceral pleura or chest wall exert a valve-like action whereby air can enter the pleural cavity but cannot escape. This condition causes a progressive rise in pressure in the pleural cavity which results in the complete collapse of the affected lung, mediastinal displacement and cardiac and respiratory failure. Moritz[71] states that if compressive pneumothorax is suspected prior to autopsy, the post-mortem opening of the thorax should be carried out under water. The skin and subcutaneous tissues are first reflected to the posterior–axillary line. Water is then run into the gutter formed between the chest wall and the reflected skin. The intercostal muscles and the pleura are incised beneath the water level and if pneumothorax is present the entrapped air will bubble up through the water. In order to find a defect in the visceral pleura it may be necessary to remove the lung and inflate it under water.

Haemothorax

A haemorrhage into a pleural cavity or a haemothorax often occurs in association with a pneumothorax. The haemorrhage may arise (a) from a penetrating wound of the lung, (b) from a penetrating wound of the heart or one of the large blood vessels or (c) from an injury to an intercostal or internal mammary vessel.*

Haemorrhage from a penetrating wound of the lung is usually limited in amount because of the relatively low pressure in the pulmonary circulation and because effective coagulation can take place in the collapsed lung tissue. Haemorrhage from a penetrating wound of the heart or a large blood vessel is usually profuse. Profuse haemorrhage may also be caused by the puncture (in a penetrating wound) or the laceration (from fractured rib ends) of an intercostal or internal mammary vessel.

Blood in the pleural cavity often remains fluid. Wilson[72] considers that two factors may be responsible for this phenomenon. In cases where tissue destruction is limited, the blood in the pleural cavity may coagulate partially or it may not coagulate at all because insufficient thrombokinase is produced. Respiratory movements of the lung by causing mechanical agitation of the escaped blood in the pleural cavity may also defibrinate it, and the separated fibrin may be deposited in the most dependent portion of the cavity.

Chylothorax

The effusion of chyle from the thoracic duct into the right pleural cavity is known as a chylothorax. This is a rare condition. The thoracic duct may be injured (a) by puncture (in a penetrating wound), (b) by laceration (from fractured rib ends) or (c) by rupture (from indirect force during extreme hyperextension of the trunk).

Interstitial emphysema

The rupture of alveoli or the laceration of the mucosa of the trachea or bronchi may result in the infiltration by air of the contiguous connective tissues. This condition is known as interstitial emphysema.

In a case where the lung is injured, air may be forced into disrupted alveolar walls during inspiration, and as the air cannot be evacuated during expiration it ultimately tracks along the interstitial tissues of the lung. In this manner the air often reaches the pleura and raises large subpleural blebs over the surface of the lungs. These subpleural blebs of air may rupture and produce a pneumothorax.

Injuries of the trachea or large bronchi may result in the infiltration of the mediastinal tissues by air. The air in the mediastinum may extend upwards into the tissues of the neck, the face and the upper limbs. Mediastinal and cervical interstitial emphysema, by compressing the large veins in the thorax and neck, may give rise to circulatory failure.

---

* On rare occasions the application of 'blunt' force to the chest has resulted in haemothorax from the laceration of a vascular pleural adhesion.

When there is a tear in the parietal pleura air may be forced through the tear into the muscular and subcutaneous tissues of the chest wall. Interstitial emphysema of this nature is most likely to occur after spasms of coughing when the air in the pleural cavity is under tension. Interstitial emphysema of the chest may extend upwards into the tissues of the neck.

Arterial air embolism

In a case of lung injury where the pulmonary veins are punctured or lacerated, air may be aspirated into the injured veins. The aspirated air may then be carried through the left atrium and left ventricle into the systemic circulation. Chase[73] has shown that in arterial air embolism, air emboli may lodge in the terminal segments of the cerebral arteries. He attributes death in these cases to the combined effects of mechanical obstruction of arterioles and widespread vasoparalysis.*

Before a post-mortem diagnosis of air embolism can be made it is necessary (a) to exclude the possibility that the bubbles of gas in the blood vessels and the heart chambers were not produced after death by gas-forming organisms; and (b) to ensure that air did not enter the blood vessels during the manipulation of the tissues in dissection.

These difficulties may be overcome by the use of regional radiological examinations carried out within a short period of death. The value of this method of diagnosis is well illustrated in a case reported by Duncan-Taylor,[76] who described a fatal case of arterial air embolism following artificial pneumothorax refill therapy. Radiography showed that the ascending aorta and its arch were distended with air. The air column extended to the innominate artery. Both domes of the diaphgram were in the cadaveric position. The heart, trachea and mediastinum were deviated to the right. (See also pulmonary air embolism, p. 372.)

Chase used post-mortem stereoscopic examinations of the skull to demonstrate the presence of air in the cranial vessels.

Cardiac tamponade

An increase in intrapericardial pressure gives rise to the condition known as cardiac tamponade. The commonest cause of cardiac tamponade is the accumulation of blood in the pericardial sac. Intrapericardial haemorrhage may be caused:

1. By penetrating wounds of the heart or large blood vessels;

2. By lacerations of the pericardium and heart from fractures of the ribs or the sternum; or

3. By ruptures of the heart or aorta from indirect force.

---

* The experimental work of Moore and Braselton[74] and Durant et al[75] suggests that death in arterial air embolism may be due to ventricular fibrillation from occlusion of the coronary arteries by air emboli.

4. By a dissecting aneurysm of the aorta or myocardial rupture at the site of a myocardial infarct (myomalacia cordis).

In cardiac tamponade the parietal pericardium may be intact, punctured or lacerated. When the parietal pericardium is punctured or lacerated, tamponade occurs if the blood accumulates in the pericardial sac faster than it can escape through the wound in the pericardium. The development of cardiac tamponade may be rapid or slow. The accumulation of blood is usually rapid in cases where the parietal pericardium is intact, e.g. in traumatic cardiac or aortic ruptures.

A collection of blood in the pericardial sac interferes with ventricular dilatation during diastole, and compresses the great veins and the right atrium. As the arterial blood pressure falls and the venous pressure rises, there is a progressive failure of the circulation.

Moritz[77] states that an accumulation of between 400 and 500 ml of blood in the pericardial sac is usually sufficient to cause death. In a case of death from cardiac tamponade a medical witness may be asked whether it would have been possible for the deceased to have performed some voluntary act after the occurrence of the injury. Unless it can be shown that the cardiac injury was such that it would have been immediately incompatible with life, it is seldom possible to state that the deceased could not have performed some voluntary act before his death.

Healing of cardiac injuries

Wilson[78] states that the changes which take place during the healing of heart wounds are similar to those which occur in other wounds. If a wound is of an extensive nature and involves branches of the coronary arteries, areas of necrosis simulating cardiac infarcts may appear in the myocardium. Ruptures of the heart may occur through these necrosed areas. A detailed account of the healing of heart wounds has been given by King.[79]

Defects in the myocardium heal by fibrosis and the resulting scars may be indistinguishable from the foci of fibrosis which replace infarcts caused by coronary artery occlusion. The clinical history and the distribution of the lesions in relation to diseased coronary vessels may serve to determine the probable origin of such myocardial scars. Extensive traumatic scarring of the myocardium may result in the formation of a cardiac aneurysm.

Thoracic trauma and coronary thrombosis

Moritz[77] considers that the probability of a blunt injury of the chest causing coronary thrombosis is remote. He states that a probable cause and effect relationship between thoracic trauma and coronary thrombosis can only be established (a) if there is objective evidence of injury of the chest wall, (b) if there is evidence of a mechanical injury of the heart, and (c) if a thrombosis of appropriate age is found in a segment of a coronary artery in the region of injury.

INJURIES TO THE ABDOMEN

Injuries to the abdomen may be divided into two groups, namely:

1. Penetrating or 'open' abdominal injuries; and
2. Non-penetrating or 'closed' abdominal injuries.

1. Penetrating or 'open' abdominal injuries

Penetrating wounds of the abdomen may be produced by bullets, but they are usually caused by punctures with pointed weapons such as knives or daggers. Penetrating wounds may result in injury to the solid and/or the hollow viscera. As a general rule, a single wound results in injury to more than one organ. Penetrating wounds of the lower chest often extend through the diaphragm and injure the liver, the spleen, the stomach or the intestines.

Penetrating wounds of the liver are relatively common and death from a wound of this nature is usually caused by shock and haemorrhage. Penetrating wounds of the spleen are less common than penetrating wounds of the liver. Haemorrhage from penetrating wounds of the spleen is usually more profuse than haemorrhage from similar wounds of the liver.

Penetrating wounds of the pancreas are uncommon. In such wounds of the abdomen the stomach is relatively protected against injury but the small intestine is often punctured. The small intestine is injured more often than the large intestine.

As the small intestine is mobile, and the abdominal wall and the hollow viscera are able to undergo considerable compression, an intestinal wound caused by a penetrating weapon may be situated at some distance from the external wound. Moreover, there may appear to be a wide discrepancy between the length of the penetrating object and the depth of the wound. This condition was seen in one of our cases when a man was stabbed in the left loin with a knife and a wound was found in the ileum close to the ileocaecal junction. The blade of the knife measured 90 mm ($3\frac{1}{2}$ in.) and the distance between the external wound and the intestinal wound as measured at autopsy was 165 mm ($6\frac{1}{2}$ in.). Penetrating wounds of the intestines may cause death through primary shock, secondary shock and haemorrhage, or through peritonitis (pp 315–316).

2. Non-penetrating or 'closed' abdominal injuries

General

In a non-penetrating or 'closed' abdominal injury there is no communication between the surface of the abdomen and the peritoneal cavity. If an external wound of the abdomen is present, the wound does not extend into the peritoneal cavity.

'Closed' abdominal injuries are caued by blunt force and occur in accidental falls, in traffic accidents and in cases of assault and homicide when
the abdomen has been kicked, or has been struck with fists or blunt
weapons.

The application of a blunt force directly to the abdomen may result in
contusions and lacerations of solid or hollow abdominal viscera. There
injuries may be accompanied by abrasions, contusions or lacerated wounds
of the skin of the abdomen, but fatal traumatic lesions of the viscera often
occur without any external evidence of injury. The symptoms and signs of
an internal abdominal injury may be clinically latent for several hours after
the injury, e.g. pain may only become manifest with the development of
complications such as peritonitis (pp 315–316).

Injuries of the abdominal wall

Injuries of the abdominal wall take the form of abrasions of the skin,
bruises of the subcutaneous tissues and haematomata or lacerations of the
abdominal muscles. These injuries are of medico-legal importance as they
indicate that a force has been applied to the abdomen. Deep-seated
contusions may track along the muscular and fascial planes and appear on
the surface several hours after the injury in a region anatomically distant
from the site of origin of the contusion, e.g. an effusion from a deep-seated
bruise of the upper abdominal wall may appear in the region of the external
orifice of an inguinal canal.

Injuries of the stomach and intestines

Injuries of the stomach and intestines may be caused by:

1. Forces of compression or 'crushing' forces;
2. Traction or 'tearing' forces; and
3. Forces of disruption or 'bursting' forces.

   1. Injuries from forces of compression. When a force is applied to the
anterior abdominal wall, the force may be absorbed by the abdominal
muscles which yield under the pressure and protect the underlying viscera.
Under certain conditions, however, a force may be transmitted through the
muscles and may compress the stomach or intestines against the rigid
posterior abdominal wall. The stomach and the large intestine are less
commonly injured by forces of compression than the small intestine.
Compression injuries of the large intestine usually involve the transverse
colon.

   Compression injuries take the form of contusions or lacerations. Contusions may occur in any of the layers of the bowel wall. Large contusions
may result in the formation of sloughs and the separation of these sloughs

can give rise to delayed perforation. Lacerations may be complete or incomplete. 'Crushing' or compression forces may injure the mesenteric blood vessels, and the occurrence of thrombosis in these vessels may give rise to infarcts of the intestine.

2. Injuries from traction forces. The mobility of the stomach and intestines affords these viscera protection from injury, as forces transmitted to them may be expended in causing their displacement rather than their distortion. A displacement of this nature, however, may stretch the attachments of the stomach or the intestines and this may result in rupture of these attachments, e.g. the mesentery may be torn as a result of displacement of the small intestine. In certain regions the intestine is partially fixed and partially mobile. When a traction force is applied to the intestine, ruptures may occur at the junction of the fixed and mobile parts, e.g. the intestine may be torn at the duodeno-jejunal junction.

The mesentery is usually torn near its intestinal attachment and the tears may extend through the mesenteric vessels and give rise to intraperitoneal haemorrhage and infarcts of the intestine.

3. Injuries from forces of disruption. Injuries of the stomach or the intestines may be caused by forces of disruption or 'bursting' forces. In these injuries a blow over the abdomen causes a violent displacement of the contents of the gastrointestinal tract. Hydrostatic forces are set up in the displaced contents and these forces may be sufficiently powerful to injure the stomach or the intestine in a region anatomically distant from the site of application of the force. The injuries may take the form of contusions or ruptures.

When the stomach is distended with food or gas an injury to this organ is particularly liable to result in rupture and the commonest site for this type of rupture is the lesser curvature. Ruptures of the intestine usually involve the ileum. The ruptures are often multiple and occur along the length of the antimesenteric border of the bowel.

The introduction of compressed air through the anus (usually done as a practical joke) may cause severe damage and rapid reflex death.

The complications and causes of death in non-penetrating injuries of the stomach and intestines are considered at pages 315–316.

Injuries of the liver

Most non-penetrating injuries of the liver are caused by forces of compression and take the form of contusions or lacerations. Contusions of the liver may be difficult to recognize at autopsy but lacerations are usually prominent. Moritz[80] states that the following six types of hepatic lacerations may result from the application of blunt force to the abdomen:

1. Transcapsular lacerations which occur over the convex surface of the liver immediately beneath the site of the external impact.

2. Subcapsular lacerations* which occur over the convex surface of the liver immediately beneath the site of the external impact.

3. Non-communicating or central lacerations which occur in the substance of the liver.

4. Coronal lacerations due to distortion involving the superior surface of the liver.

5. Lacerations of the inferior surface of the liver due to distortion.

6. So-called contrecoup lacerations involving the posterior surface of the liver.

Transcapsular lacerations may lead to rapid death from haemorrhage and shock. The immediate clinical effects of a subcapsular laceration may be minimal, but if haemorrhage from the laceration continues a large haematoma may collect under the capsule. Such a subcapsular haematoma may rupture several hours or days after the injury and give rise to fatal delayed intraperitoneal haemorrhage.

Lacerations of the liver are a common form of injury in traffic accidents. They usually occur in association with other injuries such as rib fractures, ruptures of the diaphragm, and pulmonary contusions. Lacerations of the liver often occur when a person is crushed between objects such as buffers. Lacerations may be produced by kicks or falls on the abdomen. Moritz,[81] quoting the work of Geill, observes that children are more susceptible than adults to hepatic injuries. He also states that many diseases of the liver such as malaria, bilharziasis, fatty metamorphosis and abscess formation may increase the friability of the liver to such an extent as to predispose it to injury from relatively mild degrees of external violence.

The complications and causes of death in non-penetrating injuries of the liver are considered at pages 315–316.

Injuries of the gall-bladder and the extrahepatic bile ducts are uncommon. When these structures are injured there is usually an associated injury to other abdominal viscera. The extravasation of bile into the peritoneal sac may be succeeded by peritoneal irritation and infection.

Injuries of the spleen

Injuries of the spleen may be caused by forces of compression or traction forces. Forces of compression produce lacerations of the organ, while traction forces may tear the spleen from its pedicle.

Lacerations of the spleen are usually transcapsular but the initial effect of the injury may be the production of a subcapsular laceration with haematoma formation. Vance[82] states that transcapsular lacerations may take the form of tears across the hilar or convex surfaces of the spleen. The lacerations are often multiple and assume characteristic shapes simulating the alphabetical figures Y, H or L.

---

* Subcapsular and transcapsular lacerations of the liver are sometimes responsible for the death of newly born infants. These lacerations are produced by compression of the abdomen during the process of labour, particularly in breech presentations.

Lacerations of the spleen may or may not be accompanied by fractures of the overlying ribs. In traffic accidents, lacerations of the spleen usually occur in association with other injuries, such as rib fractures, pulmonary contusions and ruptures of the diaphragm. Haemorrhage into the peritoneal cavity from a splenic laceration or a torn splenic pedicle is often profuse and usually occurs immediately after the injury. In cases where a subcapsular or perisplenic haematoma has formed, haemorrhage into the peritoneal cavity may be delayed. Delayed splenic rupture of this nature is relatively common.[83]

Wilson[84] states that the syndrome of delayed splenic rupture is characterized by a history of trauma which may be of a mild nature. The trauma is followed by a few symptoms such as vague abdominal pain and tenderness. After a latent period of hours, days or even weeks, a sudden rupture of the spleen occurs through a subcapsular or perisplenic haematoma. A delayed rupture of the spleen may give rise to profuse haemorrhage into the peritoneal cavity and death may occur from shock and the loss of blood.

Although the splenomegaly, which occurs in diseases such as malaria, kalaazar and leukaemia, may predispose the spleen to rupture from relatively mild trauma, it is doubtful whether 'spontaneous' rupture of a normal spleen occurs but fairly persuasive cases have been reported.[85,86] Moritz[87] states that ruptures of this nature might possibly occur in cases where extreme passive congestion is brought about by the sudden torsion of the pedicle of an abnormally mobile spleen.

Injuries of the pancreas

The pancreas may be injured by compression forces when the viscera are crushed against the posterior abdominal wall. Pancreatic injuries are usually accompanied by injuries to other viscera. Laceration of the pancreas may result in profuse intraperitoneal or retroperitoneal haemorrhage. The escape of pancreatic juice from ruptured ducts may give rise to retroperitoneal fat necrosis, mesenteric fat necrosis, or chemical peritonitis. The peritonitis may be confined to the lesser sac or it may be generalized.

Complications of abdominal injuries

The main complications of abdominal injuries are shock, internal haemorrhage, peritonitis and paralytic ileus.

Abdominal injuries may be followed by primary and/or secondary shock. The general features of primary and secondary shock are described at pages 234–236.

Internal haemorrhage into the peritoneal cavity is relatively common in penetrating and non-penetrating injuries of the abdomen.

The main complication of injuries to the solid viscera is intraperitoneal haemorrhage. The rate and amount of haemorrhage from solid viscera are variable. Haemorrhage from a laceration of the spleen is usually rapid and copious. Haemorrhage from a laceration of the liver is usually slow because of the relatively low pressure in the hepatic sinusoids, but the amount of blood lost over a period of time may be considerable.* Stretching of the liver capsule usually causes pain. As the capsule is not stretched in punctured or lacerated wounds unless there is subcapsular haematoma formation, the liver may be punctured or lacerated without causing pain. Pain develops when sufficient blood accumulates in the peritoneal sac to give rise to peritoneal irritation. When haemorrhage into the sac occurs slowly, several hours may elapse from the time of injury before symptoms of discomfort or signs of blood loss become manifest.

Peritonitis may occur as a complication of penetrating or non-penetrating abdominal injuries. In penetrating injuries, organisms may reach the peritoneal sac from without, or they may enter the cavity through punctured wounds of the small intestine or the large intestine. In non-penetrating injuries, peritonitis is usually caused by the extravasation of intestinal contents into the peritoneal sac through lacerations of the bowel. Owing to the relative preponderance of pathogenic organisms in the colon, peritonitis is more likely to follow ruptures of the large intestine than ruptures of the small intestine. The leakage of gastric contents into the peritoneal sac may result in a chemical irritation of the peritoneum. 'Chemical' peritonitis may also be produced by the extravasation of pancreatic juice into the peritoneal cavity in injuries of the pancreas. As the intestinal wall is sensitive to distension only, the puncture or the rupture of a loop of bowel may be unaccompanied by any pain or discomfort. For this reason the symptoms and signs of a punctured wound or a rupture of the intestine may remain clinically latent for several hours.

Multiple contusions of the intestines may give rise to paralytic ileus.

A person who has sustained an abdominal injury should be kept under observation. This is particularly important when it is suspected that the person is under the influence of alcohol, as acute alcoholic intoxication may mask the symptoms of a visceral injury. It is also important not to overlook the possibility of a visceral injury when a patient is unconscious after trauma.

INJURIES TO THE UROGENITAL TRACT

Injuries of the kidney

Penetrating injuries

Penetrating wounds of the kidney may be produced by bullets or by punctures with pointed weapons. Punctured wounds of the kidney usually result

---

* The extravastion of bile from a wound in the liver may interfere with effective coagulation and prolong bleeding.

from 'stabs' in the loin, and, as a general rule, other viscera such as the colon are injured as well as the kidney. Punctured wounds of the kidney are often accompanied by extensive retroperitoneal haemorrhage. Direct injury to the renal artery or a large intrarenal vessel, or the development of renal arterial spasm, may result in infarction of the kidney. Sepsis and the extravasation of urine into the surrounding tissues with the development of a urinary fistula may occur as sequelae of penetrating wounds of the kidney.

Non-penetrating injuries

Non-penetrating injuries of the kidneys are not common as the kidneys are situated in a relatively well-protected part of the body. These injuries usually result from blunt force applied directly to the posterior or lateral aspects of the kidneys as from blows to the loins. A relatively common kidney injury, however, which is usually associated with liver injury, is contusion about the upper pole of the right kidney. This injury is caused by a crushing of the kidney against the lower ribs by forces transmitted through the liver. Bilateral injuries of the kidneys are rare.

Certain diseases of the kidneys, e.g. pyonephrosis, may predispose the organ to injury from relatively mild degrees of external violence.

Non-penetrating injuries of the kidney take the form of contusions or lacerations. Contusions may be localized or generalized. Contusions over the posterior surface of the kidney may appear as horizontal bruises corresponding to the rib-markings overlying the kidneys.

According to Moritz[88] lacerations of the kidneys may be subcapsular (when the cortex is torn beneath an intact capsule), transcapsular (when the capsule and cortex are torn without extension into the pelvis of the kidney) and transrenal (when a tear extends from the capsule to the pelvis of the kidney). Quoting the work of Kuster, Moritz states that transcapsular and transrenal lacerations are caused by 'the explosive hydraulic effects of sudden compression of a structure whose fluid content cannot be evacuated quickly enough through normal anatomical channels.'

In transcapsular and transrenal lacerations of the kidney, ruptures of the capsule are usually multiple and often occur along lines which radiate from the hilum towards the convex border. Lacerations of this nature may cause haemorrhage into the perinephric fat with the formation of a large perirenal haematoma.* In transrenal lacerations, haemorrhage may occur into the pelvis of the kidney and urine may extravasate into the perinephric tissues. The extravasation of urine may result in infection and the development of a urinary fistula.

---

* An extensive retroperitoneal haemorrhage is usually secondary to some visceral trauma, e.g. laceration of the liver or the kidney, but such haemorrhage may occur as a primary traumatic lesion and cause death through shock.

Injury to the renal pedicle may be caused by the application of blunt force to the loin. The pedicle may be contused or lacerated. If the renal artery is severed, death may occur rapidly from haemorrhage. A partial tear of the artery may be followed by thrombosis and renal infarction. Contusion of the pedicle may give rise to renal artery spasm and this spasm may result in renal infarction. Tears of the renal artery have been described in falls from heights. It has been suggested that these tears occur when the abdominal viscera are forced caudalwards and the renal pedicle is stretched (p. 306).

Injuries of the ureters are rare and are usually accompanied by other injuries of a serious nature.

Injuries of the bladder

Penetrating injuries

Punctured wounds of the lower abdomen may penetrate the bladder. As a general rule, punctured wounds of the lower abdomen involve other viscera such as the intestine as well as the bladder. A punctured wound of the bladder may cause rapid death from haemorrhage. The puncture of a distended bladder in a lower abdominal wound may result in an extraperitoneal extravasation of urine. This complication may lead to delayed death from pelvic cellulitis.

When a distended bladder is penetrated by a high-velocity bullet, the bullet may have an explosive effect on the urine in the bladder and this may cause extensive laceration of the viscus (p. 225).

Non-penetrating injuries

The application of blunt force to the lower abdomen, e.g. from a kick or a fall, may injure the bladder. The nature of the injury depends upon whether the bladder is distended or not. When the bladder is distended the peritoneum over the dome of the viscus becomes stretched, and as it is less elastic than the muscle of the bladder the peritoneum tears in this region. The tear in the peritoneum often extends through the bladder wall and urine is extravasated into the peritoneal cavity. When the bladder is only partially distended, the application of blunt force to the lower abdomen may cause an extraperitoneal rupture of the bladder. Extraperitoneal ruptures of the bladder also occur in fractures of the pelvis when fragments of fractured bone penetrate the bladder wall. In extraperitoneal ruptures the urine may extravasate upwards to the level of the kidneys or downwards along the spermatic cord into the scrotum. The extravasation of urine into the tissues may result in cellulitis and this complication may cause death.

Moritz[89] records that a large proportion of all traumatic ruptures of the bladder occur in persons who are intoxicated. The fact that drunken persons are likely to have distended bladders is probably a predisposing factor in bladder ruptures.

Injuries of the female genital tract

Injuries of the external genitalia and the vagina caused during rape or attempted rape are described at page 359. Injuries of the vagina and the uterus produced during criminal abortion or attempted abortion are described at pages 370–373.

Penetrating wounds of the genitalia are uncommon but they may result from impalement on pointed objects during falls. Contusions and lacerations of the vulva and vagina may be produced by the application of blunt force to the genitalia, e.g. from kicks during assaults. Owing to the vascularity of the tissues, lacerated wounds of the vulva may bleed profusely. Incised and punctured wounds of the vulva may be produced by a sexual pervert (p. 360).

It is exceptional for the uterus, the ovaries or the fallopian tubes to be injured in punctured wounds of the lower abdomen, but these structures may be contused or lacerated in severe compression injuries of the pelvis.

Injuries of the male genital tract

Accidental injuries of the penis and scrotum are rare, but self-inflicted injuries may occur when mentally disordered or mentally defective persons mutilate themselves. Cases of assault and homicide have been recorded where the external genitalia have been amputated.

The urethra may be ruptured at the junction of its cavernous and membranous portions due to a 'straddle' fall whereby it is crushed against the pubic arch. Violent displacement of a full bladder, as in crushing injuries of the pelvis, may also tear the bladder away from its attachments with resultant rupture of the posterior urethra.

Injuries to the testes are uncommon. Compression or crushing of the testes may give rise to sudden reflex cardiovascular failure and death from parasympathetic cardiac inhibition (p. 154).

INJURIES TO THE LIMBS

Injuries of the limbs may be caused by bullets, but most limb injuries in civilian life are due to industrial and traffic accidents. Injuries of the limbs may be associated with injuries to the head, the chest or the abdomen, but in many cases the trauma is confined to the limbs.

An injury to a limb may have (1) local effects and (2) general effects and complications.

1. Local effects of limb injuries

An injury to a limb may result in damage to any one or any combination of its constituent tissues. Severe lacerated wounds usually extend from the skin surface to the bone and involve the subcutaneous tissues, the muscles, the vessels and the nerves. Deep-seated limb injuries affecting the muscles, the vessels, the nerves or the bones may occur without any external evidence of injury.

Injuries of the skin, the subcutaneous tissues and the muscles

Common forms of limb injury in traffic and industrial accidents are abrasions of the skin, bruises of the subcutaneous tissues and deep lacerated wounds which involve the muscles and extend down to the bone. At autopsy all 'open' wounds should be thoroughly explored, and the tissues underlying superficial injuries (abrasions and bruises) should be dissected in order to determine the nature and the extent of the limb injury. Exploration and dissection may reveal extensive laceration of adipose tissue which could give rise to fat embolism (p. 328), or it may reveal necrosis of muscle which could be complicated by acute tubular necrosis (p. 333).

Injuries of vessels

Injuries of arteries. A large artery of the limb, e.g. the brachial or femoral artery, may sustain a direct injury or the artery may be affected by an injury to the limb in its vicinity. A direct injury of a large limb artery may result in contusion or partial or complete rupture of the arterial wall and any one of these lesions can give rise to an immediate segmentary spasm of the vessel. An injury in the vicinity of a large artery may also produce an immediate segmentary spasm of the vessel, e.g. the disruptive force of a bullet passing near the femoral artery may be sufficient to induce arteriospasm in the vessel even when no lesion can be detected in the vessel wall.

Traumatic segmentary arteriospasm. Montgomery and Ireland[90] suggested that the term 'traumatic segmentary arteriospasm' should be applied to the phenomenon of localized arterial spasm which follows trauma. Traumatic segmentary arteriospasm is a common complication of fractures of the limb bones and occurs when the bone ends or fragments of a fracture contuse or lacerate an artery. Arteriospasm may occur in bullet wounds of the limbs and it is especially liable to develop when the soft tissues of the limbs are crushed, e.g. from direct compression by masonry in accidents during building operations. Crushing injuries of the soft tissues which are complicated by arteriospasm may or may not be accompanied by external signs of injury. When arteriospasm occurs, the contraction develops immediately after the arterial injury and the reaction appears to be part of the natural mechanism whereby haemorrhage from injured arteries is controlled. The spasm involves a segment of varying length of a main limb artery and this arteriospasm usually persists for at least 24 hours, but it may last as long as 3 or 4 days. The arteriospasm causes pallor, coldness and a diminution of the pulse in the affected limb. The effects on the tissues of the limbs depend upon the intensity of the spasm and the extent to which the collateral circulation is involved.

When a limb vessel undergoes segmentary spasm, associated spasm may develop (a) in the main branches of the vessel distal to the site of contraction, (b) in the trunk of the artery proximal to the site of spasm, and (c) in the vessels of the collateral circulation. In a series of experiments on rabbits, Trueta et al[91] showed that trauma applied to the main artery of one thigh of a rabbit was followed by spasm of the main artery of the contralateral limb and that the bilateral spasm often extended upwards to involve vessels such as the renal arteries. Trueta and his co-workers attributed this generalized arteriospasm to reflex sympathetic nervous effects.

The mechanism of segmentary arteriospasm and the mechanism of generalized arterial contraction have also been investigated by Kinmouth.[92] On the basis of his experimental work and on clinical observations, Kinmouth considers that traumatic arteriospasm is due to a mechanical stimulation of the vessel wall resulting in a sustained contraction of smooth muscle, in the maintenance of which nervous factors do not play a demonstrable part.* Kinmouth has also shown that the generalized arterial contraction which follows traumatic segmentary arteriospasm is due to a falling systemic blood pressure and does not depend upon reflex nervous action as claimed by Trueta and his co-workers.

The sequelae of traumatic segmentary arteriospasm are described at pages 320–321.

Arterial contusion, thrombosis and embolism. Contusions of the arteries are usually found in the intima. These lesions are often accompanied by tears of the endothelial lining of the intima and by thrombus formation. Although a vessel may be completely occluded by a thrombus, circulation to the affected part may be maintained through the collateral circulation. In some cases, however, serious interference with the blood supply of a limb may be caused by a distal extension of the thrombus or by the release of an embolus which becomes impacted at a lower level in the vessel or in one of its branches. The effects of this process may be aggravated by the development of secondary vasospasm in the vessel itself and in vessels of the collateral circulation.

Arterial contusions often result from crush injuries to the limbs, e.g. in traffic accidents.

Arterial lacerations, false aneurysms, arteriovenous fistulas and traumatic aneurysms. When an artery is lacerated or punctured, e.g. by a bone fragment in a fracture or by a bullet or sharp instrument, a perivascular haematoma may form in the tissues surounding the vessel. If the blood at

---

* Leriche[93] originally suggested that segmentary arterial spasm was initiated through a nervous reflex mechanism. He considered that when a large limb vessel was contused, spasm was induced through a local reflex in the vessel walls or through an afferent arc via the sympathetic. This theory was contested by Cohen[94] who claimed that traumatic arteriospasm was induced locally and depended upon the known properties of smooth muscle fibres which respond to sudden stretching by contraction.

the periphery of the haematoma coagulates and becomes organized, the central portion of the haematoma may remain fluid and a direct communication may be maintained between the fluid blood in the haematoma and the blood in the artery. A 'communicating' haematoma of this nature is known as a 'false' aneurysm as the collection of blood is not enclosed by any of the normal coats of the vessel. A 'false' aneurysm may pulsate and gradually increase in size. The rupture of a 'false' aneurysm may result in profuse haemorrhage and death.

A penetrating wound of a limb, e.g. from a bullet or a pointed weapon, may extend through an artery and the accompanying vein. A communication of this nature is known as an arteriovenous fistula. The communication between the artery and the vein may be direct or through an intervening false aneurysm. The development of an arteriovenous fistula results in the passage of arterial blood into the related vein, and the effect of this passage depends upon the size and the situation of the fistula. If the fistula is large and if it is situated in the proximal part of a large limb artery a considerable amount of blood may leak into the related vein. A leakage of this nature will have both local and systemic effects. The impairment in the blood supply to the limb beyond the fistula may result in muscle necrosis and gangrene (below), while the fall in arterial pressure and the rise in venous pressure may lead to progressive cardiac decompensation and death.[95]

'True' traumatic aneurysms are rare but they may occur when the outer coats only of a large limb artery are injured, e.g. a tangential bullet injury of a vessel. The inner coat of the artery protrudes through the opening in the outer coats, and by progressive 'bulging' under the influence of the intravascular pressure an aneurysm develops at the site of injury. The rupture of a 'true' traumatic aneurysm of a large vessel may lead to rapid death from haemorrhage.

The sequelae of arterial injury. Any of the syndromes and lesions described (namely, traumatic segmentary arteriospasm, arterial thrombosis and embolism, 'false' aneurysms, arteriovenous fistulas, and 'true' traumatic aneurysms) may impair the circulation in a limb. The circumstances in which arterial injuries may be followed by recovery, by ischaemic contracture or by gangrene have been well summarized by Watson-Jones.[96] Watson-Jones states that the vascular demands of the tissues of a limb are not uniform. Sensory and motor nerve endings show the greatest susceptibility to ischaemia. Muscle tissue is more susceptible to ischaemia than are the skin or bone tissues. If ischaemia persists for 6 to 8 hours, muscle tissue becomes necrosed, whereas skin can survive ischaemia for as long as 24 hours. The powers of regeneration of muscle are limited and the greater part of a zone of necrosed muscle is replaced by fibrous tissues which undergoes contraction. Watson-Jones states that:

> The fate of the tissues of a limb after vascular occlusion depends upon the
> speed with which the circulation is restored by reopening original channels

or by the development of collateral channels, and the extent to which the relative demands of tissues have been met in the interval. If a free and vigorous circulation is established within about six hours, recovery is complete. If the occlusion lasts more than six hours and the collateral circulation is not adequate, tissues with the highest vascular demands suffer most; muscles undergo necrosis and Volkmann's ischaemic contracture supervenes. If the collateral circulation is totally inadequate no tissue survives and gangrene develops.

The relationship between ischaemic muscle necrosis and acute tubular necrosis is dealt with at page 334.

Volkmann's ischaemic contracture. Volkmann's ischaemic contracture is a condition in which fibrosis of necrosed muscles results in shortening of the muscles with the production of deformities and contractures. Although most recorded cases followed occlusion of the brachial artery with resultant deformities and contractures of the forearm and hand, the condition may be caused by the occlusion of any vessel in any part of the upper or lower limbs.

Courts and juries have been inclined to regard the incidence of Volkmann's ischaemic contracture as indisputable evidence of negligence on the part of a medical practitioner, because until a few years ago it was believed that Volkmann's ischaemic contracture was caused by venous obstruction from splints, bandages or plasters which were too tightly applied in the course of treatment. Griffiths[97] and other workers have now shown that Volkmann's ischaemic contracture is not caused by venous obstruction but results from any arterial injury that reduces the blood supply of the muscles of a limb, e.g. it may be caused by traumatic segmentary arteriospasm.

Injuries of veins. Although injuries of the veins are usually associated with severe injuries to the limbs, the veins may be damaged in relatively minor limb injuries. A traumatic lesion of a vein may result in contusion of the wall of the vein and/or tearing of the intimal lining. Damage to the intima may result in the formation of a thrombus at the site of injury. Venous thrombi formed at the site of intimal wounds may become dislodged and give rise to pulmonary embolism (pp 332–333).

The laceration of a large vein in an 'open' wound of a limb may be followed by pulmonary air embolism (p. 372), while the laceration of veins in regions of extensive damage to adipose tissue may be followed by fat embolism.

Injuries of peripheral nerves

Peripheral nerves may be injured in several ways. They may be severed or partially severed in incised and punctured wounds of the limbs. Peripheral nerves may be lacerated in certain types of fractures, e.g. the musculospiral nerve (which lies in a groove in the middle third of the humerus) may be lacerated in fractures of the humeral shaft. Contusion or 'concussion' of nerves may result from compression or crushing injuries of the limbs. Peripheral nerves may also be injured by traction forces, e.g. the ulnar nerve may be stretched in fracture-dislocations of the elbow joint. As the sensory and motor nerve endings are particularly susceptible to oxygen lack, ischaemia of a limb, following an arterial injury, may result in paralysis and anaesthesia even when the peripheral nerves have not sustained direct injury.

Watson-Jones[98] defines three groups of peripheral nerve injury, namely, complete divisions of the nerve, nerve lesions in continuity, and transient nerve blocks.

When a nerve is completely divided a process known as Wallerian degeneration develops in the distal portion of the nerve. The myelin sheath becomes fragmented and absorbed, the axis cylinders disappear, and only the nerve sheath of the distal segment remains. The cells of the nerve sheath proliferate and grow out towards the proximal end of the severed nerve. After an initial limited degeneration of the proximal segment, the axis cylinders of the proximal segment begin to regenerate and extend towards the proliferating nerve sheath of the distal segment. If contact is established between the segments, some restoration of function may be effected. Spontaneous regeneration of this nature is uncommon when a peripheral nerve has been completely divided.

In a lesion in continuity the nerve is compressed or crushed but the general structure of the nerve is preserved at the site of injury. The axis cylinders of the nerve are interrupted and Wallerian degeneration occurs in the distal segment as in the case of complete division. Because the continuity of the nerve sheath is maintained, regeneration of axis cylinders in this form of injury occurs more rapidly and is more effective in restoring function than regeneration in a complete division.

A transient nerve block is caused by contusion, traction or 'concussion' of a nerve. There is no actual degeneration of axons but conduction is temporarily lost in the nerve. Normal function is usually restored within a week or ten days.

Lesions of peripheral nerves may result in paralysis and/or sensory loss. Watson-Jones states that a paralysis due to a transient nerve block recovers spontaneously—a paralysis due to a lesion in continuity usually recovers spontaneously—but a paralysis due to a complete division of a peripheral nerve seldom recovers spontaneously. Sensory loss after peripheral nerve injuries may be relatively limited owing to overlapping in the distribution of sensory fibres from other nerves.

Nerve injuries may develop some weeks or months after fractures and/or dislocations of the limb joints. As these injuries may be caused by late compression by strapping, plasters or splints, they may form the basis of an action for damages against a medical practitioner.

Fractures and injuries of joints

Fractures—general. Fractures of the bones of the limbs are common. They may be caused by direct violence, by indirect violence, or by muscular action. In a fracture caused by direct violence, the bone is broken at the site of impact of the force, e.g. a fracture of the tibia caused by the wheel of a motor car passing over the leg. Fractures caused by direct violence are always accompanied by some injury to the overlying soft tissues. They are frequently compound* and are often comminuted.† In a fracture caused by indirect violence the bone is broken in a region distant from the site of impact of the force, e.g. a fracture of the head of the radius or of the lower extremity of the humerus caused by a fall on the extended palm. Fractures caused by indirect violence are usually simple‡ fractures. A fracture caused by indirect violence may be compound when a fragment of bone pierces the skin from the inside. When injuries of the soft tissues are present, they are caused by the sharp ends of the fractured bone. Fractures caused by indirect violence are less likely to be comminuted than fractures caused by direct violence. In a fracture caused by muscular action the bone is fractured by the sudden contraction of a muscle during an unexpected movement, e.g. the olecranon or the patella may be fractured by the sudden contraction of the triceps or the quadriceps muscles respectively. Fractures caused by muscular action are usually simple fractures.‡

The presence of a fracture of a limb bone may be suspected at autopsy when there is extensive discoloration of the skin, or when abnormal mobility or crepitus is detected on palpation of the limbs. When a person dies within a short period after the injury, however, there may be insufficient time for the development of swelling or discoloration in the tissues overlying the fracture, and the presence of a fracture may be overlooked. If rigor mortis is present, the rigidity of the muscles may conceal the abnormal mobility and the crepitus. Dissection of the tissues overlying a suspected fracture should always be undertaken in order to determine whether there are any co-existing injuries to the soft parts, e.g. injuries to the vessels or the nerves. Injuries of the vessels of the limbs are dealt with at page 320. Injuries of the peripheral nerves are described at pages 323–324.

---

* A compound or 'open' fracture is a fracture which is in communication with the air through a wound.

† In a comminuted fracture there are two or more intersecting lines of fracture which divide the bone into three or more fragments.

‡ A simple or 'closed' fracture is a fracture in which there is no communication between the bone and the air. In a simple fracture the line of fracture may be transverse, oblique or spiral.

‡ In young growing persons, forces which are directly or indirectly applied to the limb bones may cause separation of the epiphyses. Such injury may lead to permanent disability due to interference with the growth of an affected bone.

An important complication of a fracture of a limb bone is infection. Spontaneous blood-borne infection of a simple or 'closed' fracture is extremely rare. The organisms which cause infection of fractures usually reach the bone through 'open' wounds. Infection of 'open' wounds may be caused by organisms which are normally present on the skin, or by organisms which invade the tissues from the environment (p. 238). Infection of bone at the site of a fracture is an important cause of delayed union. Severe infection of a fracture may result in osteomyelitis and death from pyaemia or septicaemia.

Repair of fractures—delayed union and non-union. As the occurrence of delayed union, non-union or malunion of a fracture may be the subject of legal proceedings in an action for damages against a medical practitioner, attention is directed to some of the factors which are concerned with the repair of fractures and with delayed union and non-union. These factors are described in detail by Watson-Jones.[99]

According to Watson-Jones, repair of a fracture is effected in three histological stages, namely, a stage of repair by granulation tissue, a stage of union by primary callus formation, and a stage of consolidation. The initial stage develops during the first few days after the injury and is characterized by the proliferation, between and around the fractured bone ends, of a soft granulation tissue accompanied by hyperaemia and oedema. Within a week small areas of bone are laid down around blood vessels in an irregular interwoven manner. This 'woven' bone is formed equally by parosteal, endosteal and marrow reticulum cells. The growth of 'woven' bone represents a stage of temporary repair corresponding to union by primary callus formation or 'clinical union'. The trabeculae of 'woven' bone gradually undergo resorption and are replaced by lamellae of bone which are laid down in parallel plates corresponding to the lines of stress in the bone. This period of consolidation into mature lamellar bone may take as long as a year.

During the initial stage of repair there is marked local hyperaemia at the site of fracture. Watson-Jones claims that bone reacts to hyperaemia by resorption and during the phase of hyperaemia, calcium is transferred from the fractured ends of the bone to the surrounding tissues. In a simple fracture which is protected from further injury, traumatic hyperaemia subsides within 10 days and reossification begins. If a fracture is inadequately immobilized, repeated movements of the limb result in tearing of the granulation tissue with recurring hyperaemia, continued resorption of bone and delayed union. Delayed union in compound infected fractures is accompanied by the persistence of local hyperaemia and stagnation. The importance of circulatory efficiency at the site of fracture in promoting normal healing has been emphasized by Murray.[100] Murray believes that resorption and reossification at the site of a fracture depend upon the pH of the local tissue fluid. During the first week or ten days after a fracture the haematoma shows a marked 'acid tide'. Reossification coincides with the alteration of the pH of the local tissue fluids to the alkaline side of neutral. Murray considers that calcium can only be deposited in the developing 'woven' bone within a limited pH range on the alkaline side of neutral and that this deposition can occur only while the tissue is still undifferentiated. He states that if the initial 'acid tide' is prolonged because of a circulatory status which restricts the removal of necrotic tissue, the healing tissue may become fibrous, resulting in fibrous non-union, or the deposition of calcium in the lower pH ranges may be so slow that delayed union occurs.

Watson-Jones considers that although many factors such as the imperfect apposition of fragments, the interposition of soft tissues, bone infection, osteoporosis and senile changes may influence the rate of union, the most common cause of non-union is inadequate immobilization.

Injuries of joints. Deep lacerated wounds of the limbs or punctured wounds may extend into a joint cavity, but most injuries are 'closed' injuries.

'Closed' joint injuries may be caused by blows or falls or by dislocations. Any injury to the synovial membrane, the intra-articular cartilages, the ligaments or the capsule of a joint is likely to be accompanied by a transudation of serous fluid into the joint cavity. If the synovial membrane or the joint cartilages are lacerated or if one of the bones forming the joint surface is fractured, e.g. in fracture–dislocations, haemorrhage may occur into the joint cavity.* Effusions of serous fluid are usually absorbed but blood in a joint cavity may undergo organization with resulting intra-articular adhesion formation. The possibility of a fibrous ankylosis of this nature causing the fixation of a joint must be borne in mind in cases where actions for damages are brought against a medical practitioner for alleged faulty treatment of a limb injury.

'Open' injuries of joints caused by punctured or incised wounds are very likely to become complicated by secondary infection with pyogenic organisms with resultant disorganization of the joints. Severe permanent disability may result in such cases.

2. General effects and complications of limb injuries

Haemorrhage and shock

On the basis of a study of 230 patients suffering from limb injuries (unaccompanied by injuries to the contents of the skull, the chest or the abdomen), Grant and Reeve[102] observed that there were two main types of clinical reaction. Although these reactions were alike in many respects, the

---

* Moritz[101] states that minor and even unrecognized injuries may result in massive intra-articular haemorrhage in persons suffering from disorders such as scurvy, purpura or haemophilia.

one reaction was restricted to patients who had bled profusely, while the other reaction occurred even when no blood was lost. They describe these reactions in the following terms:

> The first picture is characterized by very low blood pressure, below 70 mmHg, impalpable pulses, very rapid heart rate and cold extremities with constricted veins. To this may be added great restlessness, dyspnoea, sweating, nausea and vomiting. This picture was associated usually with large and very large wounds.† and always, so far as our observations go, with great blood loss and blood volumes well under 70 per cent normal.
>
> The second clinical picture is characterized also by low blood pressure and impalpable pulses, pallor and cold extermities, but by a slow heart rate; and though yawning, sighing respirations, sweating, nausea and vomiting may be added there is no great restlessnes nor dyspnoea. This picture was seen . . . soon after injury and was associated especially with small wounds and little or no blood loss. It presents the combination of signs commonly termed the vasovagal syndrome, which is well known to be provoked by emotional and sensory stimuli alone.

In Grant and Reeve's series of cases only a small proportion of the patients with minor wounds died, but more than half of the patients with very large wounds died. In approximately one half of the fatal cases the patients died within 24 hours of the injury and in most of these cases death was due to haemorrhage. Deaths which occurred later than 24 hours after the injury were usually caused by some complication such as infection, fat embolism or renal failure.

As there are no specific pathological changes which are characteristic of shock and haemorrhage (p. 238), the cause of death in limb injuries must be determined from the clinical findings. An autopsy is of value, however, as a thorough exploration of the limb wounds will show whether any vessels which could have bled profusely were lacerated or ruptured. An autopsy will also show whether any important visceral injury had been overlooked during life, while a histological examination of the tissues may reveal the presence of complications such as fat embolism or acute tubular necrosis.

Fat embolism and the fat embolism syndrome

Shapiro[103] has drawn attention to the fact that it is just over 100 years ago that Zenker[104,105] first described 'natural post-traumatic' fat embolism in the lungs of the victim of a crush injury of the chest and abdomen. The subject of fat embolism has attracted considerable interest in recent decades, when its medico-legal importance has been more fully appreciated.

Probably because of the early emphasis on the lungs as the site of observation of fat embolism, the view has been held that fat embolism of the lungs is *per se* a fatal condition. As long ago as 1928 Lehman and

---

† Grant and Reeve group limb injuries under four categories according to size in terms of the volume of tissue damaged as follows: small wounds, moderate wounds, large wounds and very large wounds.

McNattin[106] showed that fat embolism occurred in the lungs in a great variety of circumstances unrelated to injury or fracture of bones, and apparently did not contribute to the fatal outcome. They found fat embolism in the lungs in 50 per cent of deaths from natural causes. The finding was entirely incidental and without any pathological or clinical significance. This high incidence of fat embolism in the lungs in non-traumatic cases has been confirmed by Becker.[107] Keith Simpson[108] has reported a similar position in post-operative deaths. These are all examples of what Becker[107] has classified as *endogenous* in origin. In the *exogenous* category may be included oily abortifacients which enter the circulation or intravenously introduced oily preparations.

The most common and most important cause of fat embolism is trauma to bone. Oh and Mital[109] proposed the marrow globular theory to explain the presence of embolic fat in the circulation. The theory postulates that trauma releases fat globules from fat-laden cells in the bone marrow of fractured bones or surrounding soft tissue. These fat droplets enter the venous system and are carried to the lungs where they are trapped as emboli at the capillary level. These fat droplets may pass through the capillaries of the lungs, or traverse arterio-venous communications to reach the systemic circulation.

Three conditions are necessary for the above sequence of events to occur following a fracture:

1. Disruption of adipose tissue in the marrow space;
2. Traumatic opening up of venous channels, and
3. A transient rise in bone marrow pressure above the venous pressure.

Extensive research using radiolabelled techniques on experimental animal models has thrown doubt on this theory, and the origin of the fat globules is still uncertain.

Fat embolism has been recognized as occurring after orthopaedic surgical procedures and occasionally in the puerperium as a result of injury to the pelvic fatty tissue due to trauma during childbirth.

Sevitt[105] has recorded that fat embolism can occur in the absence of trauma to either bones or soft tissue. Embolism may occasionally occur following extensive cutaneous burns, inflammatory lesions in bones and adipose tissue, poisoning, nutritional alcoholic fatty liver, diabetes mellitus and decompression sickness.

The clinical syndrome of fat embolism may be defined as a complex alteration of homeostasis, presenting clinically as acute respiratory insufficiency. The syndrome is evident in 0.5–2% of long bone fractures and approaches an incidence of 5–10% in multiple fractures associated with pelvic injuries. The clinical syndrome is most readily quantitated by monitoring the arterial blood gases.[110]

The pathophysiology of fat embolism syndrome is indicated in Figure 12.26 adapted from Shier and Wilson.[111]

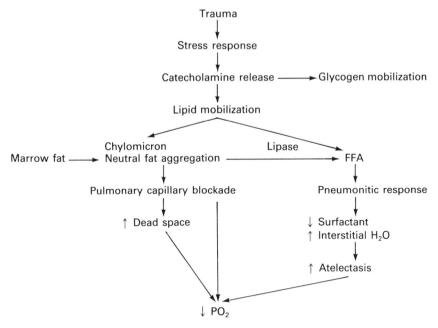

Fig. 12.26 The pathophysiology of fat embolism syndrome. (From Shier and Wilson[111].)

Arteriovenous communications in the lungs of laboratory animals have been demonstrated that allow rapid passage of glass spheres that are 20–40 times the average capillary size. Similar shunts have been demonstrated in the human lung. Bronchopulmonary venous shunting and a patent foramen ovale can be demonstrated in 20–25% of the population, as means for venous emboli to enter the systemic circulation.

Despite these two well-established bypassess, the lung maintains nearly an 80% filtering efficiency.[112]

Numerous authors[110,112–115] have highlighted the significant role of coagulation abnormalities in the fat embolism syndrome, as manifested by a rapid fall in the haematocrit value, erythrocyte aggregation, increased platelet adhesiveness, relative thrombocytopaenia, elevation of fibrin degradation products, prolonged prothrombin and partial thromboplastin times, and an increase in haptoglobin (alpha-2-macroglobulin) and alpha-l-antitrypsin.

There is increasing clinical and experimental support for the relationship of hyperlipidaemia and the alterations of coagulation as tabulated above.[110,112–115]

The fibrinolytic enzyme system may function to remove incidental fibrin deposits in animal and man, through the action of activated plasmin. A postulate is that a failure in this system after trauma results in a rise in plasma fibrinogen and fibrin, initiating intravascular clotting. It appears that neutral fats and tissue thromboplastin released from a fracture site, activate the clotting cascades and platelet aggregation. Suppression of the fibrinolytic systems in the injured patient then serves to aggravate an on-going accumulation of aggregates of fat, macroglobules, platelets, leucocytes and fibrin, which are passively concentrated in the lung, by virtue of its filtering action on venous blood before it is recycled to the systemic circulation.[110]

The acute effect of obstructive pulmonary fat embolic complexes probably have similar haemodynamic consequences to thrombo-emboli. The pulmonary circulation has an enormous compensatory capacity due to capillary recruitment, and moderate degrees of occlusion can be accommodated with only a slight rise in vascular resistance. If obstruction worsens, a raised right ventricular systolic pressure matches the increased pulmonary resistance, and maintains a near-normal blood flow. When the compensatory capabilities of the pulmonary circulation and right heart have been exceeded, however, acute cor pulmonale occurs.[113] This is manifested clinically by hypotension and a raised central venous pressure. Besides pure mechanical obstruction, pulmonary fat emboli may cause vasoconstriction via reflex and humoral means, although this has been discounted in pulmonary thromboembolism.[113]

Peltier[112] was the first to compare the pathological and physiological changes which occur after intravenous injections of neutral fat and free fatty acids. He found that neutral fat causes death as a result of pulmonary vascular obstruction, whereas fatty acids produce a chemical pneumonitis similar to that seen with a classical variant of fat embolism. In this latter case, there is a facultative increase in lipase produced by penumocytes in response to embolic neutral fat, resulting in liberation of free fatty acids that are directly toxic to the lungs.[110,112–115]

Surfactant-producing alveolar-type-2 cells have been shown to have a life cycle of five days. Ligation of the pulmonary artery in dogs produced no alterations in surface tension for 18 hours, in contrast to detergents, e.g. fatty acids, which caused immediate changes in lung compliance. Classic 'stiff' lung, which appears 24–36 hours after trauma, is postulated to be secondary to alveolar-type-2 cell inhibition, whereas the acute changes in compliance seen after severe long bone fracture are considered to be due to a chemical inactivation of existing surfactant by free fatty acids.[110]

Histopathologically, fat emboli appear as round, oval or elliptical optically clear, well-defined areas within the lumina of small arteries and arterioles. However, globular vacuoles in the kidney glomeruli as seen in a section stained with haemotoxylin and eosin are highly suggestive of fat emboli; however, for a more definitive diagnosis, positive staining of the vacuoles, using any of a variety of tinctorial methods for neutral lipids, is obligatory. The most convenient histochemical technique is that of a frozen section for fat in which either fresh or formalin-fixed tissue may be used, sections cut at 15–20 μm and then stained with oil red O.

Artefactual displacement of intravascular lipids may occur and thus great care must be taken to avoid rough handling of tissues.

After oil red O stain, emboli may appear as bright-orange to red intravascular globules. Extensive emboli may assume an elongated configuration intravascularly and may even be observed to branch at vascular bifurcations. Since the presence of occasional fat droplets may be artefactual, some observers feel that it is necessary to observe deformation of the emboli as proof of their ante-morten origin.[116]

The number of vessels involved is obviously related to the physiological effect. Sevitt[105] recommends expressing emboli per unit volume, calculated on the basis of 15 μm-thick sections using a 10 power objective, counting 20–40 fields. Less than an average of one embolus per field represents slight embolism; 1–3 moderate; and more than 3, gross embolism.

Histologically, within the first 24 hours post-embolization tissue reaction to pulmonary fat embolism may be that of a perivascular polymorphonuclear cell infiltration. This cellular response increases in intensity up to 72 hours when, in addition, eosinophils, lymphocytes and plasmacytes may be found. Peripheral scalloping of the emboli may then be observed and the emboli will gradually decrease in size, dissolving completely in about 7–10 days.

Dines et al[117] indicate that when fat has been present in the lungs for more than a few days, intra-alveolar oedema, haemorrhage, hyaline membrane formation and a bronchopneumonia will be present. Intra-alveolar macrophages with intracytoplasmic lipids may also frequently be observed.

The demonstration of fat emboli within intracerebral vessels is not necessarily an adequate explanation of the mode or cause of death. A clinical history confirming the development of symptoms referable to the site of embolization is essential for establishing the cause of death.

Conclusion. In the fat embolism syndrome, the major end organ response appears to be the lungs and the central nervous system. Fat macroglobules impair small vessel perfusion, and endothelial damage to the pulmonary capillaries leads to a ventilation/perfusion mismatch, vascular congestion, interstitial haemorrhage, alveolar wall damage, and airway collapse. The resulting clinical manifestation is a life-threatening impairment of pulmonary gas exchange.

Wound infection

Pyogenic infections, gas gangrene infections or tetanus infections may develop in limb wounds and cause death. The general features of these forms of infection are described at pages 238–240.

Pulmonary embolism

Pulmonary embolism is a serious complication of limb injuries and occurs when emboli are liberated from thrombi in the veins of a limb. The thrombi responsible for pulmonary embolism may develop in veins which have sustained direct injuries or they may form in veins which have not been injured. The main cause of spontaneous thrombosis in veins which have not been injured is stasis. Stasis may be generalized or localized. Generalized stasis occurs as part of the circulatory reaction of traumatic shock. Localized stasis may be caused by regional obstruction to the venous return through compression of veins, e.g. by displaced bone fragments or haematomas.

The effects of pulmonary embolism depend upon the size of the emboli released from the venous thrombus. When a large branch of one of the pulmonary arteries is obstructed, an infarct may develop in the lung. If smaller branches are obstructed, the collateral circulation from other branches of the pulmonary artery or from the bronchial arteries usually prevents the development of infarcts. A complete occlusion of the main stem and the right and left rami of the pulmonary artery by a so-called 'straddling embolus' may lead to sudden death. In a case of this nature death may be instantaneous, or it may occur within a few minutes. Instantaneous death is probably caused by reflex parasympathetic cardiac inhibition[118] while death which occurs after a few minutes probably results from a failure of the pulmonary circulation.[119] Young et al[120] have described the rare occurrence of paradoxical embolism by which an embolus arising in a systemic vein reaches a systemic artery by passing through a congenital defect between the right and left sides of the heart.

A diagnosis of fatal pulmonary embolism after a limb injury can be made when an embolus is found in the pulmonary artery or one of its branches, and when a part of the thrombus or the site of the thrombus can be demonstrated in one of the limb veins. Pulmonary emboli may be distinguished from post-mortem clots by the following characters: the emboli are cylindrical in shape with parallel contours, they are often branched, are frequently curled, and show no relationship in shape to the vessel in which they are found. Death from pulmonary embolism occurs most frequently about the tenth day, but may be delayed as long as three weeks after the injury.

Acute tubular necrosis

The term acute tubular necrosis is applied to a pathological lesion which is characterized by degeneration or necrosis of the convoluted tubules. Boyd[121] states that the most striking clinical manifestation of tubular necrosis is oliguria or anuria. Boyd divides such cases as regards causation into two groups: (1) a large and important group in which the pathogenesis is uncertain, but which is probably anoxic or ischaemic in nature; (2) a smaller and simpler group due to exogenous poisons such as mercuric chloride. These two groups may be termed anoxic necrosis and toxic necrosis. Included in the group of anoxic necrosis are conditions such as 'shock, burns, trauma, severe haemorrhage, the crush syndrome, intestinal obstruction, dehydration, incompatible blood transfusion and blackwater fever.' Toxic necrosis caused by such poisons as mercuric chloride and carbon tetrachloride may cause massive tubular necrosis which is most marked in the proximal convoluted tubule.

Of particular importance in forensic medicine is the so-called traumatic tubular necrosis. This condition may occur in cases of limb trauma in which muscle has undergone necrosis. Muscle may become necrosed from the ischaemia of direct compression. This form of necrosis was seen in the cases of injury described by Bywaters and Beall[122] in which the limbs of patients were compressed under fallen masonry and debris during air-raids. In traffic accidents, necrosis of muscle may occur without any prolonged crushing injury. Bywaters[123] found that dissection of the arteries of the injured limbs of persons who had been involved in traffic accidents revealed arterial ruptures, intimal lacerations with and without thromboses, arterial contusions and periarterial haematomas. As shown at page 323 any of these lesions (which may or may not be accompanied by segmentary arteriospasm) can impair the circulation of a limb and give rise to ischaemic muscle necrosis.

In a fatal case of acute tubular necrosis associated with traumatic muscle necrosis, the limb injury may have been caused by direct compression or it may have been sustained in a traffic accident. When the injury has been caused by direct compression, there may be little external evidence of injury to the limb. The clinical syndrome is characterized by the development of shock followed by oliguria or anuria. Death occurs at about the end of the first week after the injury. When the tissues of the affected limb are examined at autopsy, zones of muscle necrosis can be detected in the region of 'crushing', or in the area of distribution of the injured arteries. The naked-eye appearances of the kidney are not specific, but histological examination reveals degeneration and necrosis of focal portions of the distal part of Henle's loop and the distal convoluted tubules. The interstitial tissues around the degenerated and necrosed tubules show cellular infiltration. Casts of a haem compound are found in the lumina of the distal tubular segments and the collecting tubules. The glomeruli and proximal convoluted tubules do not show any pathological change.

The pathogenesis of the acute tubular necrosis which occurs in association with muscle necrosis has not been established. Some workers consider that the renal failure is induced by a blockage of the tubules with casts of myohaemoglobin and its derivatives. Although tubular blockage may play some part in the process, other workers believe that the renal lesion is caused by a disturbance of renal blood flow and ischaemia. According to Trueta et al[124] there are two potential routes for the circulation of arterial blood in the kidneys. The one route passes to the tubules of the medulla and the other route supplies the glomeruli in the cortex. Trueta claims that in response to sympathetic stimulation from injuries to the limbs, blood is by-passed through the medullary route without traversing the capillaries of the glomeruli in the cortex. Glomerular filtration is prevented and anuria occurs. The work of Kinmouth[125] suggests that these circulatory disturbances may be caused by some factors other than those of reflex nervous action.

The possibility of acute tubular necrosis causing death should be considered whenever a person who has received a limb injury in a traffic accident dies at about the end of the first week after the injury.

PATTERNS OF INJURY IN TRAFFIC ACCIDENTS

A large variety of injuries and a combination of injuries are sustained by persons involved in traffic accidents. These injuries often assume definite patterns in the case of a pedestrian or a driver or a passenger.

Injuries of pedestrians

In the case of pedestrians three patterns of injury are often seen:

1. In an investigation of a series of 144 pedestrian casualties. Heddy[126] found that in 30 cases the pedestrians were struck by the sides of the vehicles. In the majority of these cases the victims were either children who had run into the side of the vehicle or elderly people who had walked into the side of the vehicle as it passed.*

In cases of this nature three types of injury may be seen, namely, injuries of the head in children, and injuries of the side of the trunk in adults from the initial impact against the vehicle; injuries of the head or upper limbs† from contact with the road surface; and crushing injuries of the head, the trunk, or the limbs when the pedestrian falls and is run over by the rear wheels.

2. In the majority of pedestrian traffic fatalities the pedestrian is seen by the driver before the impact but is struck by the front of the vehicle before the driver can swerve the car to avoid the accident.

In these cases a combination of injuries may be seen at autopsy. Compound fractures of the tibia and fibula in one or both legs are often found and are caused by the impact against the bumpers. An impact against

---

* Heddy's investigation showed that many of the elderly people who were killed suffered from physical infirmities such as defects of sight and hearing. In many cases the post-mortem examination revealed unsuspected pathological lesions which would have tended to handicap the deceased as a pedestrian. The vehicles involved in the accidents were often long units such as eight-wheeler lorries, articulated vehicles or vehicles with attached trailers.

† In falling, a pedestrian may attempt to save himself by stretching out his arms, and if he falls on the extended palm of his hand he may sustain any of the fractures of the upper extremity, such as a Colles' fracture or a fracture of the clavicle, which are known to follow indirect violence of this type.

a mudguard or a headlamp may result in a fracture of the pelvis or fracture–dislocations of the sacro-iliac joints, and both these lesions may be complicated by injuries to the urogenital tract or by abdominal injuries.

The height of the pedestrian often determines the site and the nature of injuries caused by impact against the bonnet. If a pedestrian is struck from behind by the top of the bonnet, he may sustain a fracture–dislocation of the lumbar spine or a fracture–dislocation of the thoracic spine. If the pedestrian is facing the vehicle he may sustain intra-abdominal injuries and/or injuries to the chest wall and the thoracic contents. When he is lifted on to the bonnet by the force of the impact he may sustain head injuries if he strikes his head against the windscreen. When the pedestrian is thrown off the bonnet or is thrown clear of the vehicle soon after the impact he may sustain head injuries from contact with the road surface.

External injuries may be found in any region of the body which has been struck by the vehicle. The form of an abrasion or contusion may sometimes correspond with the pattern of some portion of the vehicle and this may be of significance, particularly in 'hit and run' accidents. Spilsbury[127] refers to an autopsy in which he observed a bruise shaped like a figure 8 on the thigh of the deceased. When he examined the car which was involved in the accident he found a projecting part which corresponded exactly in size and shape with the pattern of the bruise.*

3. When a pedestrian is struck by a vehicle he may fall to the ground and be run over by the wheels of the vehicle. Children are often involved in accidents of this nature.

The effects of compression or 'crushing' injuries on the limbs, the trunk and the head have been dealt with in earlier sections of this chapter.

Injuries of motor cyclists, pedal cyclists, motor drivers and passengers

When motor cycle riders or their pillion passengers are involved in collisions with other vehicles they may be thrown on to the road surface and usually sustain multiple injuries. Similar injuries are seen when motor cyclists are hurled against telegraph poles, electric standards or trees, e.g. after skids or after collisions with other vehicles. Most pedal cycle fatalities occur through collisions with other vehicles, but fatalities may occur when a cyclist loses control of his machine and crashes on to the ground or against a stationary object. The fatal injuries may be multiple but they are often confined to the head.

In a traffic accident the driver of a motor vehicle may be thrown forward on to the steering wheel. If the impact is severe, he may sustain traumatic

* In 'hit and run' accidents the clothing and hair of the victim should be carefully examined for foreign bodies such as glass, metal or paint fragments. If material of this nature is found it should be handed over to the investigating officer. It is advisable to determine the blood group of the deceased and to retain a specimen of his head hair. These examinations might be of value if blood stains or hairs are found on a seized vehicle.

lesions to the chest wall, the heart and the liver, which are often grouped together as 'the steering-wheel impact type of injury' (pp 303–306). The driver of a vehicle may sustain head injuries when he is thrown against the windscreen, the side or the roof of the vehicle.*

Passengers in open vehicles are often killed by falling from the vehicles or by being thrown from the vehicles as a result of collisions. When passengers in motor cars are thrown against the windscreen or some portion of the interior of the car they often sustain fatal head injuries. When fragments of broken glass or sharp metal penetrate the body, death may be caused by haemorrhage.

REFERENCES

1 Munro D. Cranio-cerebral injuries. Oxford: Oxford University Press. 1963: p 33.
2 Rowbotham G F. Acute Injuries of the Head, 4th ed. Edinburgh: Livingstone. 1964: pp 58–69.
3 Moritz A R. The Pathology of Trauma. Philadelphia: Lea & Febiger. 1942: p 327.
4 Rowbotham G F. op. cit. pp 60–62.
5 Rowbotham G F. op. cit. pp 62–63.
6 Gurdjian E S, Webster J E, Lissner H R. The mechanism of skull fracture. J Neurosurg 1950; 7: 106–114. See also: Gurdjian E S, Webster J E, Lissner H R. The mechanism of skull fracture, Radiology 1950; 54: 313–339. See also: Gurdjian E S, Webster J E, Lissner H R. Studies on skull fractures with particular reference to engineering factors. Am J Surg 1949; 78: 736–742. See also: Gurdjian E S, Webster J E. Head injuries. London: Churchill. 1958.
7 Kerr D J A. Forensic Medicine. 5th ed. A and C Black. 1954: p 114.
8 Rowbotham G F. op. cit. pp 69–80.
9 Holbourn A H S. Mechanics of head injuries. Lancet 1943; 245: 438–441.
10 Grundfest H. Cold Harbor Symposia on Quantitative Biology, 1936; 4:179.
11 Rowbotham G F. op. cit. p 75.
12 Rowbotham G F. Acute injuries of the head, 3rd ed. Edinburgh: Livingstone. 1949: pp 44–64.
13 Denny-Brown D, Russell W R. Experimental cerebral concussion. Brain 1941; 64: 93–164.
14 Rowbotham G F. Acute Injuries of the Head, 3rd ed. Edinburgh: Livingstone. 1949: pp 29–30.
15 Rand C W. Histological studies of the brain in cases of fatal injury to the head: a preliminary report. Arch Surg 1931; 22: 738–753.
16 Helfand M. Cerebral lesions due to vasomotor disturbances following brain trauma. J Nerv Ment Dis 1939; 90: 157–179.
17 Moritz A R. op. cit. p 305.
18 Martland H S. Punch drunk. J Am Med Assoc 1928; 91: 1103–1107.
19 Keen E N. Diffuse neuronal injury. Clin Proc 1947; 6: 49–53.

* After a motor accident the driver of a motor vehicle may be arrested upon a charge of being under the influence of alcohol. It is important for the medical practitioner to recognize that the symptoms of a head injury or the signs of traumatic shock (caused by visceral injuries) may simulate acute alcoholic intoxication (p. 419). If the medical practitioner is satisfied that the driver is under the influence of alcohol but that he has also sustained a head injury, or if the medical practitioner is uncertain as to whether or not the driver has sustained an intrathoracic or intra-abdominal injury, he must ensure that the driver is placed under medical observation. The brain or blood alcohol concentration of a person killed in a traffic accident may be of medico-legal significance. It might be of value in determining whether he was under the influence of alcohol at the time of the accident.

20 Jefferson G. The balance of life and death in cerebral lesions. Surg Gynec Obstet 1951; 93: 444–458.
21 Symonds C P. Delayed traumatic intracerebral haemorrhage. Br Med J 1940; 1: 1048–1051.
22 Moritz A R. op. cit. p 307.
23 Moritz A R. The Pathology of Trauma. 2nd ed. Philadelphia: Lea and Febiger. 1954: p 324.
24 Shapiro P, Jackson H. Swelling of the brain in cases of injury to the head. Arch Surg 1939; 38: 443–456.
25 Evans J P, Scheinker I M. Histologic studies of brain following head trauma; late changes; atrophic sclerosis of white matter. J Neurosurg 1944; 1: 306–320.
26 White J D, Brooke J R, Goldthwaite J C, Adams R D. Changes in brain volume and blood content after experimental concussion. Ann Surg 1943; 118: 619–634.
27 Strich S J. Diffuse degeneration of the cerebral white matter in severe dementia following head injury. J Neurol Neurosurg Psychiatr 1956; 19: 163–185.
28 Strich S J. Shearing of nerve fibres as a cause of brain damage due to head injury. Lancet 1961; 2: 443–448.
29 Adams J H, Genarelli T A, Graham D I. Brain damage in non-missile head injury; observation in man and subhuman primates. In: Smith W T, Cavanagh J B. eds. Recent advances in neuropathology, Vol. 2. Edinburgh: Churchill Livingstone. 1982; 7: pp 165–190.
30 Simpson R H W, Berson D S, Shapiro H A. The diagnosis of diffuse axonal injury in routine autopsy practice. Forens Sci Int 1985; 27: 229–235.
31 Rowbotham G F. Acute Injuries of the Head 3rd ed. Edinburgh: Livingstone. 1949: p 66.
32 Jamieson K G, Yelland J D N. Extradural hematoma: report of 167 cases. J Neurosurg 1968; 29: 13–23.
33 Gallagher J P, Browder E J. Extradural hematoma: experience with 167 patients. J Neurosurg 1968; 29: 1–12.
34 McLaurin R L, Ford L E. Extradural hematoma: statistical survey of 47 cases. J Neurosurg 1964; 21: 264–371.
35 McKissock W, Taylor J C, Bloom W H, et al. Extradural haematoma: observations on 125 cases. Lancet 1964; 2: 167–172.
36 Hooper R S. Observations on extradural haemorrhage. Br J Surg 1959; 47: 71–87.
37 Mendelow A D, Karmi M Z, Paul K S, et al. Extradural haematoma: effect of delayed treatment. Br Med J 1979; 1: 1240–1242.
38 Barres K P, Hamilton R D. Chronic extradural hematoma: case report. Neurosurgery 1979; 4: 60–62.
39 Blackwood W, McMenemy W H, Meyer A, Norman R M. Greenfield's Neuropathology. London: Arnold. 2nd ed. 1963: p 443.
40 Munro D. Cranio-cerebral Injuries: their Diagnosis and Treatment. Oxford: Oxford University Press. 1938: pp 127–139.
41 Perper J A, Wecht C H. Microscopic diagnosis in forensic pathology. Illinois: Charles C Thomas. 1980: p. 303.
42 Rowbotham G F. Acute Injuries of the Head, 3rd ed. Edinburgh: Livingstone. 1949: pp 72–73.
43 Gardner W J. Traumatic subdural haematoma, with particular reference to the latent interval. Arch Neurol Psychiat 1932; 27: 847–858.
44 Leary T. Subdural haemorrhages. J Am Med Assoc 1934; 103: 897–903.
45 Baker A B. Subdural haematoma. Arch Pathol 1938; 26: 535–559.
46 Rowbotham G F. Acute Injuries of the Head, 3rd ed. Edinburgh: Livingstone. 1949: pp 71–72.
47 Moritz A R, Wartman W B. Post-traumatic internal hydrocephalus. Am J Med Sci 1938; 195: 65–70.
48 Tatsuno Y, Lindenberg R. Basal subarachnoid hematomas as sole intracranial traumatic lesions. Arch Pathol 1974; 97: 211–215.
49 Drake C G. Perspectives on cerebral aneurysms. Stroke 1980; 2: p. 124.
50 Klintworth G K. Grooving of the uncus in the absence of overt intracranial disease. J Forens Med 1962; 9: pp 137–142.
51 Wilson J V. The Pathology of Traumatic Injury. Edinburgh: Livingstone. 1946: p 154.

52 Denny-Brown D, Russell W R. op. cit. pp 93–164.
53 Courville C B. Commotio cerebri. Los Angeles: San Lucas Press. 1953.
54 Pudenz R H, Shelden C H. J Neurosurg 1946; 3: 487–505.
55 Rowbotham G F. Acute Injuries of the Head. 3rd ed. Edinburgh: Livingstone. 1949: p 353.
56 Ingraham F D, Matson D D. Subdural haematoma in infancy. J Pediat 1944; 24: 1–37.
57 Moritz A R. The Pathology of Trauma. Philadelphia: Lea and Febiger. 1942: pp 332–333.
58 Schuessler W W. Self-inflicted excision of larynx and thyroid and division of trachea and oesophagus with recovery. J Am Med Assoc 1944; 125: 551–552.
59 Moritz A R. op. cit. p 188.
60 Moritz A R. op. cit. p 151.
61 Wilson J V. op. cit. p 109.
62 Wilson J V. op. cit. p 110.
63 Osborn G R. Findings in 262 fatal accidents. Lancet 1943; 245: 277–284.
64 Moritz A R. op. cit. p 147.
65 Moritz A R. op. cit. p 149.
66 Sagall E L Contusion of the heart, medical and legal considerations. In: Wecht C H. ed. Legal Medicine Annual 1971. New York: Appleton-Century-Crofts. 1971: pp 187–210.
67 Wilson J V. op. cit. pp 111 and 112.
68 Tannenbaum I, Ferguson J A. Rapid deceleration and rupture of the aorta. Arch Pathol 1948; 45: 503–505.
69 Lasky I I. Human aortic laceration secondary to impact. In: Legal medicine annual 1974. Wecht C H. ed. New York: Appleton-Century-Crofts. 1974: pp 3–29.
70 Wilson J V. op. cit. p 119.
71 Moritz A R. op. cit. p 189.
72 Wilson J V. op. cit. p 121.
73 Chase W H. Anatomical and experimental observations on air embolism. Surg Gynec Obstet 1934; 59: 569–577.
74 Moore R M, Braselton C W. Injections of air and of carbon dioxide into a pulmonary vein. Ann Surg 1940; 112: 212–218.
75 Durant T M, Oppenheimer M J, Webster M R, Long J. Arterial air embolism. Am Heart J 1949; 38: 481–500.
76 Duncan-Taylor J E. The post-mortem diagnosis of air embolism by radiography. Br Med J 1952; 1: 890–893.
77 Moritz A R. op. cit. p 145.
78 Wilson J V. op. cit. p 118.
79 King E S J. Surgery of the Heart. London: Arnold. 1941: p 297.
80 Moritz A R. op. cit. pp 220–221.
81 Moritz A R. op. cit. p 221.
82 Vance B N. Subcutaneous injuries of the abdominal viscera: anatomic and clinical characteristics. Arch Surg 1928; 16: 631–679.
83 Zabinski E J, Harkins H N. Delayed splenic rupture; a clinical syndrome following trauma; report of 4 cases with analysis of 177 cases collected from literature. Arch Surg 1943; 46: 186–213.
84 Wilson J V. op. cit. p 142.
85 Orloff M J, Peskin G W. Spontaneous rupture of the normal spleen: A surgical enigma. Surg Gynecol Obstet 1958; 106: 1–11.
86 Stewart G R, Braasch J W. Spontaneous occult rupture of a normal spleen. Med J Austral 23 January 1971: p 203.
87 Moritz A R. op. cit. p 232.
88 Moritz A R. op. cit. pp 239–246.
89 Moritz A R. op. cit. p 251.
90 Montgomery A H, Ireland J. Traumatic segmentary arteriospasm. J Am Med Assoc 1935; 105: 1741–1746.
91 Trueta J, Barclay A E, Franklin K J, Daniel P M, Pritchard M M L. Studies of the renal circulation. Oxford: Blackwell. 1947.
92 Kinmouth J B. The physiology and relief of traumatic arterial spasm. Br Med J 1952; 1: 59–64.

93 Leriche R. De l'importance en pathologié et en therapeutique des reactions vasomotrices post traumatiques. Medicine 1928; 9: 341–342.
94 Cohen S M. Traumatic arterial spasm. Lancet 1944; 1: 1–6.
95 Ellis L B, Weiss S. The local and systemic effects of arteriovenous fistula on the circulation in man. Am Heart J 1930; 5: 635–647.
96 Watson-Jones R. Fractures and Joint Injuries. 4th ed. Edinburgh: Livingstone. 1952: p 109.
97 Griffiths D L. Volkmann's ischaemic contracture. Br J Surg 1940; 28: 239–260.
98 Watson-Jones R. op. cit. p 126.
99 Watson-Jones R. op. cit. pp 3–38.
100 Murray C R. Pathology and repair of fractures. In: Christopher F. ed. A textbook of surgery, 5th ed. Philadelphia: Saunders. 1949: p 204.
101 Moritz A R. op. cit. p 357.
102 Grant R T, Reeve E B. Observations on the general effects of injury in man, with special reference to wound shock. Medical Research Council Special Report Series No. 227, London: HMSO. 1951.
103 Shapiro H A. Fat embolism. J Forens Med 1963; 10: 41–44.
104 Zenker F A. Beitrage zur Normalen und Pathologischen Anatomie der Lunge. Dresden: J Braunsdorf. 1862. Quoted by Sevitt, 1962.
105 Sevitt S. Fat Embolism. London: Butterworths. 1962.
106 Lehman E P, McNattin R F. Fat embolism: incidence at post-mortem. Arch Surg 1928; 17: 179–189.
107 Becker B J P. Fat embolism: a review of its current status. Med Proc 1961; 7: 211–217.
108 Simpson K. Fat embolism. J Forens Med 1959; 6: 19–22.
109 Oh W H, Mital M A. Fat embolism: current concepts of pathogenesis, diagnosis and treatment. Orthoped Clin N Am 1978; 9 (3): 769–779.
110 Gossling, H R, Pellegrini V D. Fat embolism syndrome. Clin Orthop 1982; 165: 68–82.
111 Shier M R, Wilson R F. Fat embolism syndrome. Surg Ann 1980; 12: 139–168.
112 Peltier L F. Fat embolism. An appraisal of the problem. Clin Orthop 1984; 187: 3–17.
113 Hagley S R. The fulminant fat embolism syndrome. Anaesth Intensive Care 1983; 11: 162–170.
114 Treiman N, et al. Lipoprotein electrophoresis in fat embolism: A preliminary report. Injury 1985; 13: 108–110.
115 Buchanan D, Mason J K. Occurrence of pulmonary fat and bone marrow embolism. Am J Forens Med Pathol 1982; 3: 73–77.
116 Allardyce D B. The post-mortem interval as a factor in fat embolism. Arch Pathol 1971; 92: 248–253.
117 Dines D E, Burgher L W, Okazaki H. The clinical and pathologic correlation of fat embolism syndrome. Mayo Clinic Proc 1975; 50: 407–411.
118 de Takats G. Embolism. In: Christopher F. ed. A textbook of surgery. 5th ed. Philadelphia: Saunders. 1949: 659.
119 Gunn F D. The lung. In: Anderson W A D. ed. Pathology. St Louis: C. V. Mosby. 1948: p 709.
120 Young R L, Derbyshire R C, Cramer O S. Parodoxic embolism. Arch Pathol 1948; 46: 43–48.
121 Boyd W B. A textbook of pathology—structure and function in disease, 8th ed. London: Kimpton. 1970: pp 646–651.
122 Bywaters E G L, Beall D. Crush injuries with impairment of renal function. Br Med J 1941; 1: 427–432.
123 Bywaters E G L. Ischaemic muscle necrosis. J Am Med Assoc 1944; 124: 1103–1109.
124 Trueta J, Barclay A E, Franklin K J, Daniel P M, Pritchard M M L. op. cit.
125 Kinmouth J B. op. cit.
126 Heddy W R H. Death on the roads. Med-Leg J 1948; 16: 16–27.
127 Spilsbury B. The medico-legal significance of bruises. Med-Leg Criminol Rev 1939; 7: 215–227.

13

Firearm wounds

An appreciation of the nature of firearm wounds depends upon a knowledge of the structure of firearms and ammunition, and upon an understanding of the mechanism of the discharge of projectiles. Internal, external and wound (terminal) ballistics are considered.

THE STRUCTURE OF FIREARMS AND CARTRIDGES

A firearm is an assembly of a barrel and an action from which a projectile or projectiles are propelled by products of combustion. Most firearms consist of three parts—the chamber, the leed, and the bore. The chamber is situated at the back or breech end of the weapon and contains the cartridge before it is fired. The chamber is connected by a short cone, known as the leed, to the bore of the weapon, and the bore extends from the leed to the muzzle or front end of the weapon. In shotguns the inner surface of the bore is smooth from end to end. In the revolver, automatic pistol, and rifle the bore is cut longitudinally into a series of spiral grooves and these weapons are therefore termed rifled weapons.

In a rifled weapon, the portions of the bore between the grooves are known as lands. The lands project into the bore between the grooves, and the calibre of the weapon is measured across the bore between the tops of a pair of lands. When a bullet is fired it passes through the bore and its surface comes into contact with the projecting spiral lands. In this way a spinning motion is imparted to the bullet and this motion keeps the projectile relatively stable in its flight.

The general features of the structure of bullet and shotgun cartridges are shown in Figs 13.1A, 13.1B and 13.1C. It will be seen that both types of cartridge contain a charge of propellant powder. In the bullet cartridge this power fills the cylinder up to the level of the base of the projectile and in the shotgun cartridge the powder is separated from the pellets by a wad or wads. A bullet or shotgun cartridge is loaded with a smokeless powder consisting of cellulose nitrate either alone or in combination with nitroglycerine. Apart from their difference in chemical composition, smokeless powders also vary in physical characteristics such as the size and shape of

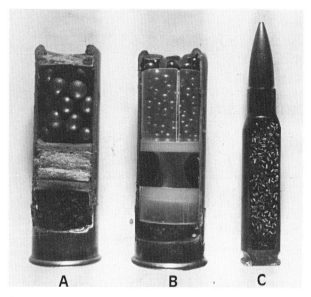

Fig. 13.1 A. Cross section through shotgun cartridge showing the charge, wad and shot;
B. Cross section through a modern shotgun cartridge, showing plastic 'Power Piston' wad;
C. Cross section through a modern high velocity rifle cartridge, showing the propellant.

the grains. All cartridges have a primer cap which is set into the flat base of the cartridge case which is also known as the head. The head of the cartridge case is frequently used to identify, not only the manufacturer but also the country of origin of a cartridge case. The primer contains a small amount of explosive mixture.

Mechanism of discharge of projectiles

When a weapon is fired, the primer is detonated by the firing pin and the explosion ignites the powder in the cartridge case. The powder burns rapidly, resulting in the evolution of a relatively large volume of gas within the confined space of the cartridge case, and the pressure of this gas forces the bullet or shot out of the cartridge and through the bore of the weapon.

The release of the projectile is accompanied by the discharge of flame, of hot compressed gases and of unburned or partially burned powder particles. The flame, discharged gases and powder grains produce effects on the skin in the region of the entrance wound if the weapon is fired at close range. The flame may burn the skin or singe the hair, while the deposit from the gases may blacken the skin surface. The flame may also be responsible for skin abrasions in relation to the entrance wound. The deposit of unburned powder particles on the skin gives rise to the condition known as tattooing. Tattooing by black powder is readily recognized on naked-eye examination but a hand-lens may be necessary to demonstrate the tattooing of smokeless powder. The degree and extent of tattooing diminishes as the range of fire increase.

Low-power rim fire cartridges such as the 6 mm BB cap and the 6 mm CB cap, particularly as manufactured in Western Europe, may not contain propellant gun powder, but only a primer compound. These cartridges, therefore, cannot produce the tattooing which is found after the discharge of cartridges containing propellant powder.

Fatal bullet wounds may be produced by rifles, revolvers or automatic pistols. In all bullet injuries there is usually an entrance wound, a bullet track in the tissues, and an exit wound. An exit wound is absent in cases where the bullet becomes lodged in the tissues after its penetration.

Tissue appearances and range of fire

Handgun wounds (revolver and semi-automatic pistol bullet wounds) are very important in medico-legal practice. As the wounds caused by pistol and revolver bullets are similar, and the calibre of the bullets used in the weapons are approximately the same, these wounds can conveniently be considered under the same heading. However, it should be noted that the muzzle velocities of magnum revolvers are higher than those of modern pistols.

Much is often made of the size of the entrance and exit wounds. In the majority of cases, the entrance wound is small and neat. However, with ultra-high velocity small bullets or bomb splinters, the entrance wound may be of the 'blowout' type.

The exit would will depend upon the shape of the local track, the temporary cavitation effect at the site of the exit, the impact velocity and type of bullet.

If the missile has remained stable in the tissues, or alternatively has expended most of its energy, a relatively small exit wound results.

Close-range and contact wounds

When a firearm is discharged very close to or in contact with the surface of the skin, the gases produced by the explosion pass into the tissues with the bullet and cause considerable laceration of the skin and subcutaneous tissues. Under these conditions the bullet entrance wound has a ragged appearance, especially over the skull where it may be stellate in appearance (Fig. 13.2).

At close range there is usually some blackening and tattooing of the skin around the bullet entrance wound (Fig. 13.3), while the hair in the region of the wound may be singed, and there may be some skin burning and abrasion in relation to the hot gases. In contact wounds, the discharge passes into the tissues through the bullet entrance opening and powder deposits as well as blackening may be observed in the depths of the wound.

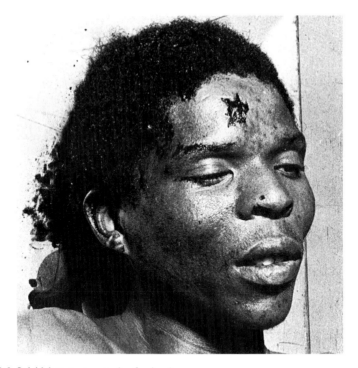

Fig. 13.2 Suicidal contact wound – forehead.

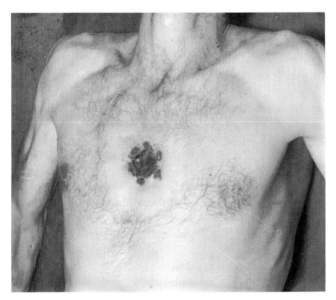

Fig. 13.3 Suicidal contact wound – chest, showing powder marks as a result of the muzzle break.

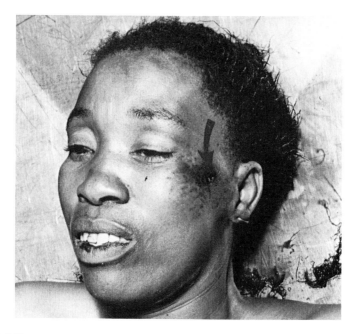

Fig. 13.4 Near-contact wound – cheek, showing eccentric entrance wound.

Range up to about 15 cm. When a firearm is discharged at a range of about 15 cm, the lacerating and burning effects of the gases are usually lost owing to the dispersion and cooling of the gases before they reach the skin. In these conditions the bullet entrance wound is circular in shape and is surrounded by a narrow zone of skin abrasion. Blackening of the skin is sometimes seen, while tattooing is invariably found at this range.

The appearance of a homicidal close-range bullet entrance wound is shown in Figure 13.4. The eccentric entrance wound indicates the direction of fire. The exit wound is demonstrated in Figure 13.5.

Range beyond 15 cm. Beyond a range of 15 cm, all traces of blackening usually disappear, while the bullet entrance opening remains circular in shape. Powder grain deposits may still be present, and are usually seen up to ranges of about 40–60 cm, but the limit within which powder grain deposits can occur varies with different weapons and different cartridges.

Factors governing the maximum range of tattooing

The amount of tattooing and the maximum distance to which the powder particles can be discharged depends upon the barrel length and the nature of the cartridge, both in its calibre and in its powder load. Under average conditions, the larger the calibre, the greater the distance to which the powder is discharged.

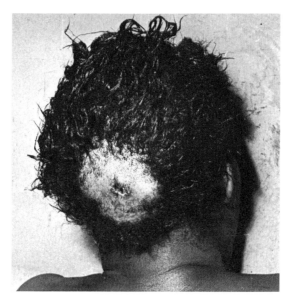

Fig. 13.5 Exit wound. (Entrance wound in Fig. 13.4.)

Tests to determine the maximum possible distance to which the powder particles can be discharged should be performed in all cases where it is important to ascertain the range of fire. If possible, these tests should be carried out with the weapon used at the crime and with similar ammunition.

Range of fire beyond the range of powder grain deposit. The range of fire of a firearm cannot be scientifically determined in cases where the weapon is discharged beyond the range of powder grain deposit.

The direction of fire

Although the direction of fire can be determined from the nature of the entrance wound and from the bullet track in the tissues, it must be appreciated that because of the potential instability of some bullets, the bullet track may bear no resemblance to the track shown by entrance and exit wounds, or the site of lodgement of the bullet where through-and-through penetration of the body has failed to occur. There can even be a sharp bend in the track within the soft tissues, without the bullet having struck bone.

The direction of fire as determined from the entrance wound

Bullets may strike the skin at right angles or at an angle and the entance wound may have a circular or oval appearance, according to the direction of fire. Under certain circumstances, a bullet entrance wound may be irregular in shape, even though the bullet was fired at right angles. The spin which is imparted to a bullet when it is fired exerts a gyroscopic effect on the bullet, and its motions are therefore comparable to those of a spinning top. Like a spinning top, a bullet has a slight wobble when first fired, it then rights itself, and may commence to wobble again when it slows down.

It the skin is struck by a wobbling bullet, the entrance wound may be irregular in shape.

As a bullet strikes the skin more obliquely, the entrance wound becomes more oval. As the obliquity of fire is increased, the wound becomes elongated in shape, and if the skin is struck at a tangent, penetration may fail to occur and only a slight linear furrowing of the skin is produced.

The direction of fire as determined from the bullet track

A bullet usually travels through the tissues in a straight line, so that the direction of fire may be determined from its track. In certain conditions, however, a bullet may be deflected from its course and this occurs most commonly when it strikes bone in its passage through the tissues. It can also occur due to the inherent instability of a bullet as it penetrates tissues, and it may undergo changes of direction within the soft tissues in its track. This is illustrated by a case in which a man was struck by a bullet which went through tissues in the following order: gall bladder, hepatic flexure of colon, duodenum, pancreas, inferior vena cava, then passing medially through the bony part of the vertebral column, to strike the left kidney, spleen and pass through the diaphragm and pericardium, before coming to rest in the chest cavity. The only part of the track of bullet which was in a straight line was through the vertebral column, and sharp bends occurred in the soft tissue track before and after.[1]

The calibre of the weapon used

If a weapon is discharged beyond contact or very close range at right angles to the skin surface, the approximate calibre of the bullet may be determined from the diameter of the entrance wound. In these conditions the diameter of the opening is slightly smaller than the calibre of the bullet because the skin is stretched at the moment of penetration. Generally, the calibre of the bullet cannot be determined if it strikes the skin surface obliquely.

The nature of the wound

As in the case of wounds in general, the nature of a firearm wound has to be determined from the circumstances of the injury taken in conjunction with the character of the wound. In most firearm wounds the circumstances are such that it is usually possible to state whether the injury was of accidental, suicidal or homicidal origin.[2]

If a revolver or pistol is found firmly grasped in the hand of the deceased it is strong presumptive evidence of suicide. The finding of a weapon beside the body, however, is not necessarily indicative of suicide as a murderer may leave a weapon at the scene of the crime to simulate suicide. Conversely a person committing suicide may have had sufficient time to dispose of the weapon provided that the wound was not immediately incompatible with life.

Suicidal bullet wounds usually occur at contact or close range. Hatcher, Jury and Weller[3] state that 'more than two-thirds of the people who shoot themselves aim for the brain, either through the roof of the mouth, at the temple or through the forehead. Almost all the rest aim for the heart.'

Fatteh[4] states:

> Based on the results of our study of 844 suicides, the sites chosen to inflict wounds, in order of frequency, are the temple area (right temple by right-handed persons and left temple by left-handed persons), heart area, mouth and the center of the forehead . . . also sometimes the area under the chin.

Canfield[5] draws attention to the rare occurrence of suicidal gunshot wounds of the abdomen.

Spitz and Fisher[6] state:

> The vast majority of suicidal shots are in the temple, the heart and the mouth. Among these the temple area is used most frequently.

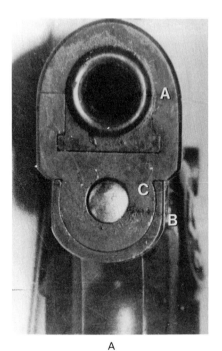 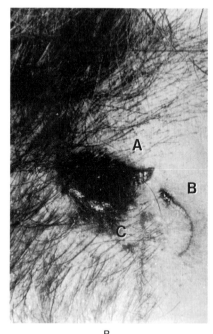

A   B

Fig. 13.6A and 13.6B The effects of a suicidal contact wound to the temple.

Figure 13.6A and 13.6B demonstrate particularly well the effects of a suicidal contact wound to the temple. The impact of the different components of the barrel and slide on the skin are indicated.

Homicidal wounds can occur at any range and may be situated in any region of the body. It is uncommon to find a suicidal bullet injury with an entrance wound in the back. The existence of several bullet wounds on the body suggests that they are of homicidal origin but does not exclude suicide.

ADDITIONAL POINTS OF MEDICO-LEGAL IMPORTANCE

Bullet exit wounds

A bullet exit would is usually irregular in shape with its edges everted and torn. Burning, blackening, and tattooing are not seen in relation to the wound. In the case of contact entrance wounds, exit wounds are smaller than such entrance wounds, but at longer ranges they are usually larger than entrance wounds. Wobbling bullets may emerge from the tissue sideways and produce considerable laceration of the skin.

The wounding potential of bullets

The wounding potential of a bullet has been described by Owen-Smith[7a] as follows:

> A wound results from the absorbtion of energy imparted by a missile when it strikes and penetrates tissue. Its available kinetic energy is calculated by the formula $KE = MV^2/2$ where M represents the mass and V the velocity. This means that doubling the mass would double the energy available, whereas doubling the velocity will quadruple the energy. When M is in kg and V is m/s, then KE is measured in joules.
>
> When a missile is stopped by the tissues it penetrates, then the energy liberated to cause damage must be equal to the total KE of the missile. If it passes through the tissues it has a remaining velocity from which can be calculated the energy released during wounding.

$$\text{The energy expended} = \frac{M(V1^2 - V2^2)}{2}$$

where V1 = strike velocity and V2 = remaining velocity.

Mechanisms of injury

A bullet can cause tissue damage in the following ways:
1. Direct effect of:

(a) bullet itself, or
(b) secondary missile effect
2. Shock waves
3. Temporary cavitaton

1(a) Direct effect of bullet itself

The physical passage of a bullet passing through the tissues causes the formation of a local track along which there is permanent tissue loss. This is an invariable effect which is exaggerated by the passage of bullets of a large calibre, as well as missiles which expand and 'mushroom' on impact.

In the case of a low-velocity handgun bullet wound, the main injury is related to the local track formation with relatively minimal surrounding tissue destruction.

1(b) Secondary missile effect

Should a bullet fragment, secondary bullet particles are set in motion and each of these secondary particles in turn becomes a missile which may cause damage away from the direction of the original missile.

Other potential sources of secondary particles may be fragments of bone, cartilage, tendon or other firm tissue to which energy has been transferred.

Secondary missile effect is most marked if a bullet fragments, or if bone is struck and the tissue destruction so produced is directly proportional to the wounding energy inherent in the secondary missile.

2. Shock waves

When bullets produce tracks in dense tissues, such as muscle, liver, spleen and blood, the tissues are compressed ahead of the track by a compression wave, in the form of a shock wave of spherical form. Tissue damage can also be produced at a considerable distance away from the original bullet track. Thus, the urinary bladder, stomach and colon may be ruptured in high velocity wounds situated at a remote distance from the abdominal cavity itself.

Intermediate tissue damage After a high-velocity missile wound has been inflicted on the tissues, several zones of tissue damage can be identified. The site of the permanent local track is marked by tissues which have been totally destroyed, and this is similar to low-velocity bullets. Surrounding this is a layer of necrotic debris caused by the temporary cavitation effect and secondary missiles, highly contaminated by micro-organisms. A variable thickness layer of live tissue surrounds the zone of necrosis, consisting of an inner portion which will prove to be non-viable as a result of the injuries sustained, and an outer portion that will remain viable provided that optimum conditions are provided for healing. Around this zone is normal tissue.

3. Temporary cavitation

Owen-Smith[7b] states that temporary cavity formation occurs predominantly with high-velocity missile injury[7] and this cavitation is responsible for the major destructive effects associated with high-velocity injuries.

High energy is absorbed by the local tissues in relation to the bullet track. These tissues are accelerated violently in both a forwards and outwards direction. The momentum gained by the tissues causes them to continue this movement, even after the passage of the bullet, thus creating a cavity which can be up to forty times the diameter of the bullet (Figs 13.7 and 13.8). A relative vacuum will be present within this temporary cavity, which may result in bacteria and debris being sucked into both entrance and exit wounds.

The cavity only exists for a few milliseconds and then collapses in a pulsatile fashion.

Bullet wounds of the head

In most of these injuries the bullet passes completely through the skull and as it enters the skull from without it produces a clean-cut hole in the outer table and a larger hole in the inner table (Fig. 13.9 and 13.10). At its point of exit from within these conditions are reversed and the hole in the outer table is larger than the hole in the inner table (Fig. 13.11). These facts are

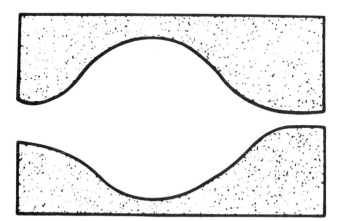

Fig. 13.7 Diagram of the maximum size of the temporary cavity in a gelatin block immediately after the passage of a high velocity bullet. (After Owen-Smith, M.S. from *High velocity missile wounds* published by kind permission of Edward Arnold (Publishers) Ltd. London)

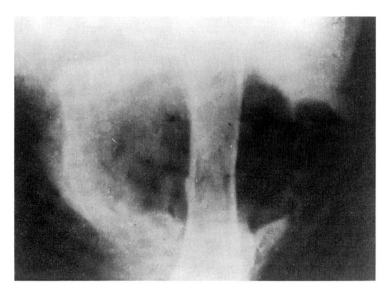

Fig. 13.8 Microsecond radiograph of a thigh of an anaesthetized sheep, showing a temporary cavity caused by a missile travelling at 770 m/s (2500 ft/s). (Crown Copyright reproduced with the permission of the Controller of Her Majesty's Stationery Office) (After Owen-Smith, M.S. from *High velocity missile wounds* published by kind permission of Edward Arnold (Publishers) Ltd. London)

often of importance in determining the direction of fire in bullet injuries of the head. The track of a bullet through the brain tissues varies greatly, depending on the range and stability of the bullet. On the other hand, if it remains high velocity at the time that it impacts with the skull, there may be considerable damage from the cavitation effect within the skull.

Fissured fractures often radiate through the vault and base of the skull from the bullet entrance and exit holes. In certain bullet injuries of the head

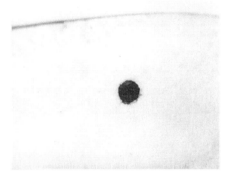

Fig. 13.9 Skull–gunshot entrance wound (outer table).

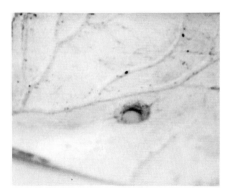

Fig. 13.10 Skull – gunshot entrance wound (inner table).

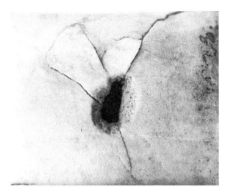

Fig. 13.11 Skull – gunshot exit wound (outer table).

the bullet may fail to emerge from the skull and in these cases an area of bony comminution is often found at the site of lodgment. When a bullet strikes the head at a tangent, penetration of the skull may fail to occur, but the force of the bullet may be sufficient to fragment the inner table at the site of impact. Delayed pressure effects and cranial oedema may be produced as a result of this.

RUBBER/PLASTIC BULLETS

Rubber bullets (baton rounds) (Fig. 13.12) were originally designed to reproduce the effects of a police baton charge in riot control. The intention is that the rubber bullet will tumble in flight and mimic the effects of a baton on contact. At recommended ranges (approximately 50 metres), the weapon is extremely effective. However, at lower ranges, and at point blank range, the rubber bullet carries sufficient momentum to become a lethal weapon. It can cause fractures of long bones or skull, massive

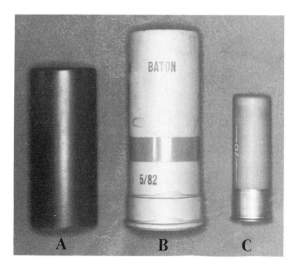

Fig. 13.12 A. Projectile from a baton round; **B.** Unfired baton round; **C.** Shotgun cartridge for comparison.

laceration and crushing injuries. The typical skin appearance is one of 'tram-track', but on a much larger scale. At this range it can also produce liver and splenic rupture.

The plastic bullet, made of polyvinyl chloride, is reputed to be more accurate and have a better striking effect than the rubber bullet.

Detailed observations of the injuries produced by rubber bullets compared to that of plastic bullets have been documented by Miller et al[8] and Rocke[9] respectively.

SHOTGUN WOUNDS

When a shotgun cartridge is fired the pellets begin to disperse soon after the cartridge has left the weapon. This dispersion increases with the range of fire but it also depends upon the degree of 'choking' of the barrel of the weapon. The term 'choking' refers to the constriction of the bores of certain shotguns at their muzzle ends. The degree of constriction is maximal in the 'full choke' weapon and is of lesser extent in the 'half choke' weapon. The purpose of the 'choking' device is to keep the charge of shot in a single mass for some distance before dispersion commences.

A contact shotgun wound is demonstrated in Figure 13.13.

At close ranges (up to about 90 cm) the shot enters the body in a single mass with all types of shotguns. In these circumstances a single large irregular lacerated wound is produced. Burning, blackening, and tattooing are seen around and in the depth of the wound. The wad is often found in the wound.

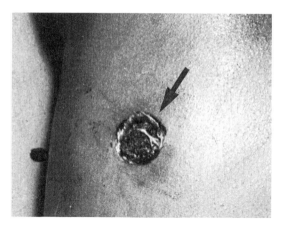

Fig. 13.13 Contact shotgun wound (buttock), showing 'cookie-cutter' effect.

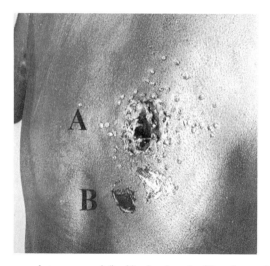

Fig. 13.14 Close range shotgun wound (back), showing: **A.** Wound caused by the shot; **B.** Wound caused by the wad.

As the range of fire increases to a few yards the burning, blackening, and tattooing disappear, while the charge of shot begins to spread so that small apertures, due to separate pellets entering the skin, appear around the central opening caused by the main mass of shot. In addition, an independent injury may be caused by the wad (Fig. 13.14). The dispersion of shot increases at greater ranges—the greater the dispersion the greater the range. The actual spread depends upon the type of boring of the weapon.

The direction of fire of a shotgun can only be determined from the entrance wound in close-range injuries.

REFERENCES

1 Boffard K. Personal communication. 1986.
2 Sellier K. Death: accident or suicide by use of firearms. Forens Sci Progress 1, Berlin: Springer-Verlag. 1986: pp 91–115.
3 Hatcher J S, Jury F J, Weller J. In: Samsworth T G. ed. Firearms investigation, identification and evidence. Harrisburg, Pennsylvania: The Stockpole Company. 1975: p 283.
4 Fatteh A. Handbook of forensic pathology. Philadelphia: J B. Lippincott. 1973: p 113.
5 Canfield T M. Suicidal gunshot wounds of the abdomen. J Forens Sci 1969; 14:445.
6 Spitz W U, Fisher R S. Medico-legal investigation of Death, 2nd ed. Springfield: Charles C Thomas. 1980: p. 256
7a Owen-Smith M S. High velocity missile wounds. London: Edward Arnold. 1981: pp 17–18.
7b Owen-Smith M S. Op. cit. pp 22–41.
8 Millar R, Rutherford W H, Johnston S, Malhotra, V J. Injuries caused by rubber bullets: a report on 90 patients. Br J Surg 1975; 62: 480–486.
9 Rocke L. Injuries caused by plastic bullets compared with those caused by rubber bullets. Lancet 1983; 1: 919–920.

14

Sexual offences, abortion, infanticide and concealment of birth, Caffey's syndrome or the battered child syndrome

SEXUAL OFFENCES

Nature of the crime of rape

Rape is committed by any male who has unlawful sexual intercourse with a female without her consent.

In the jurisdictions of some countries a boy under the age of 14 is conclusively presumed to be incapable of having sexual intercourse with a woman and can be convicted as a principal offender of indecent assault only. In such jurisdictions there seems to be no reason why a boy under the age of 14 should not be convicted of rape if he assists another to commit the offence (known in English law as a 'principal in the second degree'). In Roman–Dutch law any person (male or female and irrespective of age) who assists a male of 14 years of age or over to carry out his purpose is guilty of the crime of rape.

By sexual intercourse is meant a penetration of the external genitalia of the female by the penis. The penetration may be of any degree and a penetration of the vulva only would constitute sexual intercourse. The sexual intercourse must be unlawful.

Sexual intercourse must occur without the consent of the female. In the jurisdictions of some countries a girl under the age of 12 is held to be incapable of giving her consent, so that sexual intercourse with such a person with or without her consent is invariably rape.

In the jurisdictions of most countries consent must be full and free and it must be distinguished from submission. In some countries statutory provisions specifically define the circumstances in which it is deemed that consent cannot be said to have been given, e.g. there is no legal consent if the consent was extorted by threats or fear of bodily harm; or, if the consent was obtained by impersonating the woman's husband; or, if the consent was obtained by a fraudulent misrepresentation of the nature and the quality of the act. These statutory provisions serve to sum up the common law on rape in many countries. Thus, in an English case it was held to be rape where a man professed to treat a girl for fits, and had connection with her by pretending that he was performing an operation.[1]

There can be no consent where the woman is insensible or in a drunken stupor.

Where the accused fails in his purpose in circumstances in which success would have resulted in rape, the offence committed is that of assault with intent to commit rape, sometimes referred to as 'attempted rape'. In most jurisdictions if there is any reasonable doubt as to the intent of rape, the accused may be convicted of the lesser offence of indecent assault, or simply of assault.

Offences under girls' and mentally handicapped women's protection acts

In many countries statutory provisions exist which serve to protect girls and mentally handicapped women. In such jurisdictions a man is guilty of an offence if he has, or attempts to have, unlawful sexual intercourse with a girl under a specified age (usually 16 years). Provision is usually made in such statutes for the definition as offences of the commission with such a girl of any immoral or indecent act. It should be noted that offences are committed in these circumstances even when the girl has consented to intercourse or to the commission with her of any immoral or indecent act.

Similar statutory enactments in most countries provide that an offence is committed by a man if he has, or attempts to have, unlawful sexual intercourse with any mentally handicapped female in circumstances which do not amount to rape. As in the case of girls, provision is usually made in such statutes for the definition as offences of the commission with such a female of any immoral or indecent act.

Sexual intercourse with mentally ill female patients

In most countries it is an offence for any person to have, or to attempt to have, unlawful sexual intercourse with any female who is detained under the provisions of a Mental Disorders Act or is otherwise under care or control as a mentally disordered patient. Provision is usually made in such enactments for the definition of circumstances in which the accused may seek to prove that at the time of the act committed he did not know or had no reasonable cause to believe that the woman was so detained or was under care or control as a mentally disordered patient. It should be noted that offences are committed in these circumstances even when the woman has consented to intercourse.

Unnatural offences

The old authorities refer to many so-called 'unnatural' offences under the generic term of 'sodomy'. In modern practice the term 'sodomy' is confined to sexual intercourse between two males, and possibly, as in English law, unnatural intercourse between male and female. The term 'bestiality' is used to describe sexual connection with an animal. In these cases, proof of penetration is required, but, failing such proof, the accused may be convicted of an attempt, or of an indecent assault.

Examination of a female complainant in alleged rape

At the outset of the examination the complainant should be asked to state where and when the assault took place. Her general demeanour and mental state should be observed while she relates this information. If it appears that she is under the influence of alcohol or drugs, this fact must be noted on the report. Her general physical development should be recorded. She should be asked her menstrual history and whether she has ever been pregnant or not. She should be asked to walk, and her gait should be noted.

The complainant should then be examined for external injuries. She should be asked to remove her underclothes and to lie down on a couch. If possible she should be placed in the lithotomy position. In a good light, her thighs, external genitalia and lower abdomen should be examined for injuries and for evidence of blood and seminal stains. The labia should be separated and the hymen should be examined for evidence of injury and recent tears. The size and shape of the opening of the hymen should be noted. The type of hymen and the situation of recent tears or injuries may be recorded on a diagram. Care should be exercised in the examination of the hymen, as natural indentations along the edge of the unruptured hymen may be mistaken for recent tears.

The vagina should be examined for evidence of injury, and a vaginal speculum should be used in this examination if possible. The size of the vagina should be noted. It is convenient to record the size of the vagina as admitting one, two or three fingers, as the case may be. While the vaginal speculum is in position a swab should be taken from the posterior fornix for examination for spermatozoa. An ordinary throat swab is suitable for this purpose, but the material obtained on the swab must immediately be transferred to a microscope slide and spread out in the form of a thin film on the middle of the slide. It may be possible to aspirate the material from the vagina with a pipette.

In the case of adults, smears should be taken from the cervix and urethra for bacteriological examination of gonococci. In the case of small girls, smears should be taken from the vagina for the same purpose. These smears may be of value, particularly in the case of children, as it is found in practice that children often fail to report an initial assault, and only do so after the lapse of a period or after a repeated assault. At the time of examination, therefore, they may present a gonorrhoeal vaginal discharge. A negative smear at the time of examination may also be of value if a positive smear is obtained within a few days of the assault. It is advisable to obtain a specimen of blood for serological blood tests if consent can be obtained. An initial negative serological reaction at the time of examination and the development of a positive reaction at the end of six weeks or later may be valuable evidence.

At the conclusion of the physical examination the clothing of the complainant should be carefully examined for evidence of tears and blood or seminal stains. If seminal stains are present and are still wet at the time of the examination, they should be ringed round with chalk and marked. The complainant should always be asked if she was aware of any portions of her garments feeling wet after the assault. Stains may be found on the complainant's dress or underclothes, and in certain cases they may be present on pieces of material or handkerchiefs used by her after the assault for cleansing purposes. Clothing which is believed to contain seminal or blood stains and slides containing smears should be submitted for laboratory examination.

Interpretation of findings

The presence of a recent laceration of the hymen with injuries of the external genitalia and thighs affords valuable corroborative evidence of rape. The absence of such injuries, however, does not necessarily exclude rape. Penetration may take place through a narrow annular or semilunar hymen without any rupture occurring, while contusions of the thighs and labia may not be apparent at the time of examination. Evidence of injury is often absent in the case of married women. The rape of children, however, usually results in severe injuries with vaginal tears which may extend into the rectum.

It should be recognized that the presence of injuries is not necessarily indicative of rape. Such injuries may be self-inflicted by a woman to substantiate a false charge of rape which she has brought against a man for reasons of malice or blackmail. Children may be deliberately injured for the same reasons. Injuries may also be inflicted during intercourse which has taken place with the consent of the female. In addition, in cases of homicide, injuries may be inflicted by an accused who is a sexual pervert.

The finding of spermatozoa on examination of a vaginal smear is indicative of an ejaculation into the vagina but it affords no evidence of the time of the ejaculation. In charges of rape, therefore, particularly in the case of married women, it becomes necessary to exclude the possibility of sexual intercourse having taken place before the assault. In this connection it should be noted that spermatozoa can be recovered from the vagina three to four days after their introduction. Some authorities claim that they may be recovered after the lapse of even longer periods. On the other hand, failure to find spermatozoa does not exclude the possibility of seminal fluid having been ejaculated into the vagina because a faulty technique may have been adopted in obtaining material from the vagina. For this reason, medical practitioners should try to obtain material from the posterior vaginal fornix in the manner described at page 359. Occasionally a negative result is due to the fact that spermatozoa are absent from the seminal fluid, but this condition is rare.

The demonstration of seminal stains on the clothing of the complainant may afford some corroborative evidence of the assault. It should be noted, however, that the seminal stains may have been present on the clothing before the assault.

Examination of a male complainant in sexual offences

In a charge of sodomy or other sexual assault against a male, the practitioner may be asked to examine the passive party for evidence of injury. If much force has been used the anus may be tender and swollen while bruises and tears of the mucous membrane may be found. In addition injuries may be observed in the region of the buttocks and thighs. If the act has been performed carefully or if the passive agent is habituated no signs may be found as the anus can undergo considerable distension without injury if it is dilated slowly. The finding of spermatozoa in material taken from the anal canal would afford corroborative evidence of sodomy, but the demonstration of seminal stains on the clothing has little value, especially in adults.

Smith[2] states that habitual sodomy leads to permanent changes in the condition of the anus. The skin about the orifice becomes smooth and thickened while the anal sphincter loses its tone. The orifice is situated more deeply than usual and the mucous membrane tends to protrude. Scars may be observed in the mucous membrane and in the skin surrounding the anal margin.

The prevention of pregnancy and venereal disease after a sexual assault

It is the duty of a practitioner who examines a complainant after a sexual assault to treat any injuries which he may find and to adopt measures to prevent the occurrence of pregnancy or sexually transmitted diseases.

The medical examination of a male accused in sexual offences

At the outset, the general physical development of the accused should be noted. His mental state and general demeanour should be observed. If he appears to be under the influence of alcohol, this fact must be recorded in the report. The accused should be undressed and carefully inspected for external injuries. His penis should be examined for injuries, sores, blood or faecal or other foreign matter, while the external meatus should be examined for evidence of discharge. Smears should be taken from the meatus after pressure has been applied to the under surface of the penis along the line of the urethra. These smears may be submitted for bacteriological examination for gonococci. It is advisable to obtain a specimen of the accused's blood for a serological blood test.

At the conclusion of the examination the clothing of the accused should carefully be examined for blood stains and for evidence of tears, missing buttons, etc. These stains may be found in relation to injuries on the accused's body, or they may be found away from such injuries in the region of the lower part of his shirt or in the region of the fly of his trousers.

Loose hairs found on both the accused and the complainant or on their clothing may be of medico-legal significance if they do not resemble the hairs of the person on whom they are found, but do resemble the hairs of the accused or complainant, as the case may be. In one of our cases the accused was suffering from a skin disease which had resulted in the formation of characteristic bulbous enlargements on his pubic hairs. A hair similar in all respects to these hairs was found on the person of the complainant. If pieces of fabric which appear foreign to the clothing of the accused or complainant are found in the course of the examination, they should be retained and be submitted to the laboratory for examination. The importance of this is well illustrated by the findings in one of our cases. In this case a strand of fawn-coloured wool was removed from the vagina of the complainant, and on examination this strand appeared to have come from the tassel at the end of a scarf. The accused was arrested because he was wearing a fawn scarf and it was found that each tassel of his scarf was made up of six strands of wool. A single strand was missing from one of the tassels and the strand found in the vagina proved to be identical in structure with the wool of which the scarf was made.

In cases of bestiality, animal hairs may be found on the body of the accused. In one of our cases of bestiality several short straight greyish-white hairs were found among the pubic hairs of the accused. These hairs were not human hairs but they resembled hairs clipped from the genital region of a donkey with which the accused was found.

Spermatozoa may be found in material taken from the vagina of the animal. It is usually difficult to differentiate human spermatozoa from the spermatozoa of animals by microscopic examination, but additional tests can be carried out. A high concentration of acid phosphatase might be found in the material if it contains human semen. The material can also be examined for human semen precipitinogens by testing against a known anti-human semen precipitin serum.

The laboratory examination of clothing for seminal stains

Seminal stains on garments have a stiff consistency and are creamy-white or yellowish-white in colour. They often show up equally well on both sides of thin garments. Seminal stains show a greenish-blue fluorescence when examined under the rays of an ultra-violet lamp. This type of fluorescence is not specific for seminal stains as the same type of fluorescence may be seen in stains which have been produced by saliva, urine or vaginal secretions.

Garments submitted for medico-legal laboratory examinations are often very dirty. It is an advantage to examine such garments first under the rays of an ultra-violet lamp as the initial chemical and microscopic examinations can then be confined to those stains which fluoresce.

Before dealing with the various procedures which may be adopted to establish that a stain is a seminal stain, it is necessary to describe the composition of seminal fluid.

The composition of seminal fluid

Semen is a thick, yellowish-white, glairy secretion which contains certain cellular elements known as spermatozoa. The fluid portion is formed in the seminal vesicles and the prostate gland, and the spermatozoa are formed in the testes. The average amount of semen which is discharged at one emission is 2 to 4 ml. The ejaculate of the normal fertile male contains about 400 to 500 million spermatozoa.[3] Spermatozoa have a characteristic appearance. Each spermatozoon has a head, neck, body and tail, but only the head and tail can be recognized clearly in ordinary preparations. The head is about 5 μm long and has a flattened ovoid shape. The tail measures about 50 μm.

Seminal fluid contains a high concentration of choline and a high concentration of an enzyme known as acid phosphatase. Choline originates from the seminal vesicles and phosphatase is formed by the prostate. Certain chemical tests for seminal stains depend upon the detection of these two substances in extracts of the stains.

Aspermia

Aspermia is a condition in which spermatozoa are absent from the seminal fluid. Aspermia may be caused either by a failure in the formation of spermatozoa in the seminiferous tubules or by some obstruction of the ducts which prevents spermatozoa from reaching the urethra. Spermatozoa cannot be found in extracts of seminal stains which are caused by the seminal fluids of persons suffering from aspermia, but positive chemical tests for semen may be obtained on such extracts.

Chemical tests for seminal stains

The Florence test. The Florence test is a simple microchemical test for seminal stains. The test is carried out in the following manner:

> A portion of the stain is steeped in a 1 per cent hydrochloric acid solution. Some of the extract is placed on a clean glass slide and is covered by a clean

cover glass. A drop of a modified Wagner's reagent (1.6 g potassium iodide and 2.5 g iodine dissolved in 30 ml distilled water) is then allowed to run under the cover glass, and the preparation is examined microscopically. Dark-brown needle-shaped crystals of choline iodide develop along the line of confluence between the extract and the reagent.

The Florence test is not a specific test for semen as choline occurs in other secretions. Moreover, extracts of seminal stains which are caused by seminal fluids with a very low choline concentration may give negative reactions with the Florence test.

The Florence test may be used as a rapid preliminary test for seminal stains. If the test is positive, an opinion that the stain is a seminal stain should only be given after spermatozoa have been found in an extract of the stain. On the other hand a negative Florence test does not exclude the possibility that the stain is a seminal stain, and a direct microscopic examination for spermatozoa must always be undertaken.

Acid phosphatase tests. Hansen[4] states that in 1945 Lundquist suggested that the demonstration of a high acid phosphatase content in seminal stains might provide a means of identifying such stains on garments.

Hansen has developed a method for the rapid qualitative demonstration of high concentrations of acid phosphatase in seminal stains. This method is a ring precipitation test. Hansen claims that the test is completely specific for seminal stains.

A quantitative acid phosphatase test for seminal stains has been described by Kaye.[5] Kaye states that an acid phosphatase activity of 25 King–Armstrong units per ml of extract from an area of approximately 1 cm^2 may be considered positive for seminal stains. Details of the procedures of carrying out these two tests are given in the papers by Hansen and Kaye. We have found that the tests are relatively simple to perform and give clear-cut readings.

Hansen and Kaye state that acid phosphatase tests for seminal stains are of value in cases of aspermia and in cases where it is difficult to find complete spermatozoa.

Acid phosphatase tests may also be of value in the investigation of cases of bestiality, as a high concentration of acid phosphatase is found only in the semen of human beings and monkeys (p. 362).

In certain circumstances the blood group of a seminal stain may be determined.

Microscopic examinations of stain extracts for spermatozoa

A portion of the suspected stain measuring about 1.25 cm^2 is cut out of the garment and is placed in a clean watch-glass. A few drops of a 1% hydrochloric acid solution are added and the preparation is covered by another watch-glass to prevent evaporation.

The fabric must become thoroughly saturated with the solution. This process takes from half an hour to several hours depending upon the age of the stain and the nature of the fabric.

By means of a pair of clean forceps, the fabric is removed from the solution and is placed at one end of a clean microscope slide. A smear is then made on the slide by scraping each surface of the fabric in turn, with the edge of another clean microscope slide. The smear is allowed to dry. It is then fixed by heat and stained by Gram's method. The smear should be examined initially with a high-power objective.

If spermatozoa are present in the extract several complete spermatozoa can usually be found, although many are broken up in the process of extraction. The heads of the spermatozoa stain a reddish-purple colour. The staining reaction at the basal ends of the heads close to the neck is more intense than the staining at the proximal ends. The tails of the spermatozoa stain a greyish-pink colour.

Under certain conditions it may be difficult to find complete spermatozoa in the smear. Separated heads and tails may be seen. Difficulty in the recognition of spermatozoa often arises when the seminal stains have become mixed with blood, urine or vaginal discharges. Spermatozoa are found most readily in stains that dry rapidly and on garments that have been well protected in transit to the laboratory.

Spermatozoa may undergo disintegration in seminal stains within a few months, but in certain circumstances spermatozoa may be found in old seminal stains, e.g. we have found complete spermatozoa in a seminal stain which was deposited on clean cotton material five years before examination.

With an ultrasonic apparatus, maximum recovery of complete spermatozoa is readily obtained. This technique is to be preferred.[6,7]

General interpretation of tests for seminal stains

If complete spermatozoa are found microscopically in a stain extract, it can be positively stated that the stain is a seminal stain. The failure to find complete spermatozoa does not exclude the possibility of the stain being a seminal stain. In such cases if the chemical tests for semen are positive (particularly if the acid phosphatase tests are positive) there is a strong presumption that the stain is a seminal stain.

Examination of smears for spermatozoa

If vaginal swabs are taken properly (p. 359) in cases of rape, it may be possible to find spermatozoa as long as 72 to 96 hours after their deposit in the vagina. Willot and Allard[8] state that vaginal spermatozoa may be found up to 120 hours after intercourse.

In fatal cases of rape and assault, spermatozoa may be found in the vagina for a considerable period after death. Glaister[9] states that he has detected complete spermatozoa in a smear made from a vaginal swab, taken 85 hours after death. Smears made from vaginal swabs should be stained by Gram's method, as such smears can then be examined for spermatozoa and gonococci.

Blood stains in cases of sexual assault

The question whether a blood stain on a garment is due to menstrual blood or not is often raised in sexual charges. Menstrual blood contains epithelial cells, but the demonstration of these cells in blood stains on garments does not establish the menstrual origin of such stains because worn clothing normally contains similar epithelial cells. There is no reliable laboratory method of distinguishing a menstrual blood stain from any other type of blood stain.

ABORTION

Nature of the crime of procuring abortion

The nature of the crime of procuring an abortion varies in different countries. In some countries abortion is a common law crime and in others the crime of abortion is defined by statute or is not regarded as a crime. In general the crime is committed by any person who wilfully and unlawfully, with the intention of prematurely terminating pregnancy, does any act which causes a pregnant woman to miscarry. The act concerned usually takes such form as the administration of an ecbolic drug, the use of direct or indirect force, or the injection of some substance into the vagina or uterus.

In most countries it is established by common or statutory law that the crime may be committed by any person, including the woman herself. In many jurisdictions a woman is guilty of the crime if she permits the act to be performed upon her. In addition, anyone who obtains for a woman the means by which she can procure an abortion upon herself is guilty of aiding and abetting her, and may be convicted of the same crime as the woman herself. No crime is committed where a medical practitioner in good faith gives treatment to a patient which unexpectedly causes her to abort.

When a woman dies from a criminal abortion, in certain circumstances the person responsible may be charged with murder but as a general rule the charge is one of culpable homicide or manslaughter.

Depending upon the common law or statutory provision in different countries, no crime is committed if a medical practitioner terminates a pregnancy in order to save the life of the mother. In many countries legislative provisions have been enacted whereby, subject to varying administrative requirements, a pregnancy may be terminated lawfully if the continuation of the pregnancy constitutes a serious threat to the physical or mental health of a woman. In addition, in some countries provision is made for the lawful termination of pregnancy if there is a substantial risk that the child to be born will suffer from a physical or mental abnormality of such a nature that it will be seriously handicapped.

Shapiro[10] has summed up the religious, ethical, sociological, legal, criminal, economic and medical aspects of abortion.

Action in a case of suspected criminal abortion

A medical practitioner is placed in a difficult position when he is confronted with a case which may be one of criminal abortion. On the one hand stands his general duty to society to assist in the apprehension and punishment of a criminal; on the other stands his particular duty to his patient to concentrate on her bodily condition and to respect her confidences and observe professional secrecy in regard to her affairs. Nevertheless, it should be remembered that the professional abortionist who, often with the most rudimentary knowledge and a complete absence of precautions against injury or infection, produces dangerous miscarriages on pregnant women is a menace to society. It is the practitioner's duty wherever possible to aid in his or her apprehension. On the other hand, where a woman has attempted to terminate her own pregnancy, often in circumstances of great desperation, the general feeling of the medical profession, and in fact, of many others, is that it would be unnecessary cruelty for the practitioner to whom she comes for help to report the event to any law enforcement agency.

Bearing these considerations in mind, the following procedure is advised:

When the practitioner knows or suspects that the patient is suffering from the effects of a criminal abortion or of an attempted criminal abortion, he should endeavour to discover from the patient, if her condition allows of questioning, whether his suspicions are correct, what has been done to the patient and who has done it. He should also immediately consult a colleague who is unconnected with him professionally.

If he is satisfied that the patient herself is responsible for her condition, he should keep the information to himself. If the patient is likely to die, the practitioner should urge the woman to make a formal confession. If she seems certain to die, and realizes this fact herself, she should be urged to make a dying declaration.* If she refuses to make a confession or a dying

---

* A dying declaration is a statement made by a person who believes that he is dying and has no hope of recovery, concerning the cause of his injury or illness. It is admissible only at a trial on a charge of the murder or culpable homicide of the patient. The points for the practitioner to note are the following:

1. The practitioner should satisfy himself that the patient is in a fit mental state to make a statement and to appreciate what he is saying.

2. The declaration may be made orally, but the person receiving it should commit it to writing, either at the time it is being made or as soon as possible thereafter.

3. The actual words used by the patient should, as far as possible, be written down.

4. It may be necessary to ask questions for the elucidation or clarification of the statement, in which case the exact wording of both the questions and the answers should be recorded. (cont'd next page)

declaration, or if her condition does not permit it, there is nothing further that can or should be done by the practitioner. In case of untoward results, he will largely be protected from the danger of being accused of procuring the abortion himself or of having been an accessory to it by the fact that he has consulted a colleague otherwise unconnected with him professionally.

If, however, it appears that the abortion has been procured or attempted by a third party, the patient should be strongly urged to allow the police to be informed. If she is dying, and is aware of the fact, she should be strongly urged to make a dying declaration, or to allow a police officer or a magistrate to take a statement, or at least to allow the authorities to be told. Once again, however, if she refuses to co-operate, or if her condition does not permit it, there is nothing further that can or should be done.

In all cases, if the patient dies the practitioner will as a matter of course refuse to sign a death certificate.

Medical examination in criminal abortion

Women over the age 21 and, in most countries, married women, irrespective of their age, may be examined with their own consent, but an unmarried female under the age of 21 should not be examined without the consent of her parent or guardian. This provision may differ in different jurisdictions.

A woman or the parent or guardian of a girl may refuse to give consent for an examination. In most countries, in these circumstances, the woman or girl cannot be compelled to be examined unless she is accused of the abortion, and a judicial officer presiding at the trial or at a preliminary enquiry orders such an examination. If, after such an order has been given, the woman or girl resists medical examination, the practitioner is advised not to attempt to examine her forcibly but to report the circumstances to the Court.

Methods of procuring criminal abortions

Criminal abortions are usually produced by (1) the use of drugs; (2) the use of instruments; and (3) general violence.

(cont'd)

5. Leading questions should, as far as possible, be avoided.

6. If possible, the declaration should be read over to the patient, and he should be asked whether he adheres to it. If he is capable of signing the document he should be asked to do so, and any person present should be asked to witness his signature.

7. The practitioner must satisfy himself that the patient is convinced that he is dying and that he has no hope of recovery, and should preface his written account with a statement to this effect, and his reasons for making it.

1. The use of drugs in procuring abortions

Many drugs are used as abortifacients. Most of these drugs have no effect on the uterus or the fetus unless they are given in toxic doses. Death frequently results from the toxic effects of these drugs without abortion occurring.

The drugs which are commonly used may be classified in the following way:

(a) *Drugs acting directly on the uterus.* Ergot is the most widely used of these drugs. Quinine, which is also used occasionally as an abortifacient, may act as a uterine stimulant under certain conditions.

(b) *Drugs acting indirectly on the uterus.* Drastic purgatives and essential oils act indirectly on the uterus by causing pelvic vascular engorgement.

Purgatives. The group of resinous purgatives such as croton oil, scammony, colocynth and gamboge are often used as abortifacients.

Volatile or essential oils. Large doses of essential oils such as apiol, savin, pennyroyal, tansy and turpentine are taken to induce abortion. These drugs act as irritants of the genitourinary tract during excretion, and in toxic doses may cause extensive damage to the renal glomeruli and tubular epithelium.

Apiol is widely used in combination with ergot in the form of ergoapiol as an abortifacient. Ergoapiol contains triorthocresyl phosphate which gives rise to a form of peripheral neuritis. In one of our cases a woman took large doses of ergoapiol but failed to abort. She developed a widespread peripheral neuritis affecting all her limbs. She ultimately died of respiratory failure which was probably induced by a peripheral paralysis of the somatic nerves concerned with respiration.

Lead in the form of diachylon pills has been used extensively as an abortifacient. It is believed to have a toxic action on the trophoblastic epithelium of the ovum.

2. The use of instruments in procuring abortions

When drugs have failed to induce abortion the abortionist frequently adopts some method of mechanical interference with the uterus. The method employed depends largely upon his skill and upon his knowledge of the anatomy of the pelvic parts. Slow methods, such as the dilatation of the cervix with sea tangle or laminaria tents are occasionally employed, but as a general rule the abortionist is anxious to complete the operation quickly and a rapid method of induction is adopted.

Criminal abortion by instrumental means is usually induced: (a) by the injection of substances into the uterine cavity; or (b) by the forcible dilatation of the cervix with or without rupture of the membranes.

(a) *The injection of substances into the uterine cavity.* The ordinary enema syringe with a hand bulb is commonly employed to inject substances into the uterus, the hard nozzle being inserted into the cervix. The substances used for these injections vary. In most cases a solution of ordinary soap and water is used but solutions containing some antiseptic such as carbolic acid, lysol or mercuric perchloride are sometimes employed in the hope of preventing sepsis. These substances may be absorbed from the vaginal and uterine mucosa and this absorption occasionally results in death from poisoning.

(b) *The forcible dilatation of the cervix and rupture of the membranes.* Uterine sounds and metal and gum elastic catheters are sometimes employed to dilate the cervix while objects such as knitting needles, pieces of wire or pointed sticks are employed to rupture the membranes.

The abortionist may produce considerable damage in carrying out these methods of induction. The syringe used for the injection, or the instrument employed for the dilatation of the cervix or the rupture of the membranes, may be passed through the posterior vaginal wall. More commonly it is passed through the posterior fornix of the vagina into the peritoneal cavity in the region of the pouch of Douglas. The intestines or the rectum are often punctured in the process of penetration. If the instrument has been passed into the cervix successfully damage may still occur through penetration of the posterior wall of the cervix at its upper end or through perforation of the uterine wall. Perforation of the uterus in the region of the fundus frequently occurs in criminal abortion, as the abortionist is usually unaware of the length of the uterus at the different stages of pregnancy.

3. The use of general violence in procuring abortions

Methods of general violence, such as jumping from heights, the carrying of heavy objects, horse-riding, etc., are occasionally resorted to in the hope of procuring an abortion. In certain cases some injury is applied directly to the abdomen. These methods are often combined with hot baths or vaginal douches, but as a general rule they have no effect upon the continuation of pregnancy.

Possible causes of death in criminal abortion following upon the use of instruments

Death in criminal abortion following the use of instruments may be caused by: (1) reflex shock; (2) haemorrhage; (3) sepsis; or (4) air embolism.

1. Reflex shock

The forcible distension of the cervical canal and the uterine cavity without an anaesthetic may lead to instantaneous death through reflex nervous shock. This type of death was seen in one of our cases:

> The accused attempted to procure an abortion on a young unmarried girl by injecting an antiseptic solution containing lysol into the uterus. It was proved at the trial that the accused placed the girl on her kitchen table and without administering an anaesthetic she introduced a syringe into the lower part of the cervix without damaging the external os or the vagina. She then injected a small amount of the solution under pressure into the upper part of the cervical canal and the lower part of the uterine cavity. It was subsequently determined that the deceased collapsed as the cervical canal and uterine cavity were distended by the injected solution and death apparently occurred instantaneously.

2. Haemorrhage

Death in criminal abortion is occasionally due to haemorrhage. The haemorrhage may arise from an injury to the vagina or the uterus, or it may follow upon an incomplete separation of the membranes or the placenta from the uterine wall.

This type of death was seen in one of our cases of criminal abortion. The circumstances of this case were quite unusual:

> The accused procured an abortion on a young unmarried girl by the passage of an instrument into her cervix. The abortion was procured at the home of the accused, where the deceased died. At the trial, evidence was led which suggested that after the abortion the deceased had bled profusely per vaginam for two or three days before she died. A medical practitioner saw the deceased at the home of the accused and, when the girl died, he issued a certificate stating that death was due to haemorrhage caused by haemophilia. This extraordinary death certificate was accepted, and the deceased was buried without an autopsy being held.
>
> Some three weeks later the body was exhumed on information received by the police, and the following conditions were found at the autopsy:
>
> *General*: The body was remarkably well preserved and the tissues throughout showed an extreme degree of pallor.
>
> *The uterus*: On examination of the uterus three independent wounds were observed in the region of the fundus. In addition, a large circular-shaped wound, measuring approximately ¾ inch in diameter, was seen in the posterior wall of the cervix. Histological evidence of tissue reaction was found in this wound, but there was no vital reaction in the wounds of the fundus.
>
> It was subsequently determined that the accused had arranged for the embalming of the deceased before her burial by the introduction of preservative fluid into the peritoneal cavity by means of a trocar and cannula. In the course of the embalming the trocar was forced through the wall of the uterus in the region of the fundus. The accused was sentenced to five years' imprisonment with hard labour.

3. Sepsis

Septic infection is the commonest cause of death in criminal abortion. The infection is usually due to the introduction of unsterile instruments or solutions into the cervix or uterine cavity.

The infection of the uterus is usually complicated by extra-uterine infection such as cellulitis or peritonitis. These complications are seen particularly when the vaginal or uterine wall has been perforated. Thrombophlebitis of the uterine and other pelvic veins may occur, and in certain cases pyaemia and septicaemia develop. Tetanus following upon criminal abortion has been described, but this type of infection is uncommon.

4. Pulmonary air embolism

Pulmonary air emobolism is an uncommon cause of death in criminal abortion, but it may occur if frothy fluids are injected into the uterus. When an ordinary enema syringe is used for procuring an abortion, a considerable amount of air may be introduced with the fluid into the uterus, and if the placenta becomes detached by the pressure of the fluid, this air can readily be forced into the open uterine sinuses. This type of death was seen in one of our cases, which has been described in greater detail by one of us:[11]

> The accused attempted to procure an abortion on a young unmarried girl by injecting a soapy solution into the uterus by means of an enema syringe. The deceased collapsed during the attempt. At the autopsy air bubbles could be demonstrated in some of the veins draining the pelvic organs into the iliac veins while frothy blood was found in the common iliac veins, the inferior vena cava, the right atrium, the right ventricle and the pulmonary arteries. The placenta was detached from the uterine wall along the whole of its lower edge and a moderate amount of blood-stained fluid was found in the lower portion of the uterine cavity.

In order to diagnose pulmonary air embolism, Shennan[12] recommends that the main arterial and venous trunks should be ligated, and an incision should then be made through the parietal pericardium. The pericardial sac should be filled with water and the right ventricle should be opened *in situ*. If air is present in the right ventricle it will bubble up through the water. This method of examination presents many difficulties. As a preliminary step in the post-mortem diagnosis of air embolism we prefer to use regional radiological examinations carried out within a short period of death. Apart from their value for diagnostic purposes, such examinations provide a guide to the most advantageous dissection procedure to be followed. The advantage of this method of investigation is illustrated by the case reported by Duncan-Taylor.[13] This was a fatal case of pulmonary air embolism following upon an artificial pneumoperitoneum refill. On radiography, gas was seen to outline the right atrium, the right ventricle and the pulmonary artery. Tuberculous infiltration of the productive type was present in the left lung. The left side of the abdomen revealed the pneumoperitoneum. See also 'arterial air embolism' (p. 309).

The mechanism of death in pulmonary air embolism is obscure. Forbes[14] states that death may be caused by a mechanical interference with heart function, by a blockage of the pulmonary artery by froth with an arrest of the circulation in the lungs, or by an obstruction of the finer arterioles in the lungs by multiple emboli.

Death may occur almost immediately upon the introduction of air into the uterus under pressure, or very shortly thereafter. Death may, however, be delayed for 2 to 4 hours after the introduction of air.[15]

Signs of abortion in the living

The detection of signs of abortion in the living depends upon the time that has elapsed between the abortion and the time of examination, and upon the duration of pregnancy before the abortion. If the period that has elapsed between the abortion and the examination is long, it may be impossible to find any signs of abortion. If the period is short the signs will depend upon the duration of the pregnancy.

The signs may be indefinite in a case of abortion which has occurred within the first three months of pregnancy. Softening of the cervix with a slight enlargement of the uterus and haemorrhage or discharge from the uterus may be found, but these signs usually disappear within a few days after the abortion. In the case of a primipara the breast changes of pregnancy, which usually become manifest between the eighth and twelfth week, may be of indirect value in the diagnosis of a recent abortion. The signs will be more definite when the abortion has taken place at a later stage of pregnancy as the uterine enlargement is greater, the haemorrhage more marked, and the return to normal after the abortion more gradual.

The Xenopus (frog) test, which was originally introduced by Shapiro and Zwarenstein,[16] may afford additional evidence of pregnancy. It has been held that a positive reaction in the test animal may be obtained up to three or four days after the complete expulsion of the products of conception. In incomplete abortion a positive reaction will be obtained as long as viable chorionic tissue is present. In cases of recent abortion and incomplete abortion, therefore, a biological test of this nature may be of medico-legal value.

Animal tests have largely been replaced by quicker and more sensitive test-tube tests based on an immunological reaction for the detection of human chorionic gonadotrophin.

In all cases of suspected abortion a thorough gynaecological investigation should be made. This should include an examination for evidence of extra-uterine infection and for evidence of injury to the vagina, cervix or uterus.

The expulsion of material from the uterus during an abortion

During an abortion the whole ovum (in early pregnancy) or portions of the ovum may be expelled from the uterus. Small portions of an ovum may be expelled in blood clots, and all material passed should therefore be retained for histological examination.

The portions of ovum passed often contain chorionic villi. The naked-eye appearances of chorionic villi are readily recognizable. The microscopic structure of a chorionic villus is seen to consist of a central core of connective tissue containing blood vessels and an outer trophoblast. The trophoblast presents an inner layer of cells known as the layer of Langhans, and an outer layer of richly nucleated protoplasm without cell boundaries known as the syncytial layer. Portions of placenta in expelled material are readily recognized.

Portions of decidual membrane or decidual cells enmeshed in blood clot are often expelled in cases of abortion. Decidual cells are fairly characteristic, and appear as large pale-staining round or polygonal cells, often with eccentric nuclei. It should be noted that the decidual cells of pregnancy closely resemble the predecidual cells of menstruation.

If a complete fetus is passed during an abortion, an attempt should be made to estimate its approximate age. The rate of development of an ovum or fetus varies and only an approximate determination of age can be made. Details of development of the ovum and fetus are given in standard works on human embryology.

Signs of abortion in the dead

The pelvic organs are removed in the manner described at page 75. The vulva, vagina, vaginal fornices, cervix and body of the uterus are carefully examined for evidence of injury or haemorrhage. An examination should also be made for evidence of uterine or extra-uterine infection. It is advisable to weigh the uterus, and the cavity of the uterus should be examined for a placental site or for remains of the fetus, placenta or membranes. Histological sections should be made of all material removed from the uterus, cervix or vagina. If the vaginal or uterine wall has been injured, the tissues at the site of the injury should be excised and examined histologically for evidence of tissue reaction. The ovaries should be examined for the presence of a corpus luteum, and in primipara the expression of fluid from the breasts may be of indirect value in the diagnosis of a recent abortion.

In certain cases of abortion it may be necessary to submit specimens of the vagina or uterus for toxicological examination.

INFANTICIDE AND CONCEALMENT OF BIRTH

Nature of the crime of infanticide

The nature of the crime of infanticide varies in different countries. In most countries infanticide is a common law crime and any person, including the mother, who kills a newly born child may be charged with murder or culpable homicide (manslaughter) depending upon whether there was intent to kill or not. Apart from the common law crime, in some jurisdictions infanticide is a statutory offence as well. In some countries infanticide is defined in legislation in a manner whereby the crime is separated from murder and culpable homicide, e.g. the English Infanticide Act was framed in accordance with the view that the mental balance of a mother may be affected by the experience of labour and its after effects or by the strain of lactation.

Before a conviction for infanticide or for murder or culpable homicide can be made, it is necessary to establish that the child was born alive. Varying criteria are used in different countries for live birth. In most countries a child is deemed to have been born alive live if it is proved to have breathed. In some countries, apart from evidence of breathing, it is necessary to establish that the infant had an independent circulation and that at the time of its death, the child was entirely separated from its mother.

Nature of the crime of concealment of birth

In most countries the crime of concealment of birth is governed by legislation. The crime is committed by hiding the dead body of a child in order to conceal the fact of its birth. The legal requirements to establish the offence vary in different countries, but the following provisions are usually embodied in legislation. First, the offence can be committed by any person, including the mother, who disposes of the body of a child whether the child died before, during or after its birth. Second, the provisions are often framed in such a manner that no onus is placed on the State or prosecuting authority to prove whether the child died before, at or after its birth. Third, in most jurisdictions, a person may be found guilty of concealment of birth even if it is not proved that the child in question died before the body was disposed of.

There may be no definition of the term 'child' in enactments which define the crime of concealment of birth. In these circumstances, difficulty may be experienced in deciding what is a 'child' when delivery has taken place before the expiration of the normal period of gestation. This point was considered in the case of Rex v. Matthews.[17] This charge was laid under the provisions of an enactment which did not define the term 'child'. The accused was charged with and convicted of the concealment of the birth of her twin children. The accused gave birth to the twins at about five months after the probable time of conception. Each fetus was very small, both together weighing 1100 g ($2\frac{1}{2}$ lb). In setting aside the conviction, on review, the learned Judge pointed out that in terms of the relevant Births, Marriages and Deaths Registration Act the birth of a stillborn child must be certified and reported, but under the provisions of the Act a stillborn child is defined as a fetus of over six months of intra-uterine existence.

The learned Judge stated that he could not conceive of there being any concealment of the birth of a child where the law imposes no necessity in regard to reporting it. Quoting the opinion expressed by Gardiner and Lansdown[18] the Judge held that a fetus is not a child for the purpose of the particular statute unless it has reached a stage of development sufficient to have rendered its separate existence apart from its mother a reasonable probability.

Medical examination of women in charges of infanticide and concealment of birth

A medical practitioner may be required to examine a woman who is charged with infanticide or concealment of birth for signs of recent delivery, and if there is evidence of such delivery he may be asked to give an approximate estimate of the period that has elapsed between the birth and his examination. As he may also be required to give an opinion on the mental condition of such a woman, he should observe her general demeanour and emotional state during the examination.

The signs of recent delivery

The examination for evidence of recent delivery should include an examination for any signs which would be consistent with a precipitate or difficult labour. The detection of the signs of recent delivery in the living depend upon the period that has elapsed between the delivery and the time of examination. If the period that has elapsed is long, e.g. three to four weeks, it may be impossible to find any definite signs of delivery.

If the period is short, e.g. a few days, the uterus will be enlarged and palpable through the anterior abdominal wall. A lochial discharge will be observed and the external os of the cervix is usually torn. The labia may be swollen, and there may be evidence of recent tears of the vagina or perineum. In the case of a primipara, the expression of fluid from the breasts may be of indirect value in the diagnosis of a recent delivery.

Post-mortem examination of an infant

External examination

If the child has been found wrapped up in clothing, paper or other material, the wrapping should be retained as it may be of value in identification. The sex of the infant should be noted. The infant should then be weighed and its length should be measured.

If a placenta is found with the body it should be examined. In a case where the placenta is absent, the length of the remaining umbilical cord should be measured. The cord should be examined to see whether a ligature has been applied and to determine whether it has been cut or torn.

The body should be examined for the changes which develop after death, such as rigor mortis, putrefaction, etc. A thorough external examination of the body should be made. It should be noted whether the child has been washed or not. If there is any evidence of external injury to the body, the situation and nature of such injuries should be recorded. This limbs should be palpated for evidence of fractures.

Internal examination

In all cases the examination should commence with the dissection of the head.

Dissection of the head. Baar[19] has described a very satisfactory method for opening the skull and examining the brain. An ear-to-ear incision is first made over the vault of the skull and the two flaps of the scalp are pulled forwards and backwards. The scalp tissues are examined for haemorrhages and the bones of the vault are examined for subperiosteal haematomata and fractures.

The skull is then opened by a special dissection method which has been described in the following terms by Baar (the procedure is illustrated schematically in Fig. 14.1).

> An incision is made with a pointed knife into the anterior fontanelle at its posterior margin, approximately 5 mm from the midline. The point of the knife is pushed parallel to the inner aspect of the parietal bone for 1 to 2 mm between dura and leptomeninges and the incision is extended to the lateral angle. In a similar way the opposite side and both anterior margins are incised. One blade of a pair of strong scissors is passed beneath the parietal

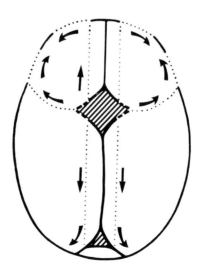

Fig. 14.1 Schematic drawing illustrating the technique for opening the skull of a newborn infant.—Primary incisions into the anterior fontanelle made with a pointed knife. . . . Extensions made with a pair of strong scissors.

dura at the medial end of the original incision and the parietal bone is cut longitudinally parallel to the sagittal suture and about 5 mm laterally to the latter. The incision is continued towards the lambdoid suture, and then laterally and downwards within the latter and finally in a similar way in the coronal suture. The same procedure is applied to the other side and two parietotemporal flaps are turned outward. In the same way flaps of the two halves of the frontal squama are prepared and turned outward. It is usually necessary to make a horizontal frontomedial extension with the help of a bone forceps, leaving only a short bridge for outward reflection of the flaps. The procedure leaves a medial strip approximately 1 cm in width with the intact superior longitudinal sinus.

After the four flaps have been reflected, the vertex of the brain and the terminations of the pial veins into the superior longitudinal sinus are inspected for haemorrhages. The falx cerebri is then examined by a gentle sideward pushing of the hemispheres. Haematomata may be found between the falx and the medial aspects of the hemispheres, or between the two dural layers of the falx. The superior longitudinal sinus in then opened and examined for ante-mortem thrombi.

The falx is separated at its antero-inferior insertion, the frontal lobes are lifted upwards and backwards, cranial nerves II to VI are cut transversely and a horizontal cut is made through the pons at the level of the incisura tentorii. The removal of the cerebral hemispheres and the upper part of the pons in this manner exposes the tentorium cerebelli. The tentorium is inspected for tears and for haematomata between its layers.

After inspection the tentorium is divided along its line of attachment at the superior petrous temporal border. The cranial nerves VII to XII are severed, the medulla is incised with a bistoury as deeply as possible, and the contents of the posterior cranial fossa are removed.

The sinuses of the dura are then opened and with a pair of forceps and the dura is detached from the base and sides of the skull. By means of a chisel the middle ear cavities and the mastoid antra are opened.

The various parts of the brain are then examined according to the procedure adopted in the examination of the adult brain (p. 71).

Chest and abdominal contents. A primary incision is made from the level of the thyroid cartilage in the midline to the pubis, avoiding the umbilicus. The abdominal cavity is then opened in the manner described at page 70 and the height of the diaphragm is noted before the thoracic cavity is opened. Before respiration the dome of the diaphragm may extend as high as the third or fourth rib. The thoracic cavity is then opened in the manner described at page 65 and the chest contents are examined *in situ*, particular note being taken of the position of the lungs.

The neck structures and the thoracic contents are then brought down to the level of the diaphragm in the manner described at pages 69–70 and the oesophagus and trachea are ligatured. The diaphragm is then divided and by dissection behind and lateral to the kidneys all the abdominal and pelvic viscera are removed in one mass with the thoracic contents.

The larynx is examined for the presence of any obstructing foreign body, and the tracha is opened down to the level of the ligature. The lungs, heart and trachea are then separated from the other viscera in a single mass, and the hydrostatic test for respiration is carried out.

The hydrostatic test for breathing. The heart, the lungs and the attached portions of the trachea and bronchi are placed in a basin of water. If there is complete expansion of the lungs, they are usually sufficiently buoyant to float and support the heart on the surface of the water.

Each lung is separated from the heart at its hilum and placed in the water to determine whether it floats. The lungs are divided into their lobes and each lobe is tested to see whether it floats. The lobes are then cut up into smaller portions, and each portion is tested in the same way. If any of these portions float, a further procedure is adopted by some authorities. Some of the floating portions are selected and placed on a flat surface such as a wooden board. Firm pressure is applied to the surface of each lung portion with the flat of a broad knife, so that the tissue becomes squeezed out. These portions of lung are again tested in the water to see if they still float.

If the body is not putrefied and all the portions of the lungs float in water after they have been compressed, it is proof that the lungs have been expanded and that respiration has been complete. If some portions of the lung float after compression and others sink, it is proof of incomplete expansion of the lungs and partial respiration. If all portions of the lungs sink it is usually held that the lungs are unexpanded and that the infant has not breathed. It should be noted, however, that cases have been recorded where respiratory movements were observed and infants were heard to cry although no portion of either lung would float.

Application of the hydrostatic test in putrefied bodies. Putrefaction of the lungs usually occurs at a late stage in the decomposition of the body of an infant. The putrefactive changes develop in stillborn and liveborn infants and in both cases the gases of putrefaction may in themselves render the lungs buoyant in water. The problem in these cases is to determine whether such floating lungs were expanded before the development of putrefaction. This problem, however, cannot be resolved by the crude manual techniques often recommended. The sinking of portions of the lungs does not exclude the possibility of the lungs having been expanded, because the putrefactive changes may have led to destruction of the lung tissue, thereby enabling the respired air to be squeezed out of the tissue together with the putrefactive gases. For this reason, when the body is putrefied, medical witnesses are often unable to give an opinion as to whether or not an infant has breathed.

The hydrostatic test and diseases of the lungs. Consolidation and oedema of the lungs is occasionally found in newly born infants. Under these conditions the affected portions of the lungs may sink in water, although the infant breathed before death. In these cases it is exceptional for the disease process to involve the whole of both lungs so that portions of expanded lung tissue can generally be found. Histological sections of the lungs will reveal the nature and extent of the disease.

Other signs of respiration. The lungs of an infant that has breathed are mottled in colour and have rounded edges. Such lungs crepitate on palpation, and when fully expanded fill the pleural cavities and overlap the heart. The lungs of an infant that has not breathed have a uniform dark-red colour, and their edges are sharp. Such lungs are solid on palpation, and when examined *in situ* are found in the posterior portions of the pleural cavities close to the vertebral column.

The heart. The heart is examined in the manner set out at page 73, special attention being paid to the foramen ovale and the ductus arteriosus.

The stomach and intestines. A double ligature is placed between the stomach and the duodenum and the gut is divided between the ligatures. This completes the isolation of the stomach, which has previously been ligatured at its oesophageal end. The stomach is placed in water to see whether it floats. It is then opened along its lesser curvature, and its contents and mucous surface examined. The contents should be examined for the presence of food, as such a finding may be of confirmatory value in establishing live birth.

A double ligature is placed at the lower end of the jejunum, and the gut is divided between the ligatures. The duodenum and jejunum are isolated and placed in water to see whether they float. The intestines are then opened along their antimesenteric border and their contents are examined.

Examination for centres of ossification. The foot is grasped in the left hand behind the heel, the toes pointing towards the dissector. With the long knife an incision is carried down between the third and fourth toes through the tissues of the foot to divide the calcaneum and the talus. An incision made at this level will generally expose the centre in the calcaneum. It is dark red in colour and quite distinct from the surrounding cartilage. If it is not seen, thin slices of cartilage should be cut until the presence or absence of the centre has been demonstrated. A similar technique is followed for the talus, which is just above the calcaneum. The centre in the cuboid is variable. It is looked for by cutting thin slices of cartilage from the cuboid, which is seen lying lateral to the original line of incision made in the foot.

To demonstrate the centre at the lower end of the femur, a cruciate incision is made through the skin over the patella. The patella is dissected free and removed. The knee joint is placed in extreme flexion so that the distal cartilaginous end of the femur presents for section. Thin plates of cartilage are then sliced off with the long knife in a proximal direction until the centre is exposed. When the centre is found, the slicing dissection must be continued so as to demonstrate a layer of cartilage between the centre and the primary centre in the shaft of the femur. In this way the primary centre will not be confused with the epiphyseal centre.

Special examinations

Occasionally it is necessary to examine portions of the lungs and the umbilical cord histologically, while in certain cases chemical tests to establish the presence of food may have to be carried out on the stomach contents.

Medico-legal applications

On the completion of a post-mortem examination on a newly born infant the following questions may be raised:

1. Was the infant born alive?
2. What was the state of maturity of the infant?
3. How long did the infant live?
4. How long has the infant been dead?
5. What was the cause of death?

1. Was the infant born alive?

In most countries, a child is deemed to have been born alive if it is proved to have breathed. The hydrostatic test is employed to establish that an infant has breathed. The interpretation of the findings of this test has been dealt with at page 379. The 'stomach-bowel test', in which the stomach and a loop of the intestine are tested for floating, is described at page 380. This test is regarded by some authorities as an additional test for respiration in non-putrefied bodies.

Other evidence of a non-medical nature, such as the hearing of a cry, is sometimes advanced in Court as proof that an infant has breathed.

Some authors have claimed that a microscopic examination of lung tissue can serve to establish whether an infant has breathed or not. They state that if respiration has not occurred, the alveoli appear as hollow gland-like structures lined by cuboidal or columnar epithelium, but if respiration has occurred, then the alveoli are well expanded and a distinct alveolar epithelial lining can no longer be seen.

Shapiro[20–22] has shown that the microscopic appearances of the lungs of stillborn infants and the lungs of liveborn infants may be indistinguishable. He states that in the course of fetal development there is a gradually evolving change in the structure of the respiratory tract, consisting of progressive branching of subsidiary ducts from the early embryonic trachea. This process goes on to the formation of alveoli consisting of well-defined alveolar spaces with fairly thin walls. This development occurs entirely during the intra-uterine existence of the fetus before term.

Figures 14.2, 14.3, 14.4 and 14.5 are taken from Shapiro's series of cases. Figure 14.2 is a section from the lung of a fetus between 4 and 5 months

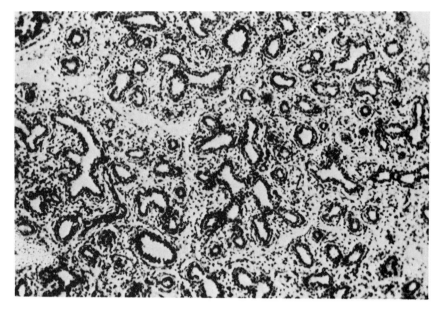

Fig. 14.2. Section from the lung of a fetus between four and five months of age. The lungs of this foetus did not float in water. Note the glandular appearance of the organ with the considerable amount of connective tissue between the ducts which are lined by cuboidal–columnar cells. Crown–rump length, 15 cm.

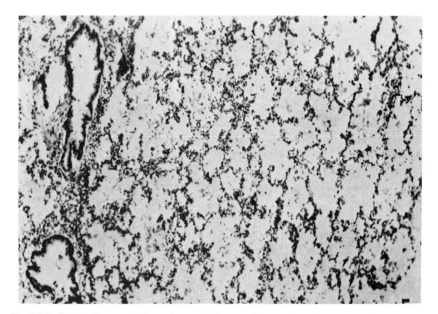

Fig. 14.3. Section from a stillborn fetus at full term. No portion of the lungs floated in water. The alveolar pattern appears almost fully developed.

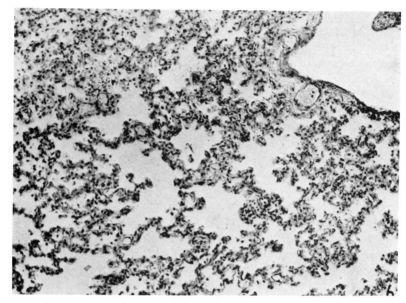

Fig. 14.4. Section from the lungs of a full-term fetus found lying free in the abdominal cavity in a case of death due to a ruptured uterus following an impacted transverse lie. No portion of the lungs floated in water.

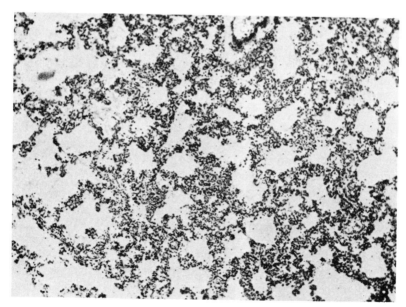

Fig. 14.5. Section from a full-term fetus which died a few minutes after birth. Death was due to a tentorial tear with intracranial haemorrhage. It is not possible to distinguish this section taken from a portion of the lung which floated, from those shown in Figs. 14.3 and 14.4, which were taken from cases of stillbirth in which no portion of the lungs floated.

of age. The section shows that the lung has a gland-like appearance with thick-walled ductules lined by cuboidal–columnar epithelial cells. In this case no portion of the lungs floated in water.

Figures 14.3 and 14.4 are sections of lungs from two stillborn full-term fetuses. In the case Figure 14.4, the full-term fetus was found lying free in the abdominal cavity in a case of death due to a ruptured uterus. The sections show that alveolar spaces have developed in the tissue and a distinct epithelial lining to these spaces cannot be seen. In both cases, no portion of the lungs floated in water.

Figure 14.5 is a section of lung from a full-term fetus which lived for a few minutes after birth. The portion of lung from which the section was taken floated in water but the microscopic appearances of this portion of lung could not be distinguished from the sections of the lungs of the still-born fetuses shown in Figures 14.3 and 14.4. As stated by Shapiro, these cases illustrate the difficulty of correlating the microscopic appearances of the lungs in cases of stillbirth and early postnatal death with the results of hydrostatic tests.

These observations have been confirmed experimentally by Ham and Baldwin.[23]

The gradual differentiation and maturation of the fetal lung during gestation, with the development of fully opened alveoli at full term, has also been confirmed by Parmentier,[24] and by Kuroda et al[25] who described expanded alveoli in a stillborn (macerated) fetus (gestational age, 36 weeks).

According to Ham,[26] the lung attains a stage of development sometime during the fifth month, when it is gland-like in character. Up to this stage of prenatal development the alveoli appear as hollow round epithelial structures lined by cuboidal to columnar epithelial cells. After the fifth month, the epithelial cells of the alveoli gradually separate from one another and the capillaries in the alveolar walls bulge into the spaces between the separating epithelial cells. The rounded alveoli become enlarged and angular and gradually the gland-like appearance of the lung changes to the alveolar pattern of the postnatal lung. This development occurs *in utero* and is independent of extra-uterine respiration. The future alveoli are filled with amniotic fluid but with the onset of extra-uterine respiration at birth, the alveoli undergo progressive expansion and the fluid is displaced by air. Ham states that part of the amniotic fluid is drained away through the upper respiratory tract after birth and part is absorbed from the alveoli.

Ham confirms the view expressed by Shapiro that microscopic examinations of the lungs are of greater value in determining fetal age than in determining live birth. If sections of a lung show that it is gland-like in character (as in Fig. 14.2), it can be assumed that not only has the fetus not breathed but it has probably not advanced beyond two-thirds of its prenatal development. On the other hand, if the alveoli are expanded it cannot be assumed that fetus has breathed, but it can be stated that is has advanced beyond two-thirds of its prenatal development.

Sequestrated lung and intra-ocular transplants. Shapiro[20] studied the microscopic appearances of a portion of a sequestrated lung removed at operation on an infant aged 4 days. The relevant operative notes of the surgeon (Mr G. R. Crawshaw) read:

> A left sided thoracotomy was performed.
>
> There was a triangular defect posteriorly in the left leaf of the diaphragm, through which the bowel, the left kidney and the left suprarenal gland had herniated into the chest. The defect was the size of about 1 in. × 1½ in. and included the aortic hiatus.
>
> After reduction, a pink pedunculated elongated tumour was seen. It was about 1 in. × ¼ in., with its narrow pedicle running down through the diaphragmatic defect and inserted into the side of the aorta above the suprarenal artery. The pedicle consisted of an artery about the size of a digital artery, and a vein. It was divided and the tumour removed.

Microscopy of this portion of the tumour (sequestrated lung which was unconnected with the respiratory tract and attached by a vascular pedicle to the aorta) revealed all the structures of fully developed lung with bronchioles, terminal bronchioles, alveolar ducts and fully expanded alveoli (Fig. 14.6 and 14.7).

Potter and Bohlender[27] describe the microscopic appearances in two cases to ectopic lung tissue as at p. 386.

Potter[28] has also described alveolar ducts and alveoli in a sequestrated lobe of lung in which respiration was never established.

Waddell[29] transplanted fetal lung tissue obtained by hysterotomy from guinea-pigs, mice and rabbits into the anterior ocular chambers of adult guinea-pigs. The transplants underwent active growth, usually filling the anterior chamber. The transplants revealed well-developed alveolar structures with terminal bronchioli and bronchi.

The additional information provided by the microscopic appearances of sequestrated lung and intra-ocular transplants, confirms the suggestion that the lung is destined to develop its fully expanded alveolar pattern before parturition, independently of intra-uterine fetal respiratory movements and probably under the influence of organizers.

2. What was the state of maturity of the infant?

Gestation extends from the time of fertilization to the onset of labour, but gestational periods are usually estimated from the beginning of the last menstrual period to the onset of labour. The average duration of the menstruation–labour interval has been given as 280 days by Kenneth[30] and as 280 to 283 days by Hollenweger-Mayr.[31] Although menstruation–labour intervals as long as 331 days are recorded by Kenneth, Hollenweger-Mayr states that only two certain cases of a duration of pregnancy greater than 302 days are to be found in the literature.

Viability. From the medical standpoint an infant is usually considered to

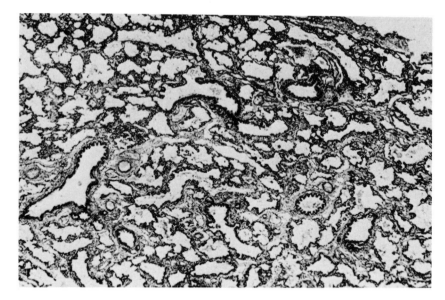

Fig. 14.6. Photomicrograph of sequestrated lung illustrating the presence of terminal bronchioles, respiratory bronchioles and alveoli. Haematoxylin and eosin (× 70) (see text).

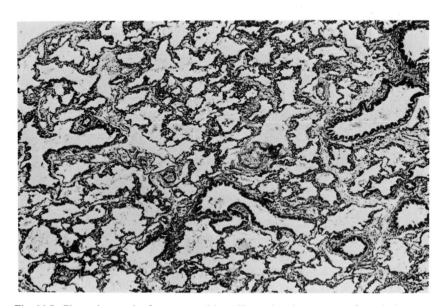

Fig. 14.7. Photomicrograph of sequestrated lung illustrating the presence of terminal bronchioles, respiratory bronchioles and alveoli. Haematoxylin and eosin (× 70) (see text).

be viable at the end of seven months of intra-uterine existence, but infants may survive if born at an earlier period.

Drugs (beta-adrenergic agents) can prolong the duration of pregnancy and postpone the onset of labour. They have rendered necessary a revision of the conventional obstetrical criteria of viability.

Estimation of maturity. An examination for the ossification centres in the bones of the foot and the lower end of the femur is the most reliable method of determining the state of maturity of a newly born infant.

The technique adopted for this examination has been described at page 380. Ossification centres usually appear in these bones at the following times: in the calcaneum at the end of the fifth month; in the talus at the end of the seventh month; in the distal epiphysis of the femur at the end of the ninth month. The centre in the distal epiphysis of the femur is about 0.6–0.8 cm in diameter at full term. The time of appearance of the centre in the cuboid is variable, but it is usually present at the end of the ninth month. The general appearance of the centres in the calcaneum, talus and lower end of the femur at full term is shown in Figure 14.8. The centres appear earlier in females. This influences the determination of fetal age.[32]

Owing to the variation in the length and weight of newly born infants, these factors cannot be relied upon in determining the state of maturity. The length of the hair or nails is of no value in the determination.

3. How long did the infant live?

The presence of food in the stomach and intestine indicates that the infant has lived long enough to be fed, and this fact may be of some value in determining the period that has elapsed since birth. The absence of meconium in the intestine suggests that an infant has probably lived for several hours. On the other hand, it should be noted that meconium may be found in the intestine up to about 48 hours after birth.

An examination of the umbilical cord may be of considerable value in determining the period that has elapsed since birth. The cord becomes desiccated about 24 hours after birth, and an area of inflammatory reaction appears at its attached end after approximately 40 hours. A zone of ulceration then appears at its attached end, and the cord is gradually separated off. This process is usually complete at the end of six days, but the time taken for complete separation may vary from about five to nine days.

4. How long has the infant been dead?

The estimation of this period is based upon the same factors that have been considered in the estimation of the post-mortem interval in adults (p. 46) subject to the modifications which occur in infants in the rate of development of post-mortem changes. These modifications have been dealt with in Chapter 1.

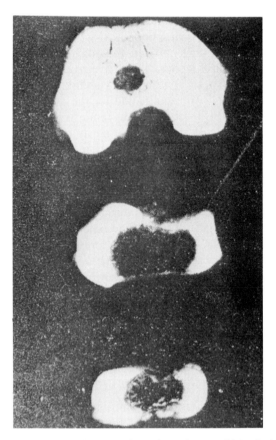

Fig. 14.8. Ossification centres at full term (from above downwards) in the lower end of the femur, in the calcaneum and in the talus.

5. What was the cause of death?

Death may be due to natural causes or to violence. Some of the causes of death from natural causes in infants have been referred to in Chapter 8. Although all types of violent death occur in infants, certain forms of homicide are seen more commonly than others. Deaths due to head injuries are seen frequently, and the features of these injuries are considered at pages 295–298.

Violent deaths in infants may be due to suffocation, throttling, strangulation, drowning, etc. The post-mortem findings in all these forms of death are essentially similar to the findings in adults and reference may be made to the descriptions of these conditions which have been given in Chapter 4.

CAFFEY'S SYNDROME OR 'THE BATTERED CHILD' SYNDROME

In 1946, Caffey[33] reported that he had found multiple fractures in the long bones in six infants suffering from chronic subdural haematoma. History of injury to the long bones as well as to the head was lacking in all cases. On the other hand there was no radiological or clinical evidence of general or localized skeletal disease which would have predisposed the bones to pathological fractures. Caffey noted that there were 23 fractures of the long bones in the six infants and Figure 14.9 taken from Caffey's paper, shows the distribution of the 23 fractures in the infants. Although Caffey stated that the long bone fractures appeared to be of traumatic origin, the traumatic episodes and the causal mechanism remained obscure.

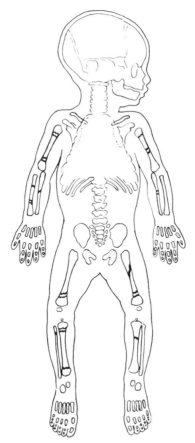

Fig. 14.9. Spot map of the skeleton showing the distribution of 23 fractures in six patients, described by Caffey[33] (see text).

Subsequent to the publication of Caffey's paper the syndrome was recognized by paediatricians and forensic pathologists, and several accounts of the condition have appeared in the literature.

In 1961, Dr Henry Kempe, at a Symposium of the American Academy of Pediatrics, proposed the term 'battered child syndrome' in order to direct attention to the seriousness of the problem. Since then, changes have been made to this denotation to include cases of neglect and emotional abuse of children. The term 'non-accidental injury' is now more generally accepted to denote the syndrome of child battering.

Describing the condition as 'the battered child' syndrome, Camps and Cameron[34] state that the condition arises:

> . . . where a child sustains injuries from one or more assaults by an adult associated with it. The more serious cases when recognized are fully investigated in life. A number, however, die from head injury and subdural haematoma with or without a fractured skull. A particular feature is the denial by the parent (or foster parent) of any injury. From recent investigations, the following facts emerge. A large proportion of the children fall within the age group 3–5 months as opposed to true infanticide when the child is new-born. In many cases there is a history of the child being 'off colour' and persistently crying. The clinical picture concerns a child, usually 3–5 months old, with slight predominance of males and often the first child and either illegitimate or unwanted. The injuries are multiple bruises on the head, trunk and limbs. Associated with them are fractures of long bones (especially femur and humerus) which should lead to X-ray of the whole body and may show old and recent fractures of the ribs and other bones including separation of metaphyseal flake fractures. The most serious lesions and hence the cause of death or disability are subdural haemorrhage, with or without fractured skull, and traumatic rupture of the liver and injuries to the viscera of the upper abdomen.

Although one of the most notable features of the battering syndrome is that it tends to be 'non-instrumental', i.e. the assaults being carried out by the unaided hands of the adult, without intervention of instruments, there are many exceptions to this, as, for example, the use of feeding bottles, pokers, belts, etc. The general rule remains, however, that direct manual violence is the most common method of injury.

Though the spectrum of injuries is very wide, certain recurrent features are of great diagnostic value:

1. Bruises, abrasions and lacerations;
2. Eye injuries;
3. Head injuries;
4. Visceral injuries; and
5. Burns.

1. Bruises, abrasions and lacerations. Soft tissue injuries are almost universal, with the head, face and neck most commonly affected. Bruises, abrasions and lacerations are frequently present. Multiplicity of bruising and bruising of differing ages are particularly significant.

Bruising of the scalp and forehead may be associated with underlying skull and brain injuries. Injury to the scalp may not be overtly apparent but extensive subaponeurotic haemorrhage may be present. The presence of bald patches on the scalp due to the hair being pulled out (traumatic alopecia), is considered by some[35] as being diagnostic of the 'battering syndrome'.

Of particular diagnostic significance is bruising of the lips, especially the upper lip, commonly with lacerations of the inner aspect. The frenulum is often ruptured and detachment of the inner surface of the lip from the gum margin is a noticeable feature, suggesting slapping or punching in the mouth region.

Bruising of the cheeks and ears is also due to slapping with the adult hand. Bruising of the neck and sides of the chest may sometimes reveal fingertip pressure marks. Symmetrical bruises beneath the angle of the jaw may be found, where the neck is held on each side, in order to immobilize the face, while the latter is being assaulted with the other hand.

If the chest is compressed while the victim is shaken violently, there may be evidence of bruising in relation to the skin of the axilla and lower ribs, often in association with multiple fractures of the posterior third of the ribs.

Bruising of the abdomen is very common and, after head injuries, rupture of abdominal organs is the second commonest fatal lesion. The bruises may be of fingertip size or larger bruises may be found, both extending from the sternum to the pubic region. Marked internal injuries may be present in the absence of overt abdominal bruising.

As the limbs form convenient 'handles' for the battering parent to grasp, the limbs may also show multiple bruising, especially over the forearms, upper arms and legs, and frequently the bruises are present bilaterally. It should be noted that delineation of the superficial bruising may be noted better the day after the performance of the autopsy.

Human bites[36] appear to be the prerogative of a battering mother. A bite mark may be considered to be analogous to a finger print, and may be used for identification purposes. Further, washings obtained within 24 hours of the bite, may provide details as to the blood group of the assailant.

The possibility that the victim was the initiator of bite marks should be considered if the marks are located such as to be compatible with having been self-inflicted. Anderson and Hudson[37] quoted such a case where the victim bit her arm, possibly to stifle her cries.

2. Eye injuries. Battering parents often ascribe black eyes as being due to an accidental fall. A fall against a flat surface would tend to produce periorbital bruising and not a bruise of the eyelids. It is most improbable for a child to sustain two black eyes in one fall. Subconjunctival haemorrhages may be present, and if the child also has a squint, the possibility of a subdural haematoma and raised intracranial pressure should be considered clinically. Other intra-ocular lesions[38] include retinal separation, lens displacement, retinal haemorrhage, subhyaloid haemorrhages and vitreous haemorrhages.

3. Head injuries. Head injuries are common and fractured skull[39] and brain damage is a most frequent cause of death. Subdural haemorrhage is common. Parenchymal brain damage also accounts for the high incidence rate of permanent cerebral dysfunction that may occur.

4. Visceral injuries. After head injuries, visceral injuries are the next most common cause of death. Rupture of the liver, intestine or mesentery, accounts for most of the fatalities and is produced by blow to the front of the abdominal wall. Extensive internal injuries may be present with minimal external signs of injury. Tears of the liver as well as rupture of the third part of the duodenum in relation to the anterior aspect of the spinal column, may occur in infants with few external signs of injury. Lacerations of the liver, most frequently present over the posterior aspect of the liver, may be associated with marked intraperitoneal haemorrhage. The latter may also occur secondary to tears of the mesentery to the small bowel, where it is stretched across the prominence of the lumbar spine.

5. Burns. Burns are commonly present and, if localized and well demarcated, a high index of suspicion should be aroused as to a battering aetiology.

Punctate burns, often accompanied by old scars, may indicate deliberate stubbing of cigarette ends upon the child's skin. A child may be punished for continually soiling its napkins by being seated on a hot stove, electric radiator, etc., or being dipped into very hot fluid. The lesions resulting from the latter method will show a distinct fluid level passing across the buttocks onto the heels. Immersion burns, distributed over the hands of an infant are highly suspicious of an abusive aetiology. Scalding burns of flung hot liquid may be difficult to disprove as having been produced as a result of an alleged accident.

In both fatal and non-fatal cases of battering, radiography is all important and in every suspect fatal case, whole body X-ray must be performed before the formal autopsy. Radiography provides information about general skeletal damage, especially as regards different times of infliction, and lesions of different ages are suggested by the stage of healing and degree of callus formation. As healing fractures are found very late in the clinical course, Galleno and Oppenheim[40] suggest that more emphasis should be placed on the specific nature of the fractures.

Characteristic radiographic lesions associated with baby battering include:

1. Separation of epiphyses, especially around the elbow and knee joint;
2. Subperiostial calcification in relation to periosteal haemorrhages;
3. Fractured ribs, frequently multiple and situated near the posterior angle of the ribs;
4. Metaphyseal fragmentation;
5. Fractures of the clavicle; and
6. Chipping of the corners of the epiphyses at large joints.

Many of these lesions are produced by rotational strains imposed upon the limbs. Fractures of the shafts of long bones may result from direct blows, either from a fist blow or from the child hitting a fixed object. Lower extremity fractures in 'non-weight-bearing' children and bilateral acute fractures (as seen in high-velocity injuries) are highly suggestive of the battered child syndrome.

Fractures of the spine and pelvis are uncommon.[41]

The differential diagnosis of the syndrome is extensive and the possibility of osteomyelitis, leukaemia, congenital syphilis, scurvy, vitamin A intoxication, rickets, juvenile osteoporosis with stress fractures, paralytic disease with fractures, congenital pain indifference and osteogenesis imperfecta may have to be considered.

Mortality and morbidity

Unfortunately, despite increasing public awareness, this syndrome still remains a major cause of death and disability among children.

Gil[42] documented that 53% of injuries were not of a serious nature, 37% were serious but without sequelae and approximately 5% produced permanent damage. According to Christoffel et al,[43] the mean death rate due to definite inflicted injury per 100 000 population in the 1–4 years of age group is 0.5 in developing countries (s.d. = 0.5) and 1 in developed countries (s.d. = 1.3).

At autopsy, it may be necessary to incise the skin in order to detect the presence of areas of deep bruising. Care should be taken not to confuse artefactual lesions with those produced by battering. As the body cools after death, the subcutaneous fat congeals, and tight clothing may produce skin identations, particularly on the neck, which may simulate features of ligature strangulation or hanging. Elastic bands may produce depressions, as well as abraded areas, resembling areas of bruising. A mongolian spot must also be distinguished from an area of bruising.

REFERENCES

1 Reg. vs. Flattery, 2 Q.B.D. 410, 1877.
2 Smith S. Forensic Medicine. 9th ed. London: Churchill. 1949: p 307.
3 Sunderman F W, Boerner F. Normal Values in Clinical Medicine. Philadelphia: Saunders. 1950: p 390.
4 Hansen P F. Determination of the prostatic acid phosphatase as a new method for the medico-legal demonstration of sperm spots. Acta Path Microbiol Scand 1946; 23: 187–214.
5 Kaye S. Acid phosphatase test for identification of seminal stain. J Lab Clin Med 949; 34: 728–732.
6 Marcinkowski T, Przybylski, Z. Seminal stains: A simple device for their determination. J Forens Med 1966; 13: 130–133.
7 Gluckman J. The study of seminal stains by means of ultrasonic apparatus. J Forens Med 1968; 15: 144–147.

8 Willot G M, Allard J E. Spermatozoa: Their persistence after sexual intercourse. Forens Sci Int 1982; 19: 135–154

9 Glaister J. Medical Jurisprudence and Toxicology. 13th ed. Edinburgh: Churchill Livingstone. 1973: p 444.

10 Shapiro H A. In: The great debate: Abortion in the South African context. Oosthuizen G C, Abbott G, Notelowitz M. eds. Human Sciences Research Council Publication Series No. 47. Cape Town: Howard Timmins. 1974: pp 231–240.

11 Gordon, I. Fatal air embolism in criminal abortion. Clin Proc Cape Town 1945; 4: 135–140.

12 Shennan T. Post-mortems and morbid anatomy. London: Arnold. 1935: p 153.

13 Duncan-Taylor J E. The post-mortem diagnosis of air embolism by radiography. Br Med J 1952: 890–893.

14 Forbes G. Air embolism as a complication of vaginal douching in pregnancy. Br Med J 1944; 2: 529–531.

15 Shapiro H A. The diagnosis of death from delayed air embolism. J Forens Med 1965; 12: 3–7.

16 Shapiro H A, Zwarenstein H. A rapid test for pregnancy on Xenopus laevis. Proc Roy Soc S Afr Oct 18;1933.

17 Rex vs. Mathews, C.P.D. 8, 1943.

18 Gardiner F G, Lansdown C W H. South African criminal law and procedure. 5th ed. Cape Town: Juta. 1946.

19 Baar H S. The post-mortem examination of the newborn infant. Br Med Bull 1946; 4: 178–188.

20 Shapiro H A. The limited value of microscopy of lung tissue in the diagnosis of live and still birth. Clin Proc 1947; 6: 149–158.

21 Shapiro H A. Medico-legal mythology: some popular forensic fallacies. J Forens Med 1954; 1: 144–169.

22 Shapiro H A. Microscopy of human foetal lung and the diagnosis of postnatal respiration. In: Legal medicine annual 1976. Wecht C H. ed. New York: Appleton-Century-Crofts. 1977: pp 34–52.

23 Ham A W, Baldwin K W. A histological study of the development of the lung with particular reference to the nature of the alveoli. Anat Rec 1941; 81: 363–379.

24 Parmentier R. L'Aeration neonatale due poumon. Revue Belge de Pathologie et de Medecine experimentale 1962; 29: 121–244.

25 Kuroda S, Nagamori H, Ebe M, Sasaki M. Medico-legal studies on the fetus and infant: with special references to histological characteristics of the lungs of liveborn and still-born infants. Tohoku J. Exp Med 1965; 85: 40–54.

26 Ham. A W. Histology. Philadelphia: Lippincott. 1950: pp 448–496.

27 Potter E L, Bohlender G P. Intra-uterine respiration in relation to development of the fetal lung. Am J Obstet Gynecol 1941; 42: 14–22.

28 Potter E L. Pathology of the fetus and the newborn. Chicago: Year Book Publishers. 1952: p 262.

29 Waddell W R. Organoid differentiation of the fetal lung: a histologic study of the differentiation of mammalian fetal lung in utero and in transplants. Arch Path 1949; 47: 227–247.

30 Kenneth J H. Gestation periods: A table and bibliography. Edinburgh: Oliver & Boyd. 1943: p 9.

31 Hollenweger-Mayr B. The upper limit of duration of pregnancy in paternity cases. Zbl Gynäk 1949; 71: 1067–1075.

32 Shapiro H A. Medico-Legal mythology. J Forens Med 1954; 1: 152–155.

33 Caffey J. Multiple fractures in the long bones of infants suffering from chronic subdural hematoma. Am J Roentgenol Rad Therapy 1946; 56: 163–173.

34 Camps F E, Cameron J M. Practical forensic medicine. London: Hutchinson. 1971: pp 191–192.

35 Neimann N, Manciaux M, Rabouille D et al. Les enfants victimes de sevices (maltreated children). Pediatrie 1968; 861–875.

36 Furness J. A general review of bite mark evidence. Am J Forens Med Path 1981; 2:49.

37 Anderson W R, Hudson R P. Self-inflicted bite marks in the battered child syndrome. Forens Sci 1976; 7:71.

38 Mushin A S. Ocular damage in the battered baby syndrome. Brit Med Jour 1971; 3:402.
39 Hobbs C J. Skull fracture and the diagnosis of abuse. Arch Dis Child 1984; 59: 246–252.
40 Galleno H, Oppenheim W L. The battered child syndrome revisited. Orthop Clin 1982; 162: 11–19.
41 Cullen J C. Spinal lesions in battered babies. J Bone J Surg 1975; 57B: 364–366.
42 Gil D G. Physical abuse of children. Findings and implications of a nationwide survey. Paediatrics 1969; 44: 857–864.
43 Christoffel K K, et al. Epidemiology of fatal child abuse: International morbidity data. J Chron Dis 1981; 34: 57–64.

15

Medico-legal aspects of acute alcoholic intoxication

The intoxicating component in alcoholic drink is ethanol (C_2H_5OH). It has a specific gravity of 0.79, i.e. 1 ml of alcohol weighs 0.79 g. The alcohol content of some common beverages is shown in Table 15.1.

When an alcohol-containing beverage is drunk, alcohol can be absorbed directly into the blood stream from the stomach (about 20%), especially if this organ does not contain food. Such alcohol as has not been absorbed from the stomach (about 80%)[1] passes through to the next part of the digestive tract (the small gut) from which it is then absorbed into the blood stream.

The alcohol in the blood draining from the stomach and intestines passes (for entirely anatomical reasons) to the liver, where it is destroyed by a specific enzyme at a constant rate. Then it flows to the venous side of the heart, whence it is directed through the lungs and back to the arterial side of the heart, from which it is delivered through the arteries to all the organs and tissues of the body, amongst other things, the brain.

From the forensic point of view, it is primarily the action of ethanol on the brain that is of practical importance. The alterations in the functions of this bodily system may interfere with the ability of a person to carry out

Table 15.1 Approximate percentages of pure alcohol in certain beverages commonly consumed

Nature of beverage	Alcohol content	
	% by volume	% by weight
Light beer (lager or pilsener)	4–6	3–5
Heavy beer (ale or stout)	6–8	5–7
Natural wines (claret or hock types)	9–14	7–12
Fortified wines (port, sherry or muscadel types)	16–20	13–16
Liqueurs	Approx. 30	24
Spirits (whisky, brandy, gin, etc.)	43*	35

* In many countries, 42.7% is the minimum legal limit of absolute alcohol in potable spirits, and is, therefore, also the maximum strength which is usually supplied commercially. From *Medical Jurisprudence*, by Gordon, Turner and Price, 3rd ed. 1953, p. 765. By permission of the publishers, E. and S. Livingstone, Ltd.

tasks which require normal judgment and normal co-ordination of muscular movements.

The action on the brain depends, among other things, on the amount of alcohol in the blood reaching the brain. This blood concentration is influenced by a variety of factors.

Absorption from the intestines

It is important to appreciate that only alcohol which has been absorbed into the blood stream has any effect on behaviour. Any alcohol which is in the cavity of the stomach or the intestines is still virtually outside the body and can, therefore, be neglected in assessing the influence of this drug on behaviour. Its only significance is the evidence it provides that alcohol has been ingested.

Alcohol in the stomach may, however, diffuse into the blood and the tissues after death, and so lead to the estimation of higher blood levels than actually existed during life, if blood samples are taken from parts into which post-mortem diffusion has taken place.

Alcohol is one of the few substances which can be absorbed directly from the stomach. Its absorption, however, is slower from the stomach than from the small gut. On the other hand, its absorption from the stomach is faster when the stomach is empty than when it contains food.

Food affects the rate of absorption in varying degree, probably by delaying the emptying time of the stomach. Starch, protein and fatty foods have all been shown to delay absorption of alcohol from the intestines into the blood. A mixed meal can depress the maximum concentration of the blood alcohol by about half.[2] Drinking milk has a similar effect.[3] Nickolls[4] states that with the presence of food in the stomach as much as 17–20% of the alcohol ingested appears to escape absorption and *never appears in the blood stream*. Alha[5] refers to convincing evidence that food ingested with alcohol may prevent 10–20% of the ingested alcohol from being absorbed.

When alcohol is ingested in man in a diluted form, it is absorbed more slowly than when taken in a concentrated form.[6] A lower maximum level is attained in these circumstances, indicating a slower rate of absorption. Not all workers agree with this observation.[5] There is also evidence that alcohol is absorbed most rapidly at concentrations of 10–20%, lower and higher concentrations being absorbed more slowly.[7] Harichaux et al[8] state that alcohol in weak concentrations (12%) accelerates gastric emptying in man, whereas high concentrations (45%) retard it.

The type of beverage also affects the rate of absorption, quite apart from the difference in alcohol concentration. When whisky is diluted to the same strength as stout, the alcohol is absorbed more rapidly and rises to a higher level in the case of the whisky. This indicates that substances are present in stout which retard absorption from the gut, probably by an effect on the emptying time of the stomach. The nature of these substances is not precisely known.[9]

This principle may be the basis for the claim that 'mixing of drinks' induces greater intoxication than would be expected from the amount consumed. In such circumstances, substances may be present or may be formed which affect the rate of emptying of the stomach, with more rapid absorption of the alcohol contained in the drinks.

However, absorption is generally complete in a matter of one to three hours, irrespective of the concentration of the alcohol and the type of beverage. After absorption is complete, there is an equilibrium between the alcohol concentration in the blood and in the tissues. It is from blood samples taken at this period that certain calculations are often made. Shortly after taking a drink, e.g. after 15 minutes, the level in arterial blood may be 40–60% higher than the level in peripheral venous blood, and this may persist for the first hour of drinking.[10] But after absorption has been completed, the alcohol level in venous blood is slightly higher than in capillary (i.e. arterial) blood.[11] Blood samples should therefore only be taken after equilibrium has been established.

Habituation or tolerance also influences absorption. Habituated heavy drinkers absorb alcohol more rapidly than do abstainers. This may partly be due to an increased rate of absorption of the alcohol as a result of a more rapid emptying of the stomach. This difference does not apply between moderate drinkers and abstainers.

The emotional state of the subject may influence the contractions of the stomach and so affect its emptying time and thus the rate of absorption.

Drugs, e.g. benzedrine or atropine, may slow the rate of absorption of alcohol, probably, in part, by retarding the emptying time of the stomach.

Alha[12] claims that alcohol is absorbed less rapidly (delayed maximum) by younger (under 35) than by older (over 35 years) subjects; but Lofthus found no difference in the tolerance of two such groups.[13]

Gastrectomy may lead to a greatly accelerated rate of absorption of alcohol.[14] Fleming et al[15] noted accelerated peak blood alcohol concentrations after truncal vagotomy and a drainage operation. They suggested that the acceleration in alcohol absorption was probably due to an increased rate of gastric emptying after surgery.

Absorption by inhalation. Blood levels may also be affected by the inhalation of alcohol. Lester and Greenberg,[16] in determinations of the percentage of alcohol absorbed from the inspired air, showed that on the average about 62% of the alcohol was absorbed. The concentration of alcohol attained in the blood is proportional to the concentration of the alcohol in the inspired air and to the rate of ventilation, and inversely proportional to the weight of the subject.

The inhalation of alcohol, under certain conditions, can result in intoxication.

The weight of the subject. When the same amount of alcohol is drunk by a group of persons, the concentration of the alcohol reached in the blood is not the same in the different persons in the experiment. This is due to an important extent to the amount of tissue in the body capable of absorbing alcohol. Bone and fat do not, apparently, absorb alcohol as the water-containing tissues do. The fatty, bony or muscular nature of the subject is therefore of great importance. It is also recognized than in the same subject the alcohol concentration after the same dose of alcohol rises to different levels on different occasions.[17-20]

Widmark attempted to calculate what fraction of the body weight can absorb alcohol. He found this fraction to be lower in women than in men and that it had a range from 0.51 to 0.85. Other investigators have found even larger ranges. Alha[21] claims that in more than 80% of his subjects the fraction had a value between 0.61 and 0.80, but the range extended from 0.52 to 0.89. The fraction may also vary in one and the same person at different times and seems to be independent of the amount of alcohol drunk.

Widmark's findings indicate that corpulent subjects have a lower fraction than have thin subjects. As it is difficult to assess the proportion of fat and bone in any person, the body weight of the subject is not necessarily a reliable guide to the amount of tissue into which the alcohol is absorbed.

It is a not uncommon practice to assume that about two-thirds of the body weight is available for the absorption of alcohol in a person of average weight, e.g. 70 kg (150 lb), under hypothetical average conditions. The results of such calculations are of interest as generalizations but do not necessarily have any application to an individual case.

McCallum and Scroggie[22] have shown that, in fact, the blood alcohol concentration does not decrease uniformly as the weight of the subject increases. These observations invalidate procedures for correcting the alcohol value obtained by adjusting it according to a formula depending on the body weight of the subject. This unwarranted adjustment is, for example, recommended in reports published by the British Medical Association.[23,24] It is also the theoretical but unjustified basis of the calculations in the Tables drawn up by Sapeika[25] for the so-called simple determination of the amount of alcohol ingested by an individual.

It is thus impossible to make accurate calculations and probably undesirable to attempt to do so.

The excretion of alcohol

Alcohol is eliminated through all the bodily routes of excretion. About 5% of ingested alcohol is excreted in the breath and about 5% in the urine. Thus, in ordinary circumstances, with the ingestion of large doses of alcohol, about 10% is eliminated in the breath and the urine. Negligible amounts are eliminated in the sweat and the faeces. The small amount excreted in the saliva is usually swallowed and therefore does not affect the position.

Newman[26] has pointed out that under extreme conditions, e.g. in the tropics or in a boiler room, the secretion of sweat may reach such proportions as to be a significant factor in the excretion of alcohol.

Factors influencing the destruction of alcohol in the body

In general, about 90% of the alcohol ingested is destroyed in the body. This is effected mainly in the liver, where the alcohol is broken down via acetaldehyde and acetic acid (vinegar) to carbon dioxide and water. From this it is clear that the accumulation of aldehydes and acetic acid in the body, from sources other than alcohol, may wrongly be estimated as representing alcohol when non-specific methods of alcohol estimation are employed.

In practice, hardly any factors influence the rate at which alcohol is destroyed in the body. Proteins and the amino acids derived from them may have a specific effect in that, when given with alcohol, a lower maximum is reached in the blood and the decline to zero is also more rapid.[27] Starches, fats, the inhalation of oxygen or carbon dioxide, the presence of a fever and drugs such as barbiturates and caffeine (contained in tea and coffee) have no appreciable effect on the rate of destruction of alcohol in the body.

There is no good evidence that habituation to alcohol increases its rate of destruction in the body of the habituated subject.

Insulin, however, may accelerate the fall of the blood alcohol concentration appreciably—a phenomenon not observed in patients with cirrhosis of the liver (an organ where presumably the main destruction of alcohol takes place and which is one of the important sites of action of insulin).[28]

Intravenous infusions of fructose have been claimed to accelerate alcohol oxidation.[29] This has been challenged by Camps and Robinson.[30]

Carpenter et al[31] have shown that muscular exercise does not have any effect on the rate of destruction of alcohol in the body, a conclusion abundantly confirmed by Nyman and Palmlov.[32]

The rate of combustion of alcohol is generally regarded as constant, but it varies in different persons and in the two sexes. Newman[33] has also postulated that this constancy does not hold above a concentration of 100 mg per 100 ml. At higher levels the rate at which alcohol is metabolized is increased. Widmark found the rate of combustion in man to vary from 4.1 to 11.1 g per hour. He gives an average of 7.3 g for males and 5.3 g for females. The regulation of the rate of metabolism of ethanol has been reviewed by Wallgren and Barry.[34]

Bonnichsen et al[35] state that the average hourly oxidation rate of alcohol is affected by the body weight of the subject. The oxidation rate increases by about 0.7 g per hour with each 10 kg of body weight.

Mellanby[36] reported in dogs an average rate of oxidation of 2.5 ml (i.e.

2 g) of alcohol per hour (i.e. 0.185 ml per kg body weight per hour); but in man this can obviously be, according to Widmark, as high as almost 14 ml per hour and as low as 5 ml per hour.

Isselbacher and Greenberger,[37] reviewing the rate of alcohol metabolism, state that alcohol can be metabolized at a rate of 100–200 mg per kg body weight per hour. This rate may be as high as 240 mg per kg per hour. The blood alcohol level can decrease between 10 and 25 mg per 100 ml per hour.

When this considerable range is taken into account, the arbitrary nature of statements can be appreciated which claim that 10–12 ml of alcohol can be destroyed per hour by 'the average man'. It is the assumption about these arithmetical averages that underlies the claim that 'the average man can destroy the equivalent of a small whisky per hour (one fluid ounce)'.[38]

The level of alcohol in the blood

As a result of the factors influencing absorption, metabolism and excretion, the alcohol concentraton rises steeply in the blood, followed by a more gradual upward slope to reach a maximum, which is more or less distinct. After this peak there is an irregularly curved fall to the period of diffusion equilibrium. This takes place over 15 to 30 minutes. Then the alcohol level in the blood falls progressively in a rectilinear fashion (elimination phase) until it has all been eliminated from the body.[39]

The typical blood alcohol pattern following the consumption of a single alcoholic drink is shown in Figure 15.1.

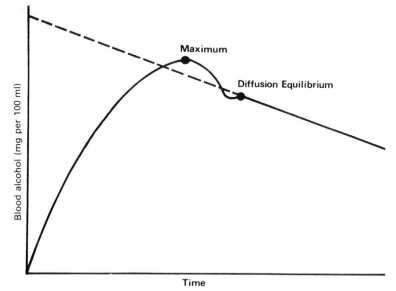

Fig. 15.1. Typical blood alcohol pattern following consumption of a single drink. (After Alha, op. cit. p. 12.)

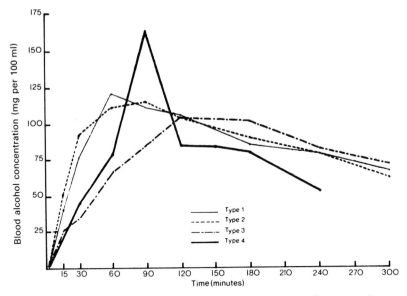

Fig. 15.2A. Variations in the type of blood alcohol curve (after Alha[40]). *Type 1.* A steep rise with a distinct peak; *Type 2.* A steep rise without a distinct peak; *Type 3.* A slow rise without a distinct peak; *Type 4.* A distinct and high peak with a subsequent depression. The curves in Figure 15.2A were obtained after an alcohol dose of 1 g per kg body weight.

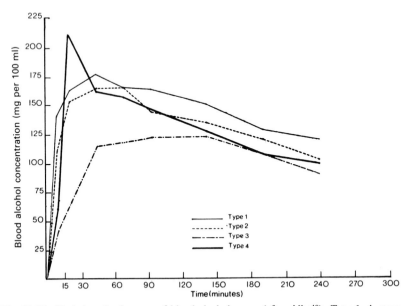

Fig. 15.2B. Variations in the type of blood alcohol curve (after Alha[40]). *Type 1.* A steep rise with a distinct peak; *Type 2.* A steep rise without a distinct peak; *Type 3.* A slow rise without a distinct peak; *Type 4.* A distinct and high peak with a subsequent depression. The curves in Figure 15.2B were obtained after an alcohol dose of 1.25 g per kg body weight.

Extensive studies by various authors have established that the peak concentration in the blood is reached within about 1 to 2 hours after ingestion. It may be reached earlier or even later; and not all persons react in the same way as is illustrated in the case of Fig. 15.1. This[40] is illustrated in Figures 15.2A and 15.2B.

Type 1: There may be a steep rise, with a distinct peak.

Type 2: There may be a steep rise, but without a distinct peak.

Type 3: There may be a slow rise without a distinct peak.

Type 4: There may be a distinct and high peak with a subsequent depression.

Alha[41] found in 12% of his blood alcohol curves, considerable irregularities in the post-absorptive phase. Shumate *et al*[42] have made similar observations. They noted repeatedly an unstable period during the first hours after ingestion of the alcohol was completed (Fig. 15.3). The steeple or peak effect observed by Alha and by Shumate *et al* is not peculiar to alcohol. It can also occur after the absorption of glucose, as may be seen when glucose tolerance tests are carried out.[43]

PERCENTAGE

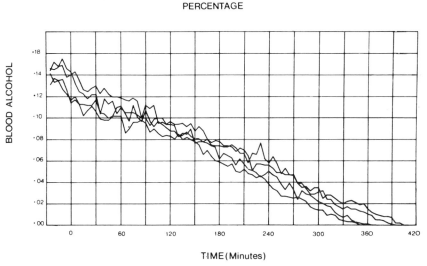

Fig. 15.3 Observed fluctuations in alcohol concentration. Data for four tests on a female subject. (After Shumate *et al*[42].)

These studies indicate that it is fallacious, in theoretical calculations derived from a known value of blood alcohol at a particular time, to apply to an individual, conclusions which are based on statistical generalizations.

Herbich and Prokop[44] emphasize the difficulty or impossibility of determining the amount of alcohol consumed or the course of the blood alcohol curve from a single subsequent estimation. Bayly and McCallum[45] also conclude that 'an accurate assessment cannot be made of the blood alcohol concentration in an individual at some time prior to the taking of a blood sample'.

Bowden,[46] reporting on the situation in Sweden, states:

> The position has been reached where scientifically it has been decided that it is not possible to determine what the blood alcohol level was at the time of driving from an analysis of the blood at a period later. This is a highly important point, properly appreciated in Sweden. It is believed at the Government laboratory in Stockholm that unsatisfactory assumptions have to be made before a scientist can start to calculate back to the time of driving, and an investigation of many cases has shown that the information produced, upon which the assumptions are made, is not reliable. In the words of the authority here: 'We will not do it; we cannot say with scientific accuracy what his blood (level) was at the time of driving'.

A report of a Special Committee of the British Medical Association entitled *The Medico-Legal Investigation of the Drinking Driver*[47] states, on the question of back calculation:

> . . . we advise strongly against the court permitting any 'back calculation' to determine how much higher the blood alcohol concentration must have been at the material time. In fact the rate of elimination of alcohol, both between different individuals and in the same individual at different times, varies to some extent and an exercise of this kind cannot, in our opinion, be justified,* although we are aware that it is the accepted practice in some other countries. Conversely, if the suspect is known to have taken alcohol just prior to being detained the possibility must be borne in mind that the blood alcohol concentration was still rising at the time the sample was taken.

THE CLINICAL CONSEQUENCES OF DRINKING TOXICATING LIQUOR

The disturbance in behaviour is due to the influence of alcohol on the central nervous system. This depends primarily on the extent to which the brain is affected.

The clinical signs and symptoms

These will, on the whole, be more marked as the alcohol concentration in the tissues increases. They will therefore vary, amongst other things: (1) with the amount of alcohol consumed; (2) with the period of time after the ingestion of the alcohol; (3) with the tolerance of the subject to alcohol.

It is claimed that the degree of intoxcation for the same level of alcohol is more marked during the phase of getting drunk than in the phase of sobering up.[48]

---

* Dubowski K M. *Unsettled Issues and Practices in Chemical Testing for Alcohol*. In: *Alcohol and Road Traffic*, London: British Medical Association. 1963: p 208.
Elbel H, Schleyer F. *Blutalkohol. 2nd ed*. Stuttgart: Georg Thieme Verlag. 1956: p 59.

The departure from normal is usually tested by a clinical examination of the subject, directed particularly to the way in which the nervous system has been affected in respect of acute mental and motor deterioration.

Non-medical evidence about the conduct of the person concerned may be extremely important and may, very properly, be considered by the Court in relation to the diagnosis, especially as it may indicate the nature of the behaviour at a time well before the clinical examination was made by the medical practitioner.

Alcohol acts pharmacologically as a depressant of the central nervous system. The normal discipline and controlled conduct of the average person is due to restraining influences which the higher centres of the brain exercise. When sufficient alcohol has been drunk to affect these higher centres, the normal restraints and inhibitions are removed. This is one of the earliest effects of alcoholic intoxication and may show itself in a variety of ways, e.g. garrulity, impairment of judgment, recklessness, etc.

As the degree of alcoholic intoxication advances, other symptoms and signs manifest themselves, mainly in relation to the effect on the nervous system.

Statutory forms are usually a guide to the medical practitioner for the examination of a person alleged to be drunk or under the influence of liquor. An analysis of such forms reveals that the observations to which the practitioner directs his attention deal largely with external appearances and the evidence of disturbances of the nervous system.

It is by now fairly generally recognized that the smell of alcohol on the breath, the pulse rate, the dilatation of the pupils and the colour of the face give no measure of the degree (if any) of intoxication.[49–52]

The smell of alcohol on the breath

Smith[52] states that one can have the odour of an alcoholic beverage on the breath at a time when there is no alcohol in the body. It is not the alcohol *per se* which imparts an odour to the breath, but the other non-alcoholic constituents in the beverage that give it the characteristic flavour of a wine, whisky, liqueur or beer. The odour of these substances can persist in the breath for many hours after the alcohol has left the body.

Reflexes

Observations on the pupils are completely subjective and consequently not of much value except in cases of coma (when the clinical problem is smallest). Kestenbaum[53] states that the normal pupil may react to light by contracting promptly or sluggishly.

Tendon reflexes may normally vary from being unobtainable to very brisk. They are therefore of no particular value in these cicumstances.

The conjunctiva

The appearance of the conjunctiva also presents difficulty as an absolute sign. It is well known that, e.g. fatigue and exposure may cause reddening of the conjunctiva. The reddened conjunctiva may also be a normal appearance.

Co-ordination

Very important observations are those made on the integrity of the nervous and the muscular systems, when tested for the co-ordination of fine movements and of grosser movements, e.g. balance, gait and speech.

There is, however, a remarkable variation in the degree of response from subject to subject. Jetter[54] states:

> When it is realized that at 0.40 per cent alcohol, a concentration close to the lethal point, an individual may show so little effects as to be adjudged sober by our criteria, or, on the other hand, that he may be in coma at this same level, it becomes evident that there exists a marked variation in the individual's reaction to alcohol.

A further study of an additional 800 cases confirmed Jetter in his views about individual tolerance.[55]

Hammond *et al*[56] report the case of a White female 23 years old, weighing 56.7 kg, who was found (15 minutes after admission to hospital) to have a blood alcohol of 780 mg per 100 ml. She was discharged 11 hours after admission with a blood alcohol level of 190 mg per 100 ml, fully coherent, with a neurological examination regarded as normal and with no evidence of alcoholic intoxication. The validity of the gas chromatographic analyses employed to determine the alcohol concentration was established by simultaneous assay of appropriate control solutions of ethanol standards of known concentration.

Van Ieperen[57] reports a case of a 55-year-old male farm worker weighing 40 kg, who was known to be a heavy drinker and who died from multiple injuries almost immediately after being knocked down by a motor car*.

Post-mortem analysis of a blood sample taken after death from the left femoral vein, and placed in a container containing an anti-coagulant and a 1% concentration of sodium fluoride, revealed a blood alcohol concentration of 850 mg per 100 ml. A gas chromatographic analysis was done, using two different columns.

The foregoing two cases illustrate the remarkable tolerance which certain persons can develop to ethanol, as measured by gas chromatography.

---

* An adult male is reported (in the Journal of the Danish Medical Association) to have drunk some 2 litres of whiskey in a suicide attempt. His blood alcohol reached 1130 mg per 100 ml. He recovered from his coma on the fifth day and was considered normal after six weeks of treatment. (*Natal Mercury*, Durban, 15 April 1982.)

The same person may also vary in his response to alcohol at different times. Rabinowitch[58,59] cites examples of intoxication at as low a level as 50 mg per 100 ml, and on another occasion no evidence of intoxication at 291 mg per 100 ml.

He also reported[18] the effects of alcohol in the original Siamese twins (Chang and Eng, born 1811; died in 1874). At the time of the initial post-mortem dissection of the twins, the post-mortem injection of a dye revealed that it passed freely from one liver into the other. It is known that Chang not only drank to excess, but was frequently 'drunk', but that, despite this, Eng never felt the effects of the drunkenness. On the basis of this initial report, Rabinowitch states that the twins provide 'unique evidence of different effects of the same amount of alcohol in the same person'. However, reference to the complete autopsy report as published in 1875 by Allen,[19] shows that a careful dissection of the injected blood vessel proved it to be a terminal twig of the portal system of Chang, did not pass, as such, across the band and broke up into minute branches before reaching the liver of Eng. There were some minor vascular anomalies in the band, but it is apparent from Allen's report that Chang and Eng had independent circulations. This fact is supported by Luckhardt[20] who states that the findings would seem to indicate 'that there was no free interchange in their circulations'. Controverting the view of Rabinowitch, Luckhardt states: 'Chang drank pretty heavily—at times getting drunk; but Eng never felt any influence from the debauch of his brother—a seemingly conclusive proof that there was no free interchange in their circulations.'

In evaluating the clinical effects of alcohol consumption, it is desirable to distinguish between evidence indicating that alcohol has been ingested and evidence indicating that the functions of the central nervous system have been affected adversely.

THE CORRELATION OF THE CLINICAL DEGREE OF INTOXICATION WITH THE BLOOD ALCOHOL LEVEL

The diagnosis of the alleged drunken state is often beset with genuine difficulty. It is generally agreed that the problem would be simplfied very considerably, in certain cases, if the blood of the accused person were examined chemically to determine its alcohol content. If the result of the chemical test is negative, or nearly so, it will substantiate the claims of the innocent; if it is positive, it may (in certain limited circumstances) assist the Court in checking the accuracy of statements made about the amount of drink alleged to have been consumed. The chemical result may also, but not always, confirm the result of the clinical examination.

Bowden[60] records the following case in a jurisdiction where breath tests were used:

> In one case in particular a driver was arrested and charged with drunk driving. This man's condition was such that he was incapable of standing

without assistance. There was an odour of alcohol on his breath, but he maintained that he had had but one drink prior to his arrest . . . [the Breathalyzer test] indicated that he had less than an ounce of whisky in his body at the time of test. This man was sent to hospital at about 9.00 p.m. that evening. About an hour later the doctor at the hospital called and questioned the Breathalyzer operator, for he was of the opinion that the man was drunk. It was not until about 5.00 a.m., after conducting various tests, that they found the man was suffering from a virus infection of the nervous system.

Except in extreme cases, a blood acohol test is unlikely to be reliable as a simple and single test for drunkenness. It is a special investigation which must be interpreted in relation to the rest of the evidence, including the medical examination.

The intoxicated state shows itself in a profound disturbance of behaviour due entirely to the influence of the alcohol on the nervous system of the subject. Therefore, any other drugs, or any disease processes affecting the same parts of the nervous system in the same way, are likely to produce disturbances in behaviour similar to those produced by alcohol. The subjects of high blood pressure, for example, may suffer transient minor strokes leading to unsteadiness and thickness of the speech, and if the victim of such a seizure happens to have the faintest smell of alcohol on his breath, he may quite unjustly be accused of drunkenness, especially by the inexperienced. The differential diagnosis must include, amongst other things, such conditions as virus infections, *petit mal*, acute carbon monoxide poisoning, head injuries, shock and the difficult problem of hypoglycaemia. The diagnosis of coma presents additional complexities (poisoning, diabetes mellitus, uraemia, head injuries, cardiovascular accidents, epilepsy, etc.).

It seems desirable for the medical examiner to make his clinical diagnosis uninfluenced by any knowledge of the results of the chemical test. Lofthus,[61] reporting on the examination of drivers detained by the police on suspicion of being under the influence of alcohol in the Oslo area during the period 1930 to 1945, states:

> At first a blood sample was taken . . . Then the suspect underwent a clinical examination according to a definite authorized schedule. The result of this examination was recorded immediately, so as to make it independent of the result of the blood analysis, which would not be known until a day or two later.

The smell of alcohol on the breath is a subjective and extremely fallible index of the amount of liquor taken or of its presence in the body. For this reason, the usual medical examination carried out by a medical practitioner cannot be dispensed with because it is designed to discover or exclude those disease conditions which may closely simulate the drunken state. There are likely to be cases, however, where the clinical investigation may not settle the matter beyond doubt. At its best, the medical practitioner's diagnosis of alcoholic intoxication is only the most reasonable inference he can draw from his *clinical* observations. It is, therefore, proper that the doctor's reasonable inference should be tested to see whether it is consistent with the independent and scientific testimony of the chemist. The doctor as an expert witness must not usurp the functions of the Court, which must assume the final responsibility of making the decision.

In some juridictions the chemical test is done on the blood and not on the breath or the urine. It is the most direct evidence obtainable in the living. It has been amply proved in animal experiments that there is a fairly constant relationship between the amount of alcohol in the blood and in the brain tissue supplied by the blood, once equilibrium has been established between the alcohol in the blood and the tissues. A blood alcohol determination, therefore, will give us a measure of the amount of alcohol in the brain itself. This is most important information to have, because the brain tissue is the site of action of the alcohol, and it is the disturbance of its functions by this drug that results in the behaviour we call 'drunken'.

There is no such simple and constant relationship between breath or urinary alcohol and blood alcohol. Haggard et al[62] instance the example of a person given 250 ml of whisky at 10 p.m. He retained his urine until 8 a.m., when his blood alcohol on direct test was zero but as calculated indirectly from the amount in the urine it was 110 mg per 100 ml. Alha and Tamminen[63] have reported high levels of alcohol (up to and even over 200 mg per 100 ml) in the urine of recently deceased persons in whom no alcohol was present in the blood.

Alcohol may pass through the bladder in either direction after death, as well as in life. The direction of diffusion is determined by the relative concentrations of alcohol in the blood and the urine at the time of death.[64]

Attempts to estimate the amount of alcohol affecting the brain, when based on analyses of breath or urine, may therefore be quite fallacious and misleading. This is unfortunate as these biological materials are easy to obtain. More recently it has been claimed that more relaible techniques have been developed for analysis of the breath, but they require skill and special training. Surveys of breath tests for alcohol have been made, among others, by Denny,[65] Landauer and Milner[66] and Milner and Landauer.[67]

A blood alcohol determination may acquaint us with the amount and concentration of alcohol circulating in the body of the subject, i.e. within the flexible range which has been established for this type of investigation. By a simple calculation it may be possible to determine (again within fairly wide limits) how much alcohol must have been imbibed within a certain period of time to produce the level found in the blood at the time of examination. This, of course, can only be attempted after absorption has stopped and equilibrium between the blood and the tissues has been attained. With the aid of simple tables (e.g. Table 15.2), this information can then be translated into terms of tots of whisky, brandy, wine or beer. This information has the advantage of being objective, although not very precise. Used with caution, it would give the Court a limited opportunity of testing

Table 15.2 Blood alcohol concentrations in relation to the amount of liquor consumed

Amount of ethanol per 100 ml of blood (tissues and blood concentrations being in equilibrium)/ml (mg)		Amount of ethanol in a man of 70 kg in weight (150 lb)/ ml (fl oz)		Minimum amount of liquor consumed, in one of the following forms, by a man weighing 70 k (150 lb)			Approximate time required for removal of alcohol from the body/hours
				Whisky[a] (fl oz)	Wine[b] (fl oz)	Beer[c] (pints)	
50	(0.063)	26.4	(0.9)	2.3	5.8	1.4	2.5
100	(0.126)	52.9	(1.8)	4.6	11.6	2.8	5.0
200	(0.252)	105.8	(3.7)	9.3	23.2	5.6	10.5
300	(0.378)	158.7	(5.5)	13.9	34.9	8.5	16.0
400	(0.504)	211.6	(7.4)	18.6	46.5	11.3	21.0
500	(0.630)	264.6	(9.3)	23.2	58.2	14.1	26.5
600	(0.756)	317.5	(11.1)	27.9	69.8	17.0	32.0

[a] Alcohol 40% by volume = 30° u.p.
[b] Alcohol 16% by volume.
[c] Alcohol 3.28% by volume.
From *Medical Jurisprudence and Toxicology* by Glaister, 11th ed., p. 601, 1962. By permission of the publishers, E. and S. Livingstone, Ltd.

the reliability of the story told by the accused. It would assist the doctor in confirming his already reasonable suspicions of what was the matter. It would also enable the Court to accept a purely clinical diagnosis of drunkenness without any reluctance. It might serve to resolve conflicting reports given by non-medical and even medical witnesses. Any such evaluation must distinguish between the general statistical probabilities and the position in a particular individual case. Data treated statistically to give average results may smooth out the many variables which may make the individual case markedly different from the average.

The collection of blood for chemical analysis

Klatzow[68] has drawn attention to the method of collecting blood. He states that it is not advisable to use McCartney bottles for collecting blood samples, as under certain circumstances it is not possible to maintain the sterility of such samples. Sodium fluoride alone is not an adequate preservative. Work has been done to show that sodium fluoride will not prevent the formation of alcohol by *Candida albicans* in the presence of certain additives, as may be found in bank blood. In certain cases, this may well influence the results of the analysis. Therefore, it is important to take the blood into a sterile container. Vac-U-Tubes are ideal for this. The skin should be swabbed with a non-alcoholic solution and the Vac-U-Tube should contain adequate amounts of sodium fluoride and potassium oxalate to prevent or to reduce fermentation and coagulation respectively. As an additional safeguard, the tubes should be refrigerated. Ideally, samples should be analysed within 2 to 3 days. This reduces to an absolute minimum the chances of contamination by endogenous alcohol formation by fermentation.

Indeed, it would be as well for the medical practitioner, as a routine, to incorporate, either in his affidavit or in his evidence, the fact that he actually observed these precautions before taking the blood sample. Hollopeter[69] records the following:

> It sometimes happens that following an accident, a blood sample is taken in hospitals at the direction of a police officer, but occasionally it is done in a crude, wholly unscientific manner.
>
> A man [was] charged with felonious drunken driving and felonious manslaughter following the death of his passenger. The defendant driver himself received serious injuries and was taken to hospital. On his admission, on the direction of the police, a sample of his blood was taken . . . the conclusion of the chemist who subsequently examined the blood was excluded because of the extreme carelessness exercised in making the withdrawal. Under cross-examination it developed that the nurse who actually withdrew the blood, under the direction of an attending doctor, first swabbed the area from which the sample was to be taken with rubbing alcohol and then inserted the syringe to withdraw the blood. Obviously any analysis for alcohol of blood so taken would be invalid.

Correlation studies

A very comprehensive study of the correlation between the blood alcohol level and the degree of intoxication has been carried out by Jetter.[70] His investigation has been quoted extensively in the literature and forms the basis of an evaluation of blood alcohol findings (Fig. 15.4).

It is important to appreciate once again that the correlations observed are based on statistical generalizations and do not apply to an individual case. For example, according to Jetter's criteria, 47% of persons may be regarded as under the influence of alcohol at a blood alcohol concentration of 150 mg per 100 ml. It other words, 53% of persons would, by the criteria employed, be sober.

Harger and Hulpieu[71] have tabulated the results of seven investigators, each of whom had his own criteria for diagnosing drunkenness (Table 15.3). The list includes the observations of Jetter.[70] The average of the combined findings of the seven investigators closely approximates the observations recorded in Jetter's series (Fig.15.4).

Even when the statistical chance of intoxication increases, it has been established that certain subjects remain sober at very high blood alcohol levels. Rabinowitch[58,59] has shown that the same subject may be intoxicated at a low blood alcohol level and, on another occasion, may be diagnosed as sober at very high levels, e.g. 273, 282 and 291 mg per 100 ml. Lofthus[72] reports a case where the subject was considered sober at a level of 257 mg per 100 ml. On the other hand, he refers to a person without any alcohol in his blood who was found to be not sober (by Kristensen) 'possibly as a result of nervousness in the test situation'.

Table 15.3 Blood alcohol level and frank intoxication

Investigator	No. of subjects		Blood alcohol (mg per 100 ml)								
			0–50	51–100	101–150	151–200	201–250	251–300	301–350	351–400	400
Widmark[a]	1942	% subjects diagnosed as drunk	0	19	50	83	93	98	100	100	—
Schwarz[b]	905		2	38	93	97	99	100	100	—	—
Harger et al[c]	140		0	46	50	92	100	100	100	100	100
Jetter[d]	1000		10	18	47	83	90	95	96	93	100
Andresen[e]	1712		10	68	81	92	97	100	—	—	—
Alha[f]	54		48	37	55	65	100	—	—	—	—
Prag[g]	100		0	14	69	90	94	94	100	100	100
Total	5853	Average	10	34	64	86	96	99	99	98	100

(a) Widmark, E. M. P. (1933): Quoted by Jungmichel, G. in *Alkoholbestimmung in Blut*, p. 109, Berlin: Carl Heymanns Verlag.
(b) Schwarz, F. (1937): *Schweiz. med Wchnschr.*, 67, 54.
(c) Harger, R. N., Lamb, E. B. and Hulpieu, H. R. (1938): *J. Amer. Med. Assoc.*, 110, 779.
Harger, R. N. (1951): In *Judge and Prosecutorin Traffic Court*, Chapter 11. Ed. by Economos, J. P. and Kreml, F. M. Amer. Bar Assoc. and Northwestern Univ. Traffic Inst., Chicago.
(d) Jetter, W. W. (1938): *Amer. J. Med. Sci.*, 196, 475.
(e) Andresen, P. H. (1950): *Medico-Legal J.*, 18, 98.
(f) Alha, A. R. (1951): *Ann. Acad. Sci. Fenn.*, Series A, V. Medica. No. 26 Helsinki.
(g) Prag, J. J. (1954): *J. Forensic Med.*, 1, 360.

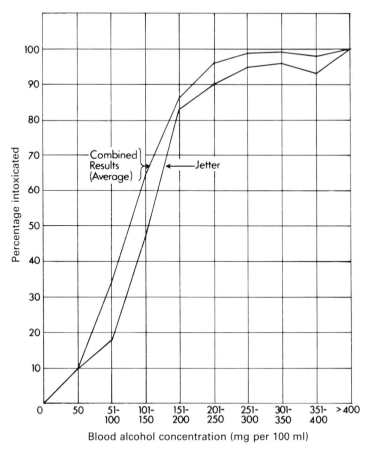

Fig. 15.4 Relationship between blood alcohol concentration and percentage of subjects intoxicated. Jetter[70] adopted the following criteria for the clinical diagnosis of acute alcoholic intoxication: (a) Gross gait abnormality; (b) In addition, at least two of the following tests must be positive: (i) abnormality of speech; (ii) flushed face; (iii) dilated pupils; (iv) alcoholic odour of the breath. Fig. 15.4 has been drawn from data published by Jetter[70] and Harger and Hulpieu.[71]

The foregoing observations indicate the fallibility of allowing the diagnosis of alcoholic intoxication to rest on the chemical determination alone. In fact, the blood level is merely one item in the evidence which must be considered in relation to other evidence about the behaviour of the subject at material times. This evidence may be medical as well as non-medical and, in this context, the blood alcohol level is only of value when it is consistent with the other non-chemical observations made.

The vagaries of the post-absorptive behaviour of alcohol in the body must make theoretical calculations of variable significance. They must not be invested with undue and unwarranted precision.

Features of the clinical examination

The time taken to complete the examination of the arrested person should be adequate for the performance of a reasonably full clinical investigation, e.g. a period of 4–5 minutes would not be adequate. It is usual for at least 15–20 minutes to be required for this type of examination, although admittedly very experienced observers may take less time.

Effect of alcohol on general behaviour

Rentoul et al[73] found that the effect of alcohol on general behaviour was:

> . . . so variable that it rapidly became apparent that no reliance can be placed on this in estimating alcohol consumption. Our subjects varied from individuals who showed no external sign of the effects of alcohol other than smell, to those who rapidly became semi-comatose and remained so for three to four hours. This was a surprise to us. We knew that a tolerance could be acquired to alcohol, but not to anything like the extent which these experiments showed. Ten ounces of whisky can be a dangerously toxic dose to someone unaccustomed to alcohol, whereas to a seasoned whisky-drinker it appears to be little more than an appetiser. An interesting observation was that no one showed any sign of exhilaration or ebullience. There appears to be no doubt that this factor in the effects of alcohol is related to companionship and surroundings. The practical importance of this is that when car accidents occur after parties, the party spirit may well be a factor in addition to the alcohol. It may even be a major factor.

The value of certain tests

The tests, especially those for the co-ordination of delicate movements, must be reasonable. A corpulent subject may have difficulty in picking up a pin from the floor, even though he is sober. The Court may well comment upon the unreasonable nature of the tests applied.[74]

In R. v. Bradley, Mr. Justice Streatfield commented on the tests given by a young, provisionally qualified doctor to a man who appeared at Worcestershire Assizes accused of being in charge of a car while under the influence of drink. The accused, aged 34, a car salesman, was found not guilty.

Dr R. said he was 23 when he carried out the tests in July, and was then awaiting his full registration as a medical practitioner, and acting as house physician. He examined the accused's reaction to light by putting his hand before Bradley's eyes, then moving it away. Bradley's reaction was slow.

Counsel defending: Do you know that the usual test in this case is to shine a torch into the eyes?

Dr R: That is a dangerous method. I was reprimanded as a student by a senior neurologist in the hospital for testing someone's reaction to light in that manner.

The doctor said he also asked Bradley to multiply seven by seven by eight. Bradley did not do it properly.

'I thought', said Dr R, 'that as he was a salesman and dealing with figures it would be a fair test'.

As another test he asked Bradley to stand on each leg alternately with his eyes shut. 'Bradley practically fell over', said the doctor. 'I came to the conclusion that he was under the influence of alcohol'.

The judge said he thought the jury would agree that the doctor was doing his best. But of the eye test he said. 'As long as I remember in this profession almost all doctors when examining people have applied the test of shining a very bright light into a man's face. This is the first time that I have heard that that was a dangerous or misleading test or an improper one. Unfortunately, this doctor adopted a different technique. He simply covered this man's eyes with his hand and then took it away in the ordinary light of the room. Then, he told me, the eyes reacted rather slowly. Well, of course they did, if there was no particularly bright light there. You may think that through no fault of his own that test somewhat misfired.'

Of the multiplication test he said: 'How many sober people could give an answer quite quickly?'

On the third test he commented, 'I wonder how many of us, unpractised, could suddenly close our eyes and without swaying stand on one leg?'

Rentoul et al[73] state (op. cit., p. 4):

> The 'picking up coins' test appears to have little value. A considerable number of completely sober people fumble the coins. Several variations on the standard test were also used, e.g. arranging matches in fixed patterns and also the finding of numbers in special patterns. None of these tests, however, showed alterations in performance sufficiently consistent to be of any use in demonstrating the effects of alcohol. In fact several people showed slight improvement at some of these tests after taking alcohol.

It should be borne in mind that a chronic alcoholic subject when sober may not be able to perform tests for co-ordination as well as when he has actually had several ounces of alcohol to drink.

French,[75] in discussing ataxia due to mental shock or fright, states:

> There are other cases of purely emotional ataxy in which there has been no traumatic factor. One speaks of 'staggering news', of having a 'staggering blow' on the exchange, and so on. Any extreme emotion, pleasant or unpleasant, may cause temporary ataxy; the worse the emotion the longer the ataxy is apt to last; and after extreme fright, panic or the like, it may be permanent though functional. These facts may become of great importance in connection with charges of drunkenness associated with motor driving accidents.

French also states that ataxia (i.e. incoordination of muscular movements) may be hysterical (with staggering as the only manifestation), traumatic, emotional (mental shock or fright), or due to chemicals or drugs (insulin, carbon monoxide, Veronal). Veronal may be followed by a staggering gait for weeks.

Fregly et al[76] have observed that maximum ataxia may occur sooner than the maximum blood alcohol level and that the ataxia may begin to improve while high blood alcohol levels are still sustained.

Alha[77] also points out that fatigue occurs in the stage of decreasing drunkenness and produces a general retardation of functions which may therefore enhance the appearance of intoxication.

Difficulties do not usually arise in extreme cases, i.e. where the subject is clearly drunk or patently sober. It is the marginal cases and those which intermediate degrees in the disturbance of behaviour that create the clinical problem.

It is important that the observations made in the medical report should be consistent. For example, a severe degree of Rombergism with a staggering gait is, *prima facie*, incompatible with a faultless performance of a delicate test for fine co-ordination of movements. Similarly, a subject with a swaying, staggering gait cannot have a weakly positive Romberg test.

It should also be appreciated that the medical examination is extremely subjective, many of the observations made being incapable of objective or quantitative record, especially under the conditions governing the examination. In any event, whether the practitioner is dealing with a case of coma or an ambulatory subject, he must consciously direct his mind to a consideration of all the other reasonable causes which may produce the same disturbance as that produced by alcohol. He must pay particular attention to the exclusion of diseases or disorders which may be present and which may be an adequate explanation of the symptons and signs observed.

A cursory and incomplete clinical examination may lead to serious error. Although the state of integrity of the nervous system is the main object of the investigation (to determine the relationship to alcohol ingestion) it is essential to conduct a complete and thorough general examination.

An arrested person is likely to be suffering from fear and acute anxiety, often complicated by fatigue states which may produce signs which may wrongfully be attributed to alcohol.[78]* A full general examination may, for example, provide evidence of liver disease. Brown,[79] in a study of liver–brain relationships, has stressed the neurological changes which may be present in a patient without coma. He found positive signs in 67.5% of his cases. The signs included inco-ordination, positive Rombergism and nystagmus.[80]

---

* State *vs*. Rosen & another (4th December 1961). In this matter the senior district surgeon examined the male accused (No. 1) at 6.30 a.m. on 15th October, 1961. The accused had been arrested at 3.40 a.m. The district surgeon found no evidence of disease.

The Romberg test was moderately positive, hand movements were slightly unco-ordinated and the pupils seemed to react rather sluggishly to light. There was a slight stagger in the gait on turning (the accused went off balance), his tongue was dry and furred and there was a somewhat sour smell on his breath which the district surgeon recorded as 'a ? faint smell of liquor'. The district surgeon stated that a state of anxiety or fatigue might show all the signs he found. Blood from accused No. 1 was examined for its alcohol content. The result was negative.

Nystagmus (alcoholic gaze nystagmus, AGN)

An undue amount of emphasis appears to have been placed on the presence of this sign (as observed clinically) by some medical examiners as evidence of alcoholic intoxication. It is by no means a constant or a common sign. Watt[81] found it present in about 10% of persons who had consumed varying quantities of alcohol. One subject who had drunk 14 tots of whisky in about four hours had no evidence of nystagmus of nystagmoid movements. Nystagmus on lateral gaze at the normal position of the head with open eyes may occur at an average blood alcohol concentration of 0.08% (range: 0.04–0.1%). It may be absent at an average concentration of 0.06% (range: 0.05–0.08%).[82] Nystagmus is thus by no means always an early sign of a disturbed nervous system and by itself it certainly cannot be regarded as enough for the clinical diagnosis of alcoholic intoxication.

Rauschke[83] regards certain types of nystagmus as having a good correlation with the clinical symptoms of intoxication; but Prestwich[84] has never found nystagmus in persons known to have taken the 'extra one or two'. He is critical of the way police surgeons produce (as if they were 'the Laws of the Medes and the Persians') nystagmus and other signs suggestive of intoxication and listed in the British Medical Association pamphlet *The Recognition of Intoxication* (1954).

A physiological nystagmus occurs in about one in five of normal persons. Nystagmus can be brought on by fatigue, emotion or postural hypotension, e.g. after or before a faint.[75] It has been reported after head injuries, and Brown[80] has found it in association with liver disease. The British Medical Association in its pamphlet *The Recognition of Intoxication*[85] describes it as a *fine* lateral nystagmus. At p. 16 of the revised (1958) edition of this pamphlet, the reference to the nystagmus as *fine* has been abandoned without any explanation. Such apparent clinical indecision may well cast doubt on the authoritative value of this pamphlet in this connection. A distinguished Mayo clinic team[86] says that sedative drugs, including alcohol, produce nystagmus of the cerebellar type. The eyes are steady on forward gaze, but nystagmus appears on looking to the sides, the quick component being in the direction of gaze.

Positional alcohol nystagmus (PAN)

Aschan *et al*[87] have demonstrated the existence of a special type of nystagmus which can be elicited after alcohol consumption with the head in certain positions. It is known as positional alcohol nystagmus (PAN) and it occurs in two phases (PAN I and PAN II). The phenomenon has more recently been reviewed by Goldberg.[88,89]

With the subject supine, and the head in the right or left lateral position, the eye movements were recorded under laboratory conditions, mainly behind closed eyelids, with special recording apparatus.

PAN I appears about half-an-hour after the intake of a single dose of alcohol, lasts for 3 to 4 hours, and its duration is independent of the dose. With the head on the right side, the slow component is upwards (anti-gravity) and the rapid component is downwards (i.e. to the right), changing to the opposite direction in the left lateral position. The second phase (PAN II) begins about 1 to 2 hours after the disappearance of PAN I and usually some 5 to 6 hours after the ingestion of the alcohol. Its beat is in the reverse direction to PAN I (i.e. the fast component beats to the left in the right lateral position and to the right in the left lateral position). The duration and intensity of PAN II, depending on the dose of alcohol taken, range from 5 to 10 hours or more. PAN II, however, lasts for many hours after alcohol has disappeared from the blood. It is claimed to be a true, objective after-effect and part of the so-called hangover syndrome.

Goldberg[88] points out that in clinical practice it may be of value to make a tentative diagnosis about the nature of an observed nystagmus, i.e. whether it is alcohol-induced or not. To assess a possible PAN, existing mostly in lateral positions behind closed eyelids, the patient will have to be put on his back, his head turned laterally to one and the other side, and the eyes closely watched. An existing PAN, even if not recorded, may disclose itself by the observer seeing, and feeling, the cornea moving behind the closed eyelids. Opening of the eyes will block the PAN if its intensity is low but will disclose it if the intensity is high.

The PAN can be differentiated from a gaze nystagmus (AGN) by testing when the eyes look forward, and not only in lateral gaze direction; also by the direction of the fast component which changes with the position of the head and with the time after intake (PAN I or PAN II respectively).

Systematic studies have to be carried out, combining clinical observations of possible nystagmus with objective recording by EOG (electro-oculography). The results have to be related to the whole course of blood alcohol in one and the same individual, and not only to single levels in different individuals.

These studies must be carried out in individuals with varying alcohol habits, i.e. in moderate consumers as well as in alcoholics, in order to serve as a basis for possible recommendations of value for clinical use.

Drugs and PAN

Goldberg[89] states:

> Whereas meprobamate, like all other CNS-depressant agents studied from antihistamines to buclozine and chlorpromazine, increases ROM (roving ocular movements) and decreases PAN, chlordiazepoxide is so far the only drug known that reduces both PAN and ROM.

The interaction between ethanol and drugs depends not only on the type of drug administered, but also on the timing with regard to the phase of alcohol metabolism.

Congeners and nystagmus (*PAN*)

Murphree *et al*[90] state that a significant nystagmus-inducing effect may be produced by the congeners in alcoholic beverages. These congeners include higher alcohols (fusel oil), organic acids, esters and aldehydes. In their experiments the nystagmus was recorded under laboratory conditions with bipolar leads from the outer canthus of each eye to the mid-forehead, permitting separate recordings for each eye.

Difficulties in the clinical examination

The difficulty of a clinical diagnosis of alcoholic intoxication, in border-line cases where the matter is not obvious, must not be under-estimated.

The medical examination is usually conducted some considerable time after the traffic accident in which the accused has been involved, and it would be extremely hazardous for the clinical examiner to dogmatize about the accused's condition and capacity at the time of the accident, with the limited amount of information at his disposal. He may not know, with any certainty, whether the accused is in the sobering-up phase or vice versa; nor can he know with any accuracy what quantity of liquor the accused has imbibed.

In discussing whether a clinical (physical) examination can assist in deciding the ability to drive a car, except when the degree of intoxication is gross, Smith and Popham[91] state that available clinical tests would not appear sensitive enough. Penner and Coldwell[92] considered that:

> The medical examination did not prove to be a sufficiently accurate method for assessing alcoholic impairment in relation to car driving. Generally, the medical examination was not sensitive enough, but this was not consistent since several subjects were considered impaired by medical examination but not on driving performance.

Indeed, in certain circumstances, e.g. where the accused has been injured, or has suffered from concussion, or is in addition suffering from emotional shock (he may have seriously injured or killed a passenger or a pedestrian), the clinical examination as a means of diagnosing alcoholic intoxication may be quite inadequate for medico-legal purposes.

The vagaries of medical examiners have not been investigated very extensively. Lofthus[93] states: 'A number of investigators have stressed the individual variation from one clinical examiner to another'. He reports Liljestrand as having found, in a group of seven observers, that the blood alcohol level at which half the subjects were diagnosed as being under the influence of alcohol, varied from 50 to 140 mg per 100 ml. Lofthus draws attention to the following individual factors in the medical examiner:

a. State of mind (temperament, overwork, called repeatedly the same night, etc.);
b. Conscious attitude towards the law and the examination (liberal–rigid);

c. Experience and confidence;
d. Incidental errors of judgment.

Lofthus also reports data showing that the diagnostic standards of medical examiners tend to change with the passage of years. He suggests that this may be due to increasing experience—not necessarily a valid hypothesis.

Andresen[94] noted that 2.9% of the 170 motorists examined by police surgeons in Denmark were found clinically to be intoxicated, although chemical analysis proved that they had no alcohol in their systems.

Penner and Coldwell[95] also found 'poor agreement between the conclusions reached by two independent medical doctors'. This disagreement consisted of differences of opinion in the various parts of the medical examination and also variations in the conclusions as to impairment drawn from similar observations.

Coldwell et al[96] analysed the results of 82 medical examinations made by each of two doctors (identified as MD1 and MD2) on the same subjects on the same days:

> . . . In 54 their opinions were identical. Of the remainder, MD1 concluded the subjects were impaired on 4 occasions and unimpaired in 24; MD2 came to exactly the opposite decision. Since the blood alcohol levels at the the time of examination by each doctor were practically identical, these differences must be due to differences in clinical opinion.

The individual variation in the conduct of medical examinations is reflected also in an analysis performed in another jurisdiction.[97]

A panel of four doctors took it in turn to be on call for the examination of persons in circumstances where there was a possibility that the subjects were under the influence of alcohol. There was no selection, therefore, of the clinical material examined by the individual doctors, and it is reasonable to assume that, over the (approximate) two-year period of the analysis, each practitioner saw a random sample of the population being examined. Drs A and B roughly coincided in having a score of about 25–30% of positive diagnoses for intoxication. Dr C, however, had a score of over 70%, and Dr D had a score approximately between these two extremes.

The foregoing factors make it clear that the medical report is only one item in the total data available to the Court from which inferences can be drawn.

Amnesia

Amnesia may be total or incomplete, i.e. there may be patchy islands of recollection. Slater and Roth state (at p. 397):[98]

> On the mental side severer degrees of intoxication are often accompanied by increased irritability, outbursts of rage and violence after solitary brooding. For most of the events and actions in this stage the subject usually remains amnesic after return to sobriety.

Frame,[99] discussing pathological alcoholic states, describes the alcoholic palimpsest as follows:

> A condition not infrequently seen amongst alcoholics and occasionally in the non-addictive drinker is the sudden onset of behaviour resembling the 'black-outs' in anoxaemia.* I have seen many authentic cases of this type but none in may experience who had committed crimes during the phase. After only moderate ingestion, without showing any signs of intoxication, the person may carry on conversation and perform fairly well-organized and elaborate acts purely on an automatic level with indication only of patchy vague memory at intervals during this period of amnesia on the following day. This patchy amnesia which is not associated with unconsciousness has been called by Bonhofer† the 'alcoholic palimpsest'. The condition has been well described by the Alcoholism Sub-Committee of the World Health Organization's Expert Committee on Mental Health.
>
> One patient of my acquaintance recently presented himself for treatment because of the onset of this symptom. Just before admission he had left an hotel, apparently perfectly sober, with the intention of driving home to the northern suburbs for dinner. About 4 hours later he found himself in open country having safely traversed the traffic of two major cities (35 miles apart) at their peak hours. He had no recollection beyond a point where he had dropped a friend on his way home.

Alcoholic palimpsests (so-called blackouts) may occur in some alcoholics 'in response to rather moderate amounts of alcohol far short of the dose sufficient to cause stupor or "passing out"'.[100]

DRIVING SKILL AND ALCOHOLIC CONSUMPTION

The main purpose of the clinical examination is to throw light on whether the examinee was competent to carry on the occupation on which he was engaged at the time of his apprehension. In practice, this usually means the ability to drive a car.[101]

One of the most comprehensive investigations of this problem was carried out at the Stanford University School of Medicine.[102] The relation of blood alcohol concentration to driving abilities was studied under controlled conditions. The performance tests used simulated driving conditions and included two tests and their combination:

The first, which was termed 'simple braking', was scored as the number of centiseconds required for the subject to apply the brakes after a red light flashed on. The second, 'simple steering', was recorded as the percentage of a one-minute period during which the subject, by manipulation of a conventional steering wheel, was able to maintain the alignment of two objects on a screen within a tolerance of 6 mm ($\frac{1}{4}$ in), one of these objects being in constant irregular motion beyond the subject's control and the

---

* *Alcoholism Sub-Committee WHO Report No. 48*. Geneva: Palais des Nations.

† Bonhofer, K. Quoted in *Alcoholism Sub-Committee WHO Report No. 48*. Geneva: Palais des Nations.

other actuated by the steering wheel. When the two tests were performed simultaneously, the procedure was termed 'vigilance steering and braking'. The braking test was designed to measure reaction time and the steering test eye-to-hand co-ordination, while the combined test introduced complexity and the factor of attention. A certain amount of judgment was involved in all, but particularly in the combined test. Nevertheless, the investigators were well aware of the desirability of a better test of judgment, and acknowledged the handicap involved by the lack of such a test.

A period of practice on a day prior to the examination was found to control fairly adequately the effect of practice, subsequent scores not varying more than 5% on either side of the base line. Thus, changes greater than this in magnitude must have been due to the effect of alcohol. On the day of the examination the subject presented himself at the laboratory, having not eaten for at least three hours, and a control score on the tests was secured. He was then give a dose of alcohol varying from 0.5 to 2 ml per kg of either Scotch or Bourbon whisky diluted with soda water and cooled with ice, which he was expected to ingest within 15 minutes. In the great majority of cases the dose was 1 ml per kg, the other doses being given in repetitions of the test on the same subjects. At the end of an hour after the start of imbibition the tests were given again, and a sample of venous blood from a cubital vein was obtained for analysis for alcohol by the method described by Newman. The blood alcohol concentrations at the time of the test varied from 45 to 185 mg per 100 ml, the peak of the distribution curve being at 100 mg per 100 ml.

In spite of the homogeneity of the group tested, the scores on the tests varied rather widely, this variation being slightly less in the more complex steering tests than in the braking reaction time. Thus, in the steering test the range of scores before alcohol was from 99.2 to 65.5%, a spread of 33.7%, while the greatest drop recorded after alcohol was slightly less than this, from 78.5 to 48%, or 30.5%. In the braking test the range of scores before alcohol was from 36.1 to 53.3 centiseconds, a spread of 17.2 centiseconds, while the greatest decrease in performance after alcohol was slightly more than this, 18.4 centiseconds. Because of this very considerable variation in performance from person to person, which probably correlates well with their skill if not necessarily with their safeness as operators of motor vehicles, it must at once be obvious that even if all the subjects were affected in the same degree by a given concentration of alcohol in the blood, their performance after alcohol would vary much as it had before, the general level being lowered but the variations from one individual to another remaining. This is merely another expression of the commonly accepted fact that drivers vary in their skill, so that if all were to suffer an equal loss of skill some would be reduced below the accepted minimum standard while others, although less skilful than formerly, would still be above average.

In addition, to this, it was found that the loss in skill by different individuals at the same blood alcohol concentration was not equal, but varied within wide limits, as had been indicated by other workers already quoted. In demonstrating this fact, the data from 98 trials on 65 subjects were considered. The test of 'vigilance steering and braking' was used as the criterion of driving skill, since it embodied more factors common to this than either test taken separately, although the same conclusions could be reached by the use of the data on either 'simple steering' or 'simple braking'. Drop in performance after alcohol in each component of the test was calculated as the percentage of the original score represented by the difference in the scores before and after alcohol. The percentage drop in the two components was averaged to give the final figure used in the survey. It should be noted that this value gave a valid measure of loss of skill for comparison within the members of the group, but did not in any way represent any concrete 'amount of skill', if such could be conceived. To illustrate: a man showing, for example, a drop of 50% would be affected twice as much as one showing a drop of 25%, but one could not by any means say that this meant that he had exactly 50% of his original skill remaining after alcohol.

The correlation between this loss of skill on the tests and the blood alcohol concentration at the time of the test was calculated for the whole group by the Pearson correlation-coefficient formula, in which a coefficient of 1.0 indicates perfect and 0 no correlation. The value determined was 0.485. When it is recalled that a similar correlation, namely 0.5, exists between the height and weight of a population, it readily will be seen that the correlation between blood alcohol concentration and loss of ability in the tests was far from perfect. True, those with high blood alcohol concentrations did tend to show the greatest losses, just as tall people tend to weigh more than short ones; yet we must admit that a yardstick makes a rather crude weighing machine. So also we must consider blood alcohol concentration a crude indicator of the degree of intoxication.

No attempt was made to deduce from the data the blood alcohol concentration at which an individual, or even the average individual, could be considered under the influence of alcohol so far as motor vehicle operation is concerned. In order to apply the findings to this problem, we must first accept one of the various definitions of the terms 'under the influence' or 'intoxicated', and then satisfy ourselves concerning the validity of the tests used in gauging the ability to safely conduct a motor vehicle. As to the definition, if the Arizona definition is used, all the tests need show is that some impairment, however slight, has occurred due to alcohol and it can be safely assumed that any change in score beyond the maximum chance variation of 5% indicated such impairment. Then the blood alcohol concentration at which all subjects tested showed impairment in excess of this 5% should constitute definitive evidence of being under the influence of alcohol. The data of Newman and Fletcher show this to occur at approximately 105 mg per 100 ml. We may therefore say without fear of contradiction that this work indicates that when the blood alcohol concentration exceeds 105 mg per 100 ml all individuals are in some degree affected by alcohol. That this concentration might well be placed considerably lower by the use of more sensitive tests is quite possible; and it must further be borne in mind that many individuals would show this degree of impairment at concentrations of half this magnitude. Thus, it is seen that the evidence of this work supports the validity of a blood alcohol concentration considerably lower than that laid down by the National Safety Council as prima facie evidence of being 'under the influence' in those states subscribing to the Arizona type definition. As for the states interpreting the term in the California fashion, the problem is not so simple. To be of positive value in this regard, the tests employed must be capable of determining whether or not an individual can drive a motor vehicle in the manner in which an ordinarily prudent and cautious person would operate a similar vehicle under the same circumstances. We believe the tests capable of evaluating skill in certain restricted activities necessary to motor-vehicle operation, but certainly proficiency in this restricted sphere of activity is no guarantee of safe conduct of a car. As a matter of fact, one individual with half the skill of another as recorded by the tests may be the safer driver, if he recognizes his limitations and remains within them. Also, the tests are not adequate in the evaluation of the more abstract factors contributing to safe driving, such as judgment and caution. Thus we cannot say that there is a certain score on these tests which represents the minimum skill compatible with safe driving, and that the blood alcohol concentration at which all subjects fell below this minimum should be considered *prima facie* evidence of intoxication. Should it be possible to develop such a test, which could be shown to correlate with ability to drive a car with safety, then the problem of licensing drivers would be solved, and when an individual showed himself to fall below the standard set, because of the presence of alcohol in his blood in any significant amount, a conviction for drunken driving could easily be obtained under the California ruling. In the absence of such a test we must rely on the behaviour of the individual as indicated by the evidence of how he was driving at the time of the accident, supported by the usual clinical examination for drunkenness, which might well be improved by the use of testing equipment such as was employed in this study, incomplete as is the information so obtained.

Rentoul[103] described prolongation of the reaction time as the blood alcohol increased, in a experiment on ten subjects. This effect, he claimed, may continue even after the alcohol concentration is falling, and in most cases this is due to nausea. The author concludes: 'To what extent this affects car drivers is controversial'.

The application of this limited experiment to driving conditions must be evaluated in the light of the Stanford University experiments (p. 421) on simulated driving which showed that the loss of skill on the tests, which included a measurement of the reaction time (the simple braking test), correlated with the blood alcohol concentration only to the extent of 0.485.

The results of the Stanford University experiments on the relationship between blood alcohol concentration and driving skill (in simulated driving situations) thus clearly controverts the claims that at a given blood alcohol level (in the range 45–185 mg per 100 ml) all persons are so affected as to be unable to drive a car properly.

Bjerver and Goldberg[104] have also investigated the effect of drinking alcohol on driving ability, using six practical road tests. Their experiment was done with very small numbers, seven subjects being tested in the beer-drinking group and ten subjects in the spirit-drinking group. There were 20 subjects in the control group.

By statistical treatment of the results the authors conclude that alcohol impairs driving ability by between 25 and 30% at very low concentrations of blood alcohol, e.g. 40–60 mg per 100 ml. But when the individual data are scrutinized, it is seen that this is by no means a uniform effect, some of the alcohol subjects showing, in fact, a considerable improvement in performance, as compared with the controls.

Drew et al[101] studied, under laboratory conditions, the effects of small amounts of alcohol in experiments which, in a simplified form, resembled driving a vehicle. They concluded that, in general:

> . . . performance begins to deteriorate with very low blood alcohol levels and that deterioration progresses as the blood alcohol rises. There was, however, a wide variation in the effect of alcohol on different individuals, and about a quarter of those tested showed reduced error after alcohol, although most of these did so only by a compensatory reduction of speed.

Some subjects actually improved after alcohol 'in that they drove more slowly, more consistently and made less error' (op. cit., p. 52). See also at page 1602 of Newman and Fletcher.[102]

The experiments illustrate the danger of applying statistical generalizations to individual cases. Moreover, smoothing out the scatter of the results of observations and basing inferences on mere averages may well hide the great variability in the results.

The Law Reform Commission Report No. 4 (1976)[105] has summarized the correlation between blood alcohol concentration and driving impairment as follows:

'(a) For blood alcohol levels of 0.05 per cent, and below, some individuals are impaired by alcohol but most drivers, even if affected, are affected only slightly. While deterioration in performances of tasks related to driving can be demonstrated 0.05 per cent increased liability to accident appears first somewhat above 0.05 per cent. It is therefore, reasonable to say that at blood alcohol levels of 0.05 per cent or less the person concerned is unaffected, *in a practical sense*, as regards road safety.

(b) Blood alcohol levels in the range 0.05 to 0.10 per cent. All individuals are affected at or before 0.10 per cent is reached. In some people this may be largely compensated by slower or more careful driving—but even in these cases the person concerned is less able to cope with the demands made on his driving ability in emergency situations which often precede accidents and to this extent alcohol in this range is a contributing factor towards accidents. It is in this range that measurable increased liability to accident appears, taking drivers as a group.

(c) Drivers with blood alcohol levels above 0.10 per cent are affected to the extent that their driving becomes distinctly impaired. The impairment increased progressively as the blood alcohol level rises until at levels of 0.15 per cent there is substantially increased liability to accident.

(d) At levels of 0.20 per cent and above most people are obviously intoxicated. The increased risk of accidents is now severe.'

ALCOHOL AND DRUGS

1. *Barbiturates.* Both alcohol and barbiturates are depressants of the nervous system. When taken together (or soon after each other) the one enhances the effect of the other.

Jetter and McLean[106] have reported experimental evidence suggesting a synergistic effect when alcohol and a barbiturate (phenobarbital) are administered together, i.e. the combined effect of the two drugs is greater than can be accounted for by the sum of the effects of the two drugs acting separately.

This synergism may explain the occasional lethal nature of this 'deadly combination' in man,[107] even though only non-fatal amounts of each drug may have been taken.

A rapidly fatal course is a feature of these cases, death occurring in a matter of hours. In one case described by Jetter and McLean death occurred after half an hour. This rapid course is quite unlike the prolonged coma that characteristically follows lethal doses of alcohol or barbiturates taken separately. Similar cases have been reported elsewhere.[108,109] Teare[110] has reported on the additive effects of alcohol and barbiturates.

Barbiturates have a pharmacological action closely paralleling that of alcohol. Their effects may therefore simulate those of acute alcoholic intoxication.

2. *Other drugs.* In general, drugs capable of producing sedation or depression of the nervous system will simulate or enhance the effects of alcohol. Some of the these drugs are in very common use, e.g. antihistamine (for hay-fever), tranquillizers (which may produce fatigue and a reckless or indifferent attitude).[111]

In small doses stimulating drugs, e.g. amphetamines, delay fatigue without causing any serious disturbance of behaviour. Weatherall,[112] in a very useful survey entitled *Drugs and the Motorist*, in dealing with amphetamine (Benzedrine), states that 'a night driver will probably be all the safer for consuming a dose of 5 mg'.

The amphetamines may, however, produce gross disturbances of mental processes and reflexes, when taken in large doses.

Loomis[113] states that, ordinarily, clinical doses of some of the sedatives and tranquillizers do not produce measurable impairment of function and do not appear to influence the simultaneous effects of alcohol. Loomis's experiments were designed to mimic some of the physical conditions involved in driving.

Carpenter and Varley[114] have reviewed the literature on the joint action of tranquillizers and alcohol on driving. Forney and Hughes[115] have reviewed the combined effect of alcohol and drugs.

THE ESTIMATION OF ALCOHOL IN THE BLOOD OF DECEASED PERSONS

This problem was investigated by Bowden and McCallum.[116] These authors described a method of chemical analysis based on the standard principles involved in chemical methods for the determination of alcohol. They point out that there is an experimental error in the chemical estimation amounting to 4 mg per 100 ml of blood.

They also state that the use of the technique described by them, when applied to a post-mortem sample of blood for its alcohol content, will include (in the value obtained) a figure of up to 20 mg per 100 ml of blood of volatile reducing substances in the case of many disease states, including diabetes mellitus.

They make the specific point in their paper:

> If the dual condition existed, diabetes and alcoholism, a small allowance (20 mg) would be necessary for the interfering substances in the interpretation of the result.

It is therefore necessary to establish that the deceased was not a diabetic.

Bowden and McCallum also record the fact that after death substances are produced which behave as alcohol when their method of chemical analysis is employed. They conclude as follows:

> In the present state of our knowledge, and in the light of the survey which we have made in this field, no volatile reducing substances behaving as alcohol are produced in the body in sufficiently large amounts to alter the blood alcohol level by more than 20 milligrammes either before death or within a period of three days after it.

If the deceased was not a diabetic it would therefore appear to be perfectly proper to deduct from the value obtained an amount of 24 mg.

Alha[117] states that substances occurring in fruit that has been eaten may produce errors in the determination of the blood alcohol. The diet of the deceased at the material time is therefore important.

Before the significance of the true alcohol value is assessed, certain other important factors must be borne in mind. The first of these is the source of the blood sample on which the analysis was done.

Bowden and McCallum recognize that neither the odour of alcohol nor the amount of alcohol present in the stomach at autopsy is a reliable indication of the amount of alcohol that has been consumed. They point out that alcohol diffuses through the wall of the stomach after death, and their investigations make it clear that even after a post-mortem interval of six to eight hours it is probably unreliable to do an analysis on blood taken from the heart.

They also assert that it is unsafe to take blood from a pool in the chest or the abdominal cavity at autopsy for a blood alcohol estimation, whether there is alcohol in the stomach at autopsy or not.

They found that blood taken from a large vein in the chest or from the heart at autopsy 'is not suitable for a quantitative blood alcohol estimation if any appreciable time interval has elapsed between death and the autopsy. The result is too high, and this is probably due to the diffusion of alcohol from the stomach after death'.

If alcohol was present in the stomach at the time of death, then the alcohol level found in such a sample 'would be too high and should not be used in medico-legal cases except qualitatively, or to say that the deceased had taken alcohol before death'.

Their ultimate opinion is that a post-mortem sample of blood for alcohol estimation should only be taken from a peripheral vein, i.e. a vein in the leg, the thigh or the arm. The recommendation to employ femoral vessels for taking blood samples is endorsed by Plueckhahn,[118] who agrees that alcohol can diffuse through the intact stomach wall after death into the surrounding tissues, including the pericardial fluid and the pleural fluid. He is of the view, however, that the alcohol levels in blood taken from within the intact chambers of the heart, were virtually unaltered for 48 hours after death, even in the presence of alcohol in the stomach contents.

Bowden and McCallum also advise that the blood should be subjected to analysis without delay. It is, however, probably quite safe to keep it in a full-stoppered test-tube for some days in a refrigerator, if a preservative has been added to the blood.

Although Bowden and McCallum emphasize that blood for alcohol analysis should only be taken from a peripheral vein, they admit that 'any change in the alcohol level of the peripheral blood within this period of death (i.e. 48–72 hours) is towards a slight rise, and in no case did we obtain figures showing a fall of practical significance'.

However, if Table II (p. 78 of their paper), on which this conclusion is based, is examined, it will be seen that in three of the seven cases studied by these authors the alcohol in the blood taken from a peripheral vein after death rose as follows, indicating more than a *slight* rise:

In Case III there was an increase from 81 to 93 mg per 100 ml within 9 hours after death.

In Case VI there was an increase from 7 to 15 mg per 100 ml within 24 hours after death.

In Case VII these was an incease from 24 to 38 mg per 100 ml within about 24 hours after death.

Gifford and Turkel[119] have confirmed the observations of Bowden and McCallum on the post-mortem diffusion of alcohol from the stomach into the blood. They introduced whisky into the stomachs of cadavers and found that sufficient diffusion could then occur to produce thoracic blood levels as high as 312 mg per 100 ml. Their findings also support the desirability of taking cadaver blood from peripheral veins, e.g. the femoral veins in the lower limb.

Turkel and Gifford[120] observed (in experiments with heart blood samples obtained *post mortem*):

> Taking a level of 0.150 per cent (i.e. 150 mg per 100 c.c.) as the basis for legal presumption that a person is clearly under the influence of alcohol, let us arbitrarily assume that a person actually had a level of 0.110 per cent at the instant of death. As has been shown, a false elevation of either 0.05 or 0.09 percentage points in the heart blood alcohol can occur, and would give an erroneous blood alcohol level of 0.16 per cent or 0.200 per cent, respectively, thus clearly but improperly establishing that person as intoxicated.

Harger[121] has criticized the claim that blood diffuses from the stomach to the heart after death. He wrongly states that Turkel and Gifford[120] based their claim on finding higher alcohol levels in the heart than in the femoral vein *post mortem*. This claim is, in fact, based on the actual experimental demonstration of this diffusion by Gifford and Turkel[119] in an earlier paper, which is referred to in the paper by Turkel and Gifford quoted by Harger.

In dealing with embalmed bodies, the possibility of alcohol in the embalming fluid must be considered.

The blood sample tested should be pure blood not mixed with other body fluids, e.g. cerebrospinal fluid.

Newman[122] reviews the alcohol concentration in the cerebrospinal fluid as follows:

The alcohol level in the lumbar spinal fluid lags behind that in the blood while the blood alcohol concentration is rising. During the fall of the blood level the spinal fluid concentration first equals and then rises above that of the blood. When fluid was taken from the upper end of the spinal system (near the brain) these differences were less marked. In other experiments in which the blood concentration of alcohol was kept constant over a period of five hours, at the end of this period the cerebrospinal fluid concentrations were more or less equal, but were higher than the levels in the blood plasma by an appreciable amount.

In experiments on cadavers, the spinal fluid concentration was always greater than the brain concentration, the ratio in intoxicated individuals being 1.4:1.0, but at low concentrations it was as high as 3:1.

Plueckhahn[123] states that mixtures of cerebrospinal fluid and blood from the cranial cavity may have an alcohol concentration up to 35% higher than blood samples from the heart or leg.

These experiments illustrate the great difficulty that exists in interpreting the significance of an alcohol estimation on a post-mortem sample of blood not taken immediately and properly after death.

It is therefore important to know from what part of the body the sample was taken, under what conditions it was transmitted to the laboratory, the time taken for its transmission to the laboratory, the time taken by the laboratory before the estimation was begun, as well as the conditions of storage in the laboratory.

In dead bodies that best evidence is to be obtained from an analysis of brain tissue.

Gonzales et al[124] state that putrefaction reduces the amount of alcohol in alcohol-containing tissues (including blood) when putrefaction proceeds in the test-tube.

They make the point that:

> No experiments have been performed to determine whether changes in the ingested alcohol content of tissue occurring in the body during ordinary putrefaction are comparable to *in vitro* findings, but available evidence suggests that, when changes occur, the ingested alcohol concentration will always decrease in value.

On the other hand the general consensus is that tissues not containing alcohol may produce substances which will be measured as alcohol when they undergo putrefaction.

These authors also point out:

> Unfortunately, no data are available on the changes that occur during putrefacion of tissue containing borderline concentrations of alcohol but the consistent loss of higher concentrations and the failure of non-alcoholic tissue to exceed the lower range of borderline values suggests that there would be no increase in the alcohol values which might result in an unjust interpretation.

These observations may be criticised on the basis that no bacteriological studies were done to establish the particular types of organism associated with the putrefactive processes. Plueckhahn and Ballard[125] have shown that bacteria and yeasts can produce significant amounts of alcohol if they contaminate post-mortem blood samples. This post-mortem production of alcohol in blood can be prevented by the addition of sodium fluoride in a concentration of 1% in all blood samples stored at room temperature for 10 days. It is thus the most efficient and suitable preservative for autopsy blood samples.

Gormsen[126] records the fact that false-positive alcohol reactions may be obtained when the blood contains alcohol-producing micro-organisms. He states:

> Should putrefaction have set in and alcohol is found in the blood and the organs, but *not* in the urine, the alcohol reaction in the blood is probably false due to putrefaction.
>
> If urine is not available and putrefaction has commenced and alcohol is found by means of a specific method in the blood and the organs, it is necessary—especially if the distribution of alcohol in blood and organs is uneven—to carry out further bacteriological examinations of the blood as well as in vitro examinations of the ability of the isolated micro-organisms to produce alcohol. This is necessary if errors are to be avoided.

It seems clear from Gormsen's work that certain precautions should be taken in connection with the analysis of blood from dead bodies which have undergone putrefaction:

1. Samples of blood *and of urine* should be tested.
2. Bacteriological examination of the blood should be carried out.
3. Special investigations should be done to test the alcohol-producing ability of the micro-organisms isolated from the blood.

It is also important to evaluate the alcohol concentration found in relation to whether the deceased at the time of the accident was still absorbing alcohol (i.e. in the phase of increasing intoxication) or whether he was already sobering up after the alcohol concentration had reached equilibrium between the blood, the brain and other tissues.

There is evidence that the clinical symptoms are considerably more marked in the phase of increasing than in that of decreasing drunkenness.

Under average conditions equilibrium is in most cases attained within one to two hours, but it may take longer, e.g. two to three hours. If the deceased was therefore in a sobering-up phase at the time of the accident, the percentage change of his having been intoxicated would be further diminished.

Luvoni and Marozzi[127] conclude that the calculation of the blood alcohol concentration from that found in organs or other body fluids can lead to serious error if it is not known whether the deceased, at the time of death, was in the absorption or the post-absorption phase.

REFERENCES

1 Smith H. Drinking and driving. Crim Law Quart 1960; 3: 65–122.
2 Haggard H W, Greenberg L A, Lolli G. Absorption of alcohol with special reference to its influence on concentration of alcohol appearing in blood. Quart J Stud Alcoh 1941; 1: 684–726.
3 Miller D S, Stirling J L, Yudkin J. Effect of ingestion of milk on concentrations of blood alcohol. Nature London 1966; 212:1051.
4 Nickolls L C. The Scientific Investigation of Crime. London: Butterworths. 1956: p 332.

5 Alha A R. Blood alcohol and clinical inebriation in Finnish men. Ann Acad Sci Fen Series A, V, Medica. 1951: p 36.
6 Miles W R. Comparative concentrations of alcohol in human blood and urine at intervals after ingestion. J Pharmacol Exp Ther 1922; 20: 265–319.
7 Newman H W. Acute alcoholic intoxication. Stanford University Press. 1941: p 5.
8 Harichaux P, Capron J P, Lienard J, Freville M. Influence de l'éthanol sur l'evacuation gastrique: étude clinique et experimentale. Lille Med 1970; 15: 1059–1065. Abstracted in Quart J Stud Alcoh Part B 1972; 33:550.
9 Newman H W. op. cit. pp 5–6.
10 MacDonald J M. Psychiatry and the Criminal. Springfield: Thomas. 1958: p 132.
11 Alha A R. op. cit. p 23.
12 Alha A R. op. cit. p 35.
13 Lofthus J. Blood alcohol test and clinical examination of automobile drivers in Oslo. Quart J Stud Alcoh 1957; 18: 217–228.
14 Betetto D, Cristina F, Cappelletti S. Per una valutazione del danno epatico nel gastroresecato. III. Aspetti del metabolismo alcoolico nel gastroresecato. (Studio della curva alcoolemica da carico). Arch Pat Clin Med 1964; 41:36–47. Abstracted in Quart J Stud Alcoh 1966; 27: 551.
15 Fleming J A, Haynes S, Le Quesne L P. The effect of vagotomy and a drainage procedure on alcohol tolerance. Br J Surg 1971; 58: 92, 96.
16 Lester D, Greenberg L H. Inhalation of ethyl alcohol by man. Quart J Stud Alcoh 1951; 12: 167–178.
17 Alha A R. op. cit. p 34.
18 Rabinowitch I M. Effects of alcohol on Siamese twins. Can Med Assoc J 1960; 82: 551–552.
19 Allen H. Report of an autopsy on the bodies of Chang and Eng Bunker, commonly known as the Siamese Twins. Trans Coll Phys Philadelphia, Third Series. 1875; 1: 3–46.
20 Luckhardt A B. Report of the autopsy of the Siamese Twins together with other interesting information covering their life. Surg Gynecol Obst 1941; 72: 116–125.
21 Alha A R. op. cit. pp 49–50.
22 McCallum N E W, Scroggie J G. A study of blood alcohol concentrations in subjects within various weight ranges. Quart J Stud Alcoh 1963; 24: 195–202.
23 B M A Report. The Recognition of Intoxication, Rev. ed. B M A House, Tavistock Square, London, 1958: p 28.
24 B M A Report. Relation of Alcohol to Road Accidents. B M A House, Tavistock Square, London. 1960: p 36.
25 Sapeika N. Simple determination of the amount of alcohol ingested by an individual. J Forens Med 1960; 7: 106–108.
26 Newman H W. op. cit. p 36.
27 Newman H W. op. cit. p 71.
28 Newman H W. op. cit. p 79.
29 Forney R B, Hughes F W. The combined effect of alcohol and other drugs. Springfield: Thomas. 1968: p 22.
30 Camps F E, Robinson A E. Influence of fructose on blood alcohol levels in social drinkers. Med Sci Law 1968; 8: 161–167.
31 Carpenter T M, Lee R C, Budett M. Influence of glucose and of fructose on effective dead space in human respiration. Am J Physiol (Proc) 1933; 104:17.
32 Nyman E, Palmlov A. On effect of muscular exercise on metabolism of ethyl alcohol. Skand Arch Physiol 1934; 68: 271–291. Quoted by Newman H W. op. cit. p 68.
33 Newman H W. op. cit. p 57.
34 Wallgren H, Barry, III, H. Actions of alcohol, Vol. 1. Amsterdam: Elsevier. 1970: p. 95 et seq.
35 Bonnichsen R, Dimberg R, Sjoberg L. Oxidation of alcohol. Stockholm Institutit för Maltdryck-forskning. 1964: Publ. No. 12. Abstracted in Quart J Stud Alcoh 1966; 27:554.
36 Mellanby E. Alcohol: Its absorption into and disappearance from the blood under different conditions. M R C Special Report Series No. 31, London: H M S O. 1919: p 14.

37 Isselbacher K J, Greenberger N J. Metabolic effects of alcohol on the liver. New Eng J Med 1964; 270: 351–356.
38 Nickolls L C. op. cit. p 334.
39 Alha A R. op. cit. p 11.
40 Alha A R. op. cit. pp 30–31.
41 Alha A R. op. cit. p 38.
42 Shumate R P, Crowther R F, Zarafshan M. A study of the metabolism rates of alcohol in the human body. J Froens Med 1967; 14: 83–100.
43 Scott R B. ed. Price's textbook of the practice of medicine, 10th ed. London: Oxford University Press. 1966: p 376.
44 Herbich J, Prokop L. Studies on the influence of food and fluid ingestion on the blood alcohol level. Wien Klin Wschr 1963; 75: 421–427. Abstracted in the Medico-Legal Journal 1964; 32:47.
45 Bayly R C, McCallum N E W. Some aspects of alcohol in body fluids. II. The change in blood alcohol concentration following alcohol consumption. Med J Austral 1959; 2: 173–176.
46 Bowden K M. Driving under the influence of alcohol: A report. Department of Forens. Med., University of Melbourne, privately published, p. 29. This report has also been published (in part) in J Forens Med 1963; 10: 148–156.
47 Report of a Special Committee of the British Medical Association, The medico-legal investigation of the drinking driver. London: British Medical Association. 1965: p 33.
48 Alha A R. op. cit. p 14.
49 Alha A R. op. cit. p 86.
50 Jetter W W. Studies in alcohol; diagnosis of acute alcoholic intoxication by correlation of clinical and chemical findings. Am J Med Sci 1938; 196: 475–487.
51 Lofthus J. op. cit. p 223.
52 Ward Smith H. op. cit. p 80.
53 Kestenbaum A. Clinical methods of neuro-opthalmologic examination. New York: Grune and Stratton. 1947: p 285.
54 Jetter W W. op. cit. p 486.
55 Jetter W W. Studies in alcohol; experimental feeding of alcohol to non-alcoholic individuals. Am J Med Sci 1938; 196: 487–493.
56 Hammond K B, Rumack B H, Rodgerson D O. Blood ethanol: A report of unusually high levels in a living patient. J Am Med Assoc 1973; 226: 63–64.
57 van Ieperen L. Blood alcohol levels. S Afr Med J 1980; 57:522.
58 Rabinowitch I M. Chemical tests for alcoholic intoxication. Can Bar Rev 1953; 31: 1069–1074.
59 Rabinowitch I M. Chemical tests for alcoholic intoxication. Can Bar Rev 1954; 32: 243–244.
60 Bowden K M. op. cit. pp 88–89.
61 Lofthus J. op. cit. p 219.
62 Haggard H W, Greenberg L A, Carroll R P, Miller D P. Use of urine in chemical test for intoxication; possible errors and their avoidance. J Am Med Assoc 1940; 115: 1680–1683.
63 Alha A R, Tamminen V. Fatal cases with an elevated urine alcohol but without alcohol in the blood. J Forens Med 1964; 11: 3–5.
64 Moritz A R, Jetter W W. Antemortem and postmortem diffusion of alcohol through mucosa of bladder. Arch Path. 1942; 33: 939–948.
65 Denny R C. The truth about breath tests. London: Nelson. 1970.
66 Landauer A A, Milner G. Breathalyzer test and the blood alcohol level. Austral Law J 1971; 45: 360–362.
67 Milner G, Landauer A A. Breathalyzer faults: principles and practice. Med J Austral 1971; 1: 1280–1284.
68 Klatzow D. Personal communication.
69 Hollopeter C. The practical lawyer, December 1957: p 58.
70 Jetter W W. Studies in alcohol. I. The diagnosis of acute alcoholic intoxication by a correlation of clinical and chemical findings. pp 475–487. II. Experimental feeding of alcohol to non-alcoholic individuals. pp 487–493. Am J Med Sci 1938; 196.

71 Harger R N, Hulpieu H R. In: Thompson G N. ed. Alcoholism. Springfield: Thomas. 1956: p 171.

72 Lofthus J. op. cit. p 227.

73 Rentoul E, Smith H, Beavers R. Some observations on the effects of the consumption of alcohol and its relation to road traffic. Forens Sci Soc J 1962; 3: 2–10.

74 Smith S, Simpson K. eds. Taylor's principles and practice of medical jurisprudence, 11th ed. Vol. 2, London: Churchill. 1957: P 432.

75 French H. ed. An index of differential diagnosis of main symptoms, 6th ed. Bristol: Wright. 1945: p 90.

76 Fregly A R, Bergstedt M, Graybiel A. Relationships between blood alcohol, positional alcohol nystagmus and postural equilibrium. Quart J Stud Alcoh 1967; 28: 11–21.

77 Alha A R. op. cit. p 79.

78 State vs. Rosen & another, 4th December 1961. (See footnote on p 416.)

79 Brown I A. Liver-brain relationships. Springfield: Thomas. 1957: p 61.

80 Brown I A, op. cit. p 62.

81 Watt A C. Personal communication: 1959.

82 Aschan G. Different types of alcohol nystagmus. Acta oto-laryngol Suppl 1958; 140: 69–78.

83 Rauschke J. Alkohol-nystagmus und leistungsschädigung: experimentelle Untersuchungen zur Brauchbarkeit der nystagmusprüfung beim nachweis der alkoholbeeinflussung. Medizinische 1958; 12: 460–465. Abstracted in Quart J Stud Alcoh 1960; 21: 143–144. (Alcohol nystagmus and impairment of performance: experimental investigation on the utility of nystagmus tests in assessing the effects of alcohol.)

84 Prestwich J C. Recognition of intoxication. Br Med J 1960; 2: 1521–1522.

85 British Medical Association. The Recognition of Intoxication. BMA House, Tavistock Square, London, 1954: p 15.

86 Mayo Clinic Staff. Clinical examination in neurology. Philadelphia: Saunders. 1957: pp 94, 96.

87 Aschan G, Bergstedt M, Goldberg L, Laurell L. Positional nystagmus in man during and after alcohol intoxication. Quart J Stud Alcoh 1956; 17: 381–405.

88 Goldberg L. In: Alcohol and road traffic. London: British Medical Association. 1963: p 128.

89 Goldberg L. In: Popham R E. ed. Alcohol and alcoholism. Toronto: University of Toronto Press, 1970: pp 45–48, 51.

90 Murphree H B, Price L M, Greenberg L A. Effect of congeners in alcoholic beverages on the incidence of nystagmus. Quart J Stud Alcoh 1966; 27: 201–213.

91 Ward Smith H, Popham R E. Blood alcohol levels in relation to driving. Can Med Assoc J 1951; 65: 325–328.

92 Penner D W, Coldwell B B. Car driving and alcohol consumption: medical observations on an experiment. Can Med Assoc J 1958; 79: 793–800.

93 Lofthus J. op. cit. p 218.

94 Andresen P H. Traffic and alcohol. Medico-legal J 1950; 18: 98–105.

95 Penner D W, Coldwell B B. op. cit. Quoted by H. Ward Smith[1] at p 90.

96 Coldwell B B, Penner D W, Smith H W, Lucas G H, Rodgers R F. Effect of ingestion of distilled spirits on automobile driving skill. Quart J Stud Alcoh 1958; 19: 590–616. Quoted by Smith[1] at p 83.

97 Meltzer L. Personal communication: 1958.

98 Slater E, Roth M. Mayer-Gross. In: Mayer-Gross, Slater and Roth's Clinical Psychiatry, 3rd ed. Baltimore: Williams & Wilkins. 1969.

99 Frame M C. Alcoholism—some medico-legal aspects. J Forens Med 1955; 2: 151–163.

100 Wallgren H, Barry III, H. Actions of alcohol, Vol. 2, Amsterdam: Elsevier. 1970: p 808.

101 Drew G C, Colquhoun W P, Long H A. Effect of small doses of alcohol on a skill resembling driving. M R C Memorandum 38. London: HMSO. 1959.

102 Newman H W, Fletcher E. The effect of alcohol on driving skill. J Am Med Assoc 1940; 115: 1600–1602.

103 Rentoul E. Alcohol and road traffic. London: BMA 1963: p 149.

104 Bjerver K, Goldberg L. Effect of alcohol ingestion on driving ability; results of practical road tests and laboratory experiments. Quart J Stud Alcoh 1950; 11: 1–30.

105 Law Reform Commission Report No. 4 1976. Alcohol, drugs and driving. Canberra: Australian Government Publishing Service.
106 Jetter W W, McLean R. Poisoning by the synergistic effect of phenobarbital and ethyl alcohol. Arch Path. 1943; 36: 112–122.
107 Coroner's Cases, Barbiturates and alcohol. Br Med J 1960; 1:1578.
108 Koppanyi T. In: Himwich H E. ed. Alcoholism: basic aspects and treatment. American Association for the Advancement of Science. Washington, 1957: pp 93–113. Quoted by Weatherby J H, Clements E L. Quart J Stud Alcoh 1960 21: 394–399. (Concerning the synergism between paraldehyde and ethyl alcohol.)
109 Koppanyi T, Canary J J, Maengwyn-Davies G D. Problems in acute alcohol poisoning. Quart J Stud Alcoh 1961; Suppl. 1: 24–36.
110 Teare R D. Some problems of barbiturate and alcoholic intoxication. Medico-legal J 1966; 34: 4–10.
111 Laubenthal F. Zschr Verkehrsmed 1958; 4:67.
112 Weatherall M. Drugs and the motorist. Medico-legal journal 1959; 27: 44–56.
113 Loomis T A. Alcohol and road traffic. London: B M A. 1963: p 119.
114 Carpenter J A, Varley M E. Alcohol and road traffic. London: B M A. 1963: p 156.
115 Forney R B, Hughes F W. The combined effect of alcohol and other drugs. Springfield: Thomas. 1968.
116 Bowden K M, McCallum N E W. Blood alcohol content: some aspects of its post-mortem uses. Med J Austral 1949; 76–81.
117 Alha A R. op. cit. p 26.
118 Pleuckhahn, V D. The significance of blood alcohol levels at autopsy. Med J Austral 1967; 2: 118–124.
119 Gifford H, Turkel H W. Diffusion of alcohol through stomach wall after death. A cause of erroneous post mortem blood alcohol levels. J Am Med Assoc 1956; 161: 866–868.
120 Turkel H W, Gifford H. Erroneous blood alcohol findings at autopsy. Avoidance by proper sampling technique. J Am Med Assoc 1957; 164: 1077–1079.
121 Harger R N. Alcohol and road traffic. B M A House, Tavistock Square, London, 1963: p 218.
122 Newman H W. op. cit. pp 22, 154.
123 Plueckhahn V D. op. cit. p 118.
124 Gonzales T A, Vance M, Helpern M, Umberger C J. Legal medicine, pathology and toxicology, 2nd ed. New York: Appleton-Century-Crofts: 1954: p 1184.
125 Plueckhahn V D, Ballard B. Factors influencing the significance of alcohol concentrations in autopsy blood samples. Med J Austral 1968; 1: 939–943.
126 Gormsen H. Yeasts and the production of alcohol post mortem. J Forens Med 1954; 1: 170–171. See also: Alcohol production in the dead body—further investigations. J Forens Med 1954 1: 314–315.
127 Luvoni B, Marozzi E. Ethyl alcohol distribution in the various organs and fluids of cadavers. J Forens Med 1968; 15: 67–70.

Index